Handbook of Ultrasound Imaging

Handbook of Ultrasound Imaging

Editor: Michelle Skinner

AMERICAN
MEDICAL PUBLISHERS
www.americanmedicalpublishers.com

AMERICAN
MEDICAL PUBLISHERS
www.americanmedicalpublishers.com

Cataloging-in-Publication Data

Handbook of ultrasound imaging / edited by Michelle Skinner.
p. cm.
Includes bibliographical references and index.
ISBN 979-8-88740-163-8
1. Diagnostic ultrasonic imaging. 2. Diagnostic imaging. 3. Ultrasonic imaging.
4. Ultrasonics in medicine. I. Skinner, Michelle.
RC78.7.U4 H36 2023
616.075 43--dc23

American Medical Publishers,
41 Flatbush Avenue,
1st Floor, New York,
NY 11217, USA

ISBN 979-8-88740-163-8 (Hardback)

Contents

Preface

This book was inspired by the evolution of our times; to answer the curiosity of inquisitive minds. Many developments have occurred across the globe in the recent past which has transformed the progress in the field.

Ultrasound imaging is a clinical imaging technique that provides real-time, quantitative anatomical and physiological information in humans. It can serve both diagnostic and therapeutic functions. The diagnostic ultrasound is a non-invasive technique that uses sound waves to scan the structures or parts within the body. Ultrasound images can capture the movement of the internal organs, fetus and blood flow through the vessels inside the body. There are several medical applications of ultrasound, which include monitoring the development and health of the fetus during pregnancy. A Doppler ultrasound is used to assess the movement of blood to parts of body such as the heart, placenta and testes. Therapeutic ultrasound can be used to alleviate pain from the spread of cancer into the bones (bone metastases). Some other applications of ultrasound imaging include treatment of uterine fibroids and prostate surgery. Various studies that are constantly contributing towards advancing technologies and evolution of this field have been examined in detail within this book. It brings forth some of the most innovative concepts and elucidates the unexplored aspects of ultrasound imaging. The book will provide comprehensive knowledge to the readers.

This book was developed from a mere concept to drafts to chapters and finally compiled together as a complete text to benefit the readers across all nations. To ensure the quality of the content we instilled two significant steps in our procedure. The first was to appoint an editorial team that would verify the data and statistics provided in the book and also select the most appropriate and valuable contributions from the plentiful contributions we received from authors worldwide. The next step was to appoint an expert of the topic as the Editor-in-Chief, who would head the project and finally make the necessary amendments and modifications to make the text reader-friendly. I was then commissioned to examine all the material to present the topics in the most comprehensible and productive format.

I would like to take this opportunity to thank all the contributing authors who were supportive enough to contribute their time and knowledge to this project. I also wish to convey my regards to my family who have been extremely supportive during the entire project.

Editor

1

Interpretation errors in focused cardiac ultrasound by novice pediatric emergency medicine fellow sonologists

Rosemary Thomas-Mohtat[1,6*], Craig Sable[2,6], Kristen Breslin[1,6], Jacqueline G. Weinberg[3], Aparna Prasad[4], Lauren Zinns[5] and Joanna S. Cohen[1,6]

Abstract

Background: Focused cardiac ultrasound (FOCUS) is a core competency for pediatric emergency medicine (PEM) fellows. The objectives of this study were (1) to evaluate test characteristics of PEM-fellow-performed FOCUS for pericardial effusion and diminished cardiac function and (2) to assess image interpretation independent of image acquisition.

Methods: PEM fellows performed and interpreted FOCUS on patients who also received cardiology service echocardiograms, the reference standard. Subsequently, eight different PEM fellows remotely interpreted a subset of the PEM-acquired and cardiology-acquired echocardiograms.

Results: Eight PEM fellows performed 54 FOCUS exams, of which two had pericardial effusion and four had diminished function. PEM fellow FOCUS had a sensitivity of 50.0% (95% CI 9.19–90.8) and specificity of 100.0% (95% CI 91.1–100.0) for detecting diminished function, and sensitivity of 50.0% (95% CI 2.67–97.33) and specificity of 98.1% (95% CI 88.42–99.9) for detecting pericardial effusions. When PEM fellows remotely interpreted 15 echocardiograms, the sensitivity was 81.3% (95% CI 70.7–88.8) and specificity 75% (95% CI 67.0–81.0) for detecting diminished function, and sensitivity of 76.3% (95% CI 65.0–85.0) and specificity 94.4% (95% CI 89.0–97.0) for detecting pericardial effusion. There were no differences in sensitivity and specificity of PEM fellows' interpretation of FOCUS studies compared to their interpretation of cardiology echocardiograms. Interrater reliability for interpretation of remote images (kappa) was 0.66 (95% CI 0.59–0.73) for effusion and 0.31 (95% CI 0.24–0.38) for function among the fellows.

Conclusion: Novice PEM fellow sonologists (a physician who performs and interprets ultrasound) in the majority of instances were able to acquire and remotely interpret FOCUS images with limited training. However, they made real-time interpretation errors and likely need further training to incorporate real-time image acquisition and interpretation into their practice.

Keywords: Point of care ultrasound, Focused cardiac ultrasound, Education, Pediatric emergency medicine

*Correspondence: rthomasm@cnmc.org
[1] Department of Emergency Medicine and Trauma Services, Children's National Medical Center, Washington, DC, USA
Full list of author information is available at the end of the article

Introduction

In 2010, the American Society of Echocardiography and the American College of Emergency Physicians released a consensus statement on the importance of focused cardiac ultrasound (FOCUS) on patient care and treatment in an emergency setting [1]. Subsequently, the American Academy of Pediatrics and the American College of Emergency Physicians have released policy statements stressing the importance of training for pediatric emergency medicine (PEM) fellows in point of care ultrasound (POCUS). They recommend a structured POCUS curriculum and competency assessment for PEM fellows [2]. An expert panel of PEM physicians trained in POCUS, included FOCUS as one of the core ultrasound exams for this curriculum [3].

PEM providers who have completed a dedicated extra year of POCUS fellowship training can diagnose pericardial effusion and abnormalities of function with high sensitivity and specificity [4–6]. However, there are limited data on competency assessment of PEM fellows with routine training in POCUS during their PEM fellowships. Our primary objective was to assess PEM fellows' accuracy in assessing cardiac function and the presence of pericardial effusions while performing FOCUS exams with limited training. Our secondary objective was to assess the accuracy of PEM fellows' interpretive skills of both FOCUS and complete echocardiograms in a remote classroom setting. We hypothesized that PEM fellows would perform better on interpretation of remotely acquired images than on images acquired in real time.

Materials and methods

This study took place at a freestanding tertiary care children's hospital with approximately 90,000 emergency department (ED) visits per year and with a cardiology service that performs 21,000 echocardiograms a year. PEM fellows completed FOCUS training, consisting of a 1 h lecture on echocardiography, a month of basic POCUS training with regular supervised ultrasound scans, and quality assurance sessions with PEM POCUS-trained faculty. In addition, each PEM fellow competed a minimum of 10 FOCUS exams reviewed by PEM POCUS-trained faculty. The fellows were taught to determine function by qualitatively evaluating how closely the anterior leaflet of the mitral value approached the interventricular septum in the parasternal long axis view. They were taught to evaluate pericardial effusion in all four views. FOCUS exams included four standard cardiac views: the parasternal long, parasternal short, apical 4 chamber, and subxiphoid views. Specifically in the parasternal long axis view, they were taught to note any anechoic structures above the descending aorta, within the pericardium.

A convenience sample of patients' ages 1 month to 21 years, with an indication for an echocardiogram as determined by a pediatric cardiologist, were enrolled between April 2014 and June 2015. The patients were enrolled in the pediatric ED, cardiology clinic, or the inpatient service. The indications for the echocardiograms included chest pain, syncope, altered mental status, hypoxia, and follow-up of known cardiac disease. Premature infants with post-conception age less than 36 weeks and patients who were less than 8 day post-sternotomy were excluded. Because the cardiology echocardiogram was the reference standard, we also excluded patients if they experienced significant therapeutic interventions or changes in clinical conditions between the FOCUS exam and the cardiology echocardiogram. This included progression of illness requiring transfer of the patient to a higher level of care, need for emergent surgery, initiation of ECMO, intubation, or the initiation of intravenous vasopressor agents.

Eight PEM fellows performed FOCUS, using a Sonosite M-Turbo® ultrasound system (Bothell, WA). Within 24 h of FOCUS, a cardiologist or echocardiography technician performed an echocardiogram with a Phillips IE 33 ultrasound system (Andover, MA). PEM fellows were blinded to the results of the cardiology echocardiogram and vice versa. The PEM fellows were blinded to the clinical status of the patient to the extent possible; the PEM fellow performing the FOCUS did not access the medical record or discuss the clinical case with the patient or with the provider caring for the patient. However, we could not blind the fact that a patient was in the resuscitation bay or the ICU, for example.

The PEM fellows performing FOCUS completed a case report form (CRF) immediately following the performance of the FOCUS. The CRF included the fellows' interpretation of the presence or absence of significant pericardial effusion and the qualitative global systolic function as either normal or depressed. We used dichotomous qualitative variables for pericardial effusion (absent/trivial versus present) and cardiac function (normal versus depressed) rather than attempting to quantify amount of fluid or ejection fraction.

A board-certified pediatric cardiologist, blinded to the patient's clinical presentation, chief complaint, cardiac history and PEM fellow interpretation of FOCUS, reviewed and interpreted the recorded clips of each FOCUS and cardiology echocardiogram. This cardiologist used a CRF with a similar format to the PEM fellows to subjectively note the presence or absence of significant effusion, the qualitative global function and if the quality of the study was adequate to perform these assessments.

The blinded interpretation of the cardiology-performed echocardiogram was used as the reference standard for subsequent analysis.

In the second phase of the study, PEM fellow interpretation skills were assessed remotely in a classroom setting. Thirty matched studies were compiled: 15 FOCUS exams performed by PEM fellows and 15 cardiology-acquired echocardiograms on the same patients. We selected studies, so that 5 of these sets had pericardial effusions, 5 had diminished function, and 5 were normal. Eight PEM fellows were shown these studies in random order and were asked to comment on the presence or absence of pericardial effusion and global cardiac function. PEM fellows were not given any clinical information about the patients. Only the four standard views were presented. Only one of these eight PEM fellows had acquired images in the first phase of the study.

IBM SPSS version 24 (Armonk NY) and Microsoft Excel (Microsoft, Inc, Redmond, WA) were used to calculate test characteristics of PEM fellow FOCUS exams, with cardiology echocardiograms as the reference standard. Similar methodology was used to calculate test characteristics of PEM fellows' interpretation of both FOCUS and cardiology studies in the remote setting.

Results

Eight PEM fellows enrolled a convenience sample of 54 patients (Table 1).

Two (4%) patients had pericardial effusions and 4 (8%) had diminished function. The median time to complete the FOCUS was 6 min (IQR 5, 9). The median time difference between the two ultrasounds (PEM and cardiology) was 34 min (IQR 17.5, 58.8). No patients were excluded for changes in clinical status or interventions. The expert cardiologist did not find any PEM FOCUS studies with technical limitations precluding the determination of the two variables of interest.

Phase 1

Results of the bedside FOCUS studies compared with the cardiology echocardiograms for our two variables of interest are shown in Tables 2 (diminished function) and 3 (pericardial effusion). The distributions of test characteristics of PEM fellow performed and interpreted FOCUS are shown in Fig. 1. Video clips of the four errors are available in Additional file 1: Phase S1, Phase S2, Phase S3, Phase S4.

The sensitivity of PEM fellow performed and interpreted FOCUS was 50.0% (95% CI 9.19–90.8) with a specificity of 100.0% (95% CI 91.1–100.0) for detecting diminished function. The sensitivity was 50.0% (95% CI 2.67–97.33) and specificity of 98.1% (95% CI 88.42–99.9) for detecting pericardial effusions (Table 4).

All three cases of missed pathology were by a single 2nd year fellow. The one missed pericardial effusion was in an inpatient with a structurally normal heart with a clinically significant effusion. One of the patients with missed diminished function was a clinic patient with a structurally normal heart with mild to moderately diminished left systolic function. The second patient with missed diminished function was an ED patient with known congenital heart disease and moderately decreased right and left systolic function.

Phase 2

The test characteristics of remote interpretation of 15 sets of images by a different set of similarly trained eight PEM fellows are shown in Table 5. The sensitivity was 81.3% (95% CI 70.7–88.8) and specificity was 75% (95% CI 67.0–81.0) for detecting diminished function. The sensitivity was 76.3% (95% CI 65.0–85.0) and specificity was 94.4% (95% CI 89.0–97.0) for detecting pericardial effusion. Individual performance of each fellow remotely is detailed in Fig. 2.

There was no statistical significant difference between the sensitivity of detecting diminished function ($p=0.13$) or pericardial effusion ($p=0.48$) during real-time

Table 1 Demographics of recruited patients ($N=54$)

Male	29 (54%)
Location	
ED	18 (33%)
Cardiology clinic	28 (52%)
Inpatient	4 (7%)
ICU	4 (7%)
Congenital heart disease, present	16 (30%)
Age in years [median (IQR)]	8 (1.75, 14.25)

Table 2 Results of FOCUS compared with cardiology echocardiograms for diminished function

	Cards+	Cards−
FOCUS+	2	0
FOCUS−	2	50

Table 3 Results of FOCUS compared with cardiology echocardiograms for pericardial effusion

	Cards+	Cards−
FOCUS+	1	1
FOCUS−	1	51

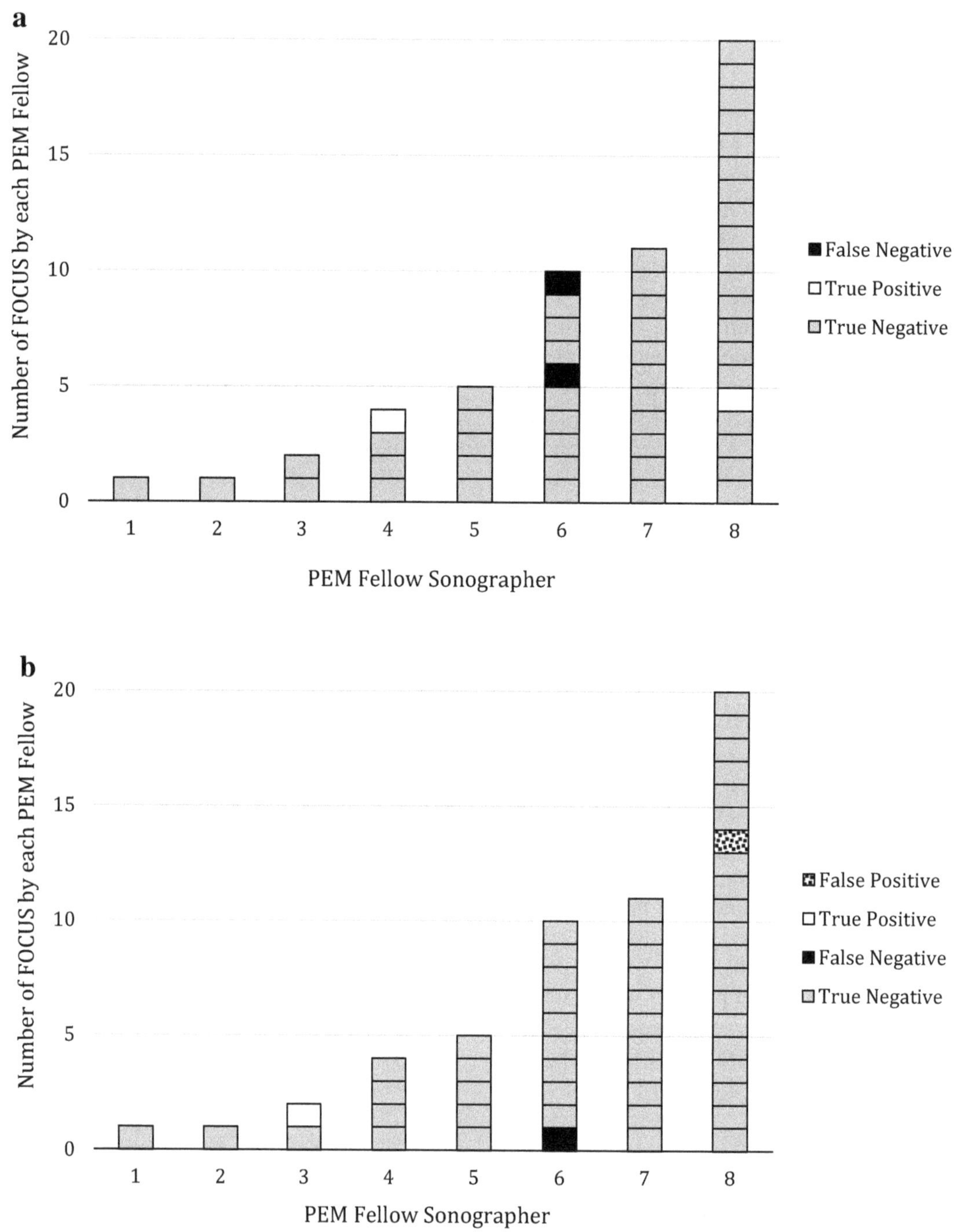

Fig. 1 Test characteristics of FOCUS performed by PEM fellows

interpretation and classroom interpretation. There was also no significant difference between specificity during real-time interpretation and remote interpretation for detecting effusion ($p = 0.3$). There was, however, a statistically significant improvement in specificity when interpreting function in real time (100%) as compared to the remote interpretation (75%) ($p < 0.01$).

We calculated the interobserver reliability of fellows' interpretation of effusion and diminished function among each other in Phase 2. The kappa for effusion was 0.66 (95% CI 0.59–0.73) and the kappa for function was 0.31 (95% CI 0.24–0.38).

There was no statistically significant difference in the sensitivity or specificity of detection of diminished

Table 4 Performance metrics of real-time interpretation of FOCUS (Phase 1)

	Diminished function	Pericardial effusion
Sensitivity, % (95% CI)	50.0 (9.19–90.8)	50.0 (2.67–97.33)
Specificity, % (95% CI)	100.0 (91.1.0–100.0)	98.1 (88.42–99.9)

Table 5 Performance metrics of overall classroom interpretation of combined FOCUS and cardiology echocardiograms (Phase 2)

	Diminished function	Pericardial effusion
Sensitivity, % (95% CI)	81.3 (70.7–88.8)	76.3 (65.0–85.0)
Specificity, % (95% CI)	75.0 (67.0–81.0)	94.4 (89.0–97.0)

function or pericardial effusion when comparing PEM fellows' remote interpretations of FOCUS images to the same PEM fellows' remote interpretations of cardiology-acquired echocardiograms (Tables 6 and 7). Performance metrics of classroom interpretation of individual fellows is presented in Figs. 3 (sensitivity) and 4 (specificity). Select videos of errors made in Phase 2 are included in Additional file 2: Phase S5, Phase S6, Phase S7, Phase S8.

Discussion

This is the first study that has evaluated PEM fellow performance of FOCUS and specifically evaluated remote interpretation of FOCUS distinctly from acquisition. We demonstrated that with limited training, PEM fellows are able to acquire FOCUS images of sufficient quality to allow interpretation of the presence or absence of pericardial effusion and the presence or absence of significantly diminished cardiac function. The reviewing cardiologist found all FOCUS to be of sufficient technical quality to make these determinations. PEM fellows in our study had improved sensitivity when interpreting FOCUS images remotely in a classroom setting, suggesting that some fellows may face challenges of simultaneous acquisition and interpretation while at the bedside. When remotely evaluating echocardiograms, PEM fellows showed similar ability to interpret FOCUS exams and cardiology obtained exams, also suggesting that the deficit in interpreting the FOCUS exams, while obtaining them was less related to the quality of the image acquired. In addition, the interpretation of pericardial effusion had greater interobserver agreement among the fellows than determination of diminished function, as it is an easier assessment to make.

These findings suggest that novice PEM fellow sonographers may need more training in real-time interpretation while scanning at the bedside. Prior research showing more accurate interpretation of FOCUS has involved a larger number of training scans. Current recommendations from the American College of Physicians are for 25–50 scans per application, but the exact number is still debated [7]. Emergency medicine faculty with 10 h of mixed didactic and hands on scanning and more than 45 ultrasounds and adult non-cardiology residents with 12 h of mixed didactic and hands on scanning with a mean of 33 ultrasounds showed increased competency in FOCUS [8, 9]. Blehar et al. [10] evaluated learning curves of acquisition and interpretation of POCUS by emergency medicine residents; they found that acquisition of FOCUS had no plateau point on the learning curve (i.e., that it was consistently difficult to achieve mastery), and the interpretation learning curve did not plateau for FOCUS until the learners had performed about 30 scans.

In addition, we found that novice PEM fellow sonographers were able to more accurately interpret their own images remotely, suggesting that the fact of being at the bedside during interpretation added a layer of complexity. This may be due to perceived time or performance pressure at the bedside, which could be exacerbated in real-time resuscitation situations. For this reason, we think that real-time image interpretation is a critical skill for PEM fellow sonographers.

Given the low prevalence of pericardial effusion and depressed cardiac function in the pediatric patient population overall, other modes of encountering pathology such as via simulation or review of image banks may be necessary to improve interpretation by novice sonologists. Both low and high fidelity ultrasound simulation modalities are available [11]. A 1-day workshop using multi-faceted simulation based education and assessment of focused cardiac ultrasound in the evaluation of the hypotensive patient, showed improved competency in emergency medicine residents [12].

When PEM fellows performed and interpreted FOCUS at the bedside, the study had high specificity but poor sensitivity for identifying pericardial effusion and diminished cardiac function. Eliminating the data of the one fellow who had the 3 misses from the analysis would yield a sensitivity of 100% for both correct identification of pericardial effusion and diminished function by PEM fellows.

This study has several limitations. First, this was performed at a single institution. Results at other hospitals may be different. Second, there were few patients with cardiac disease. Therefore, the point estimates of sensitivity and specificity can be skewed by one or two incorrect readings, with the resultant wide confidence intervals

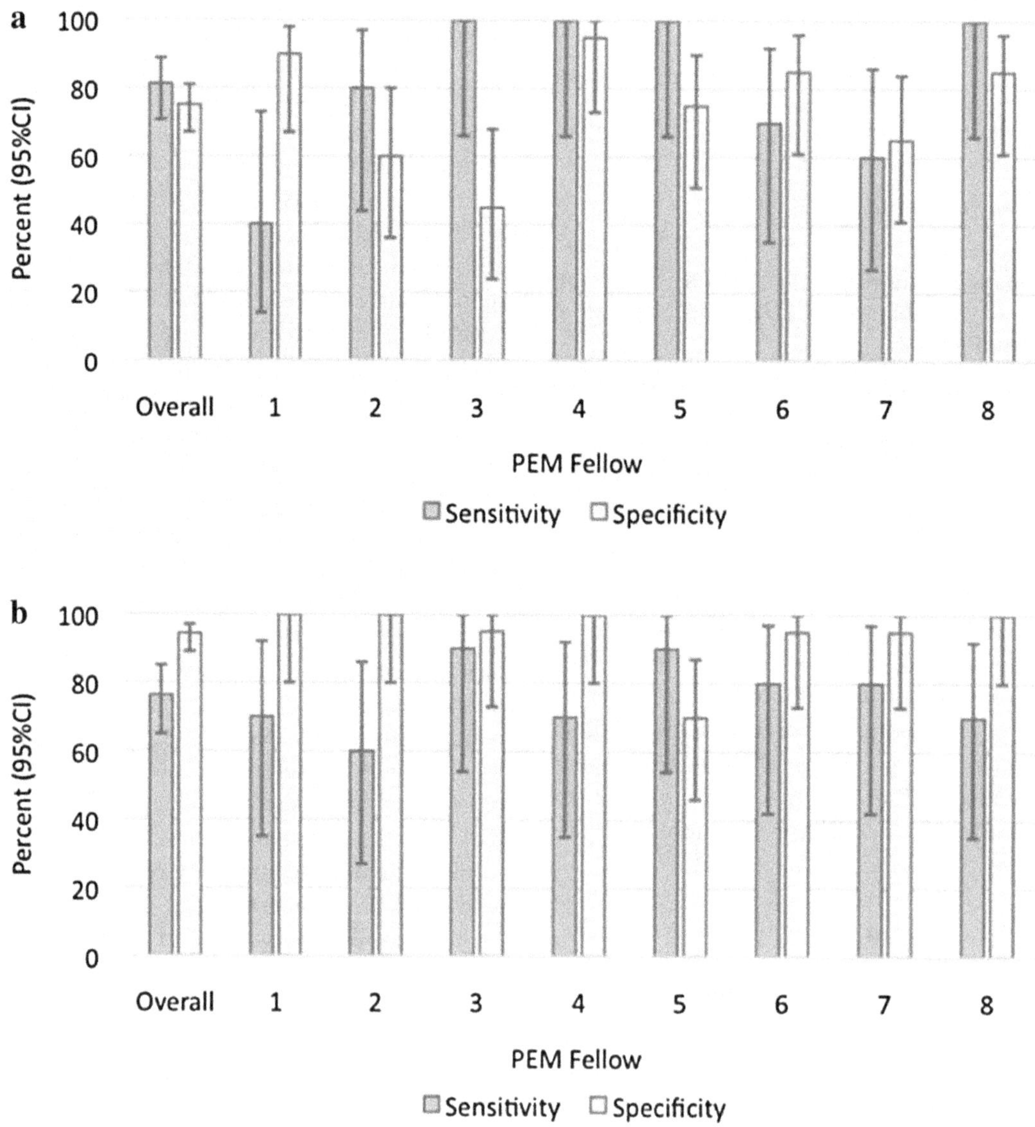

Fig. 2 Classroom test of images (Phase 2). Overall sensitivity and specificity of interpretation of abnormal studies by 8 PEM fellows for function (**a**) and effusion (**b**)

Table 6 Performance metrics of classroom interpretation of FOCUS of diminished function (Phase 2)

	FOCUS	Cardiology echo	*p*
Sensitivity, % (95% CI)	77.5 (61.0–89.0)	85.0 (69.0–94.0)	0.57
Specificity, % (95% CI)	73.8 (63.0–83.0)	76.3 (65.0–85.0)	0.86

Table 7 Performance metrics of classroom interpretation of FOCUS of pericardial effusion (Phase 2)

	FOCUS	Cardiology echo	*p*
Sensitivity, % (95% CI)	80.0 (64.0–90.0)	72.5 (56.0–85.0)	0.60
Specificity, % (95% CI)	95.0 (87.0–98.0)	93.8 (85.0–98.0)	0.60

for these estimates. Most of the incorrect interpretations were obtained by one fellow, which suggests a need for individual remediation rather than a more global problem. FOCUS image acquisition and interpretation may or may not be generalizable to other novice FOCUS learners, but reviewing errors or misclassification is an

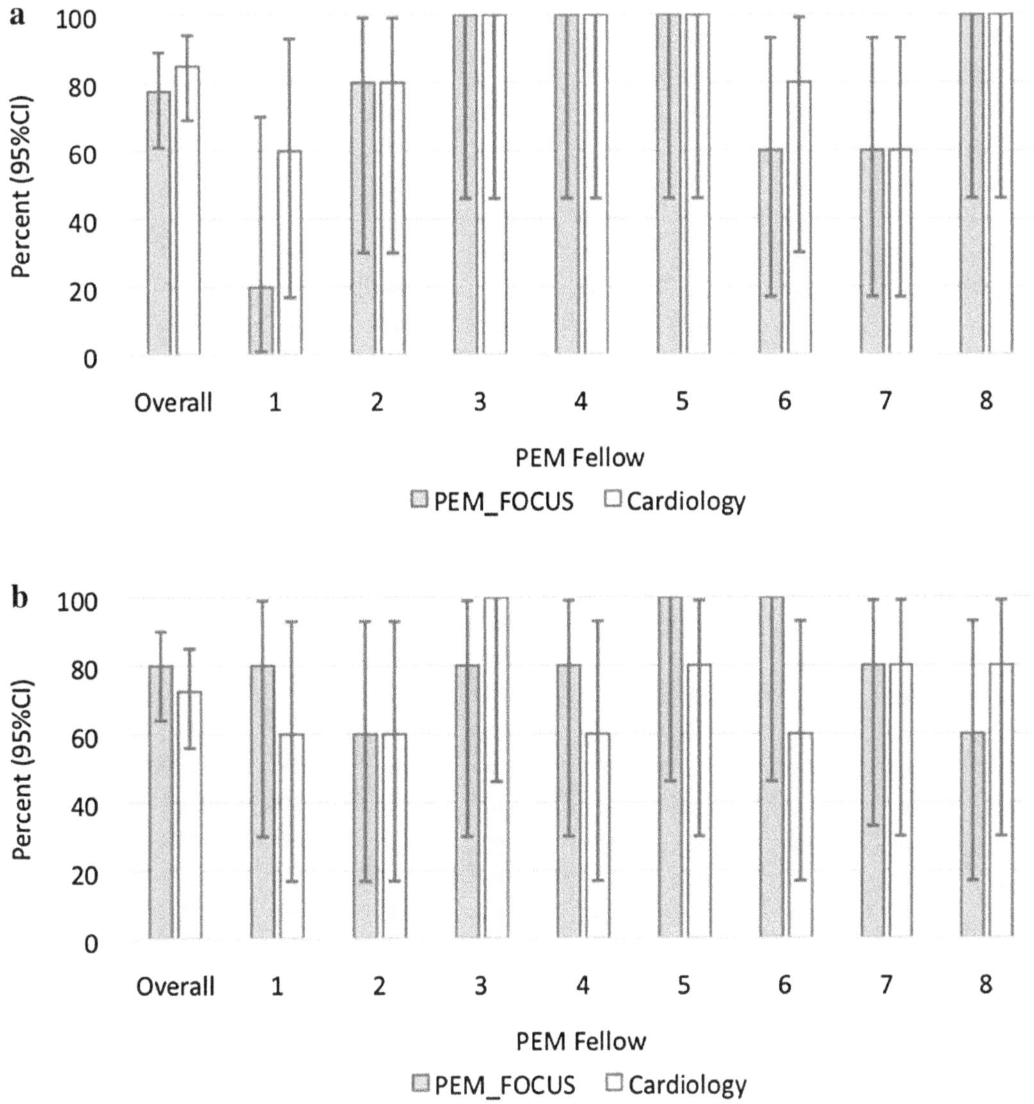

Fig. 3 Sensitivity of interpretation of classroom test of images of PEM FOCUS versus cardiology images by 8 PEM fellows for function (**a**) and effusion (**b**)

integral part of any quality assurance program. We did not study implementation of a FOCUS protocol in the emergency room [13].

In addition, by design and due to logistic issues, we did not study chamber size abnormalities, cardiac standstill, or determination of cardiac arrest. International recommendations have been made for the use of FOCUS in cardiac arrest; while feasibility of using FOCUS in cases of pediatric cardiac arrest has been published, adult studies have noted challenges in agreement of interpretation of cardiac standstill among different levels of providers [14–16].

Conclusion

In this small study, PEM fellows for the most part were able to obtain ultrasound images of sufficient quality to allow interpretation of diminished cardiac function and pericardial effusion. However, interpretation was better performed remotely than at the bedside by PEM fellows. There was greater interrater agreement for pericardial effusion than diminished function by the novice PEM sonographer. Prior to completion of the current recommendation of 25 scans, novice PEM fellow sonologists are likely to make real-time acquisition and interpretation errors, and therefore, supervision and quality assurance are necessary. We recommend more extensive training in

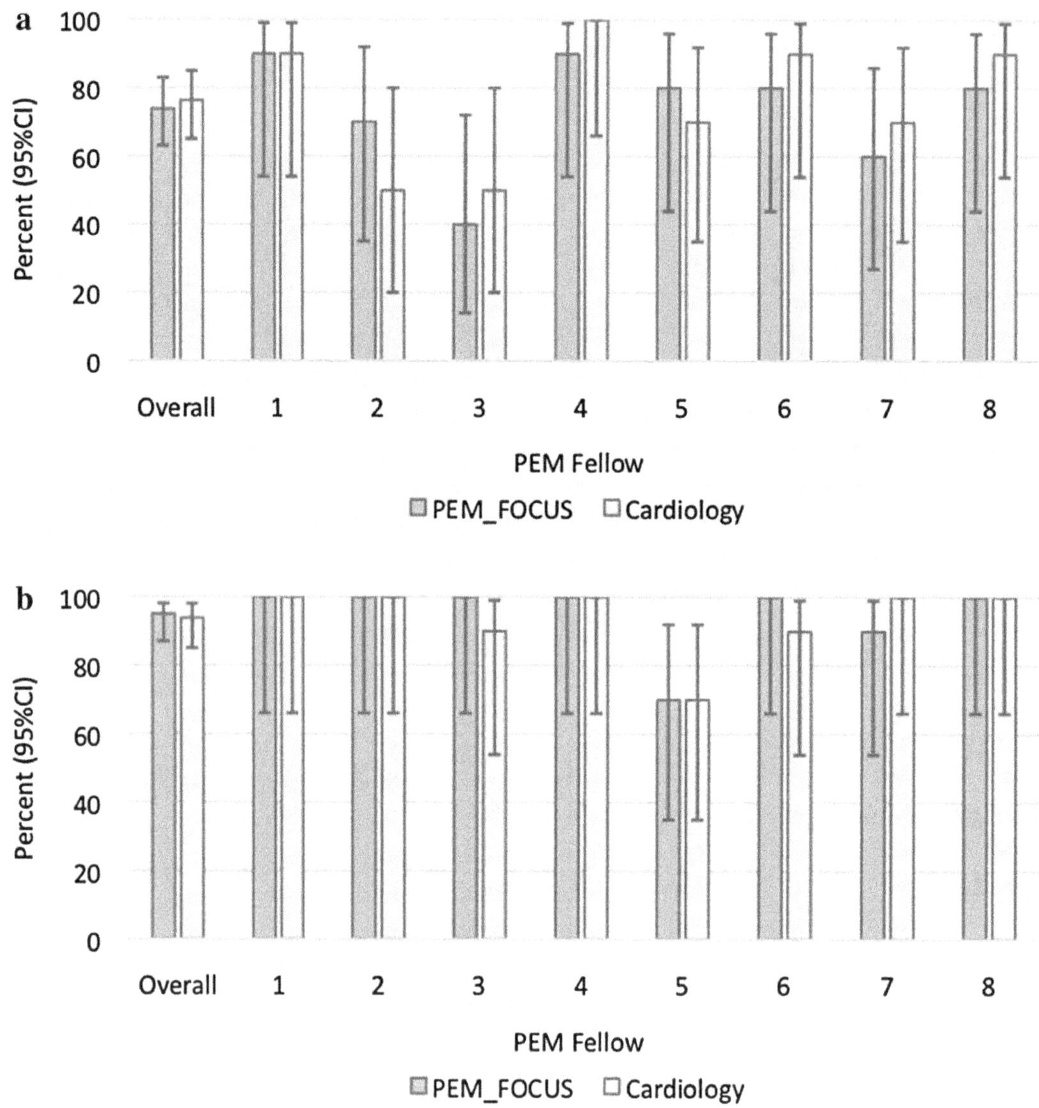

Fig. 4 Specificity of interpretation of classroom test of images of PEM FOCUS versus cardiology images by 8 PEM fellows for function (**a**) and effusion (**b**)

focused cardiac ultrasound. Future studies may wish to incorporate a severity-enriched patient population or use other modes of presenting pathology such as pediatric ultrasound image banks that are being developed.

Additional files

Additional file 1: Phase S1. Missed diminished function (False Negative). Parasternal long axis view. Image acquisition made interpretation difficult. The gain setting is a bit dark to visualize the interventricular septum and the anterior leaflet of the mitral valve. The captured video would be improved by including the inferior portion of left ventricle and apex. **Phase S2**. Missed diminished function (False Negative). Parasternal long axis view. Image acquisition made interpretation difficult. Similar to Additional file Phase 1(a) gain setting is a bit dark and the left ventricle is not well imaged. **Phase S3**. Normal interpreted as effusion (False Positive). Subxiphoid view. Image acquisition made interpretation difficult, again with the gain setting too dark. Trace or trivial amount of pericardial effusion was considered negative for our study; it was listed as "None/ Trivial" on the data collection form. **Phase S4**. Missed pericardial effusion (False Negative). Parasternal long axis view. Image acquisition was adequate, while gain could be increased. This was a gross operator interpretation error.

Additional file 2: Phase S5. Missed pericardial effusion (False Negative). Parasternal long axis view. Image acquisition is good. This was an interpretation error. A pericardial effusion is seen above the descending thoracic aorta and pericardium. Also of note, there is also a small pleural effusion present, seen as the anechoic strip below the pericardium and lateral to the descending aorta. Phase S6. Missed pericardial effusion (False Negative). Parasternal long axis view. Small pericardial effusion is visible in this view. This was an interpretation error. Phase S7. Normal function called abnormal (False Positive). Parasternal long axis view. Images acquisition is acceptable. This was an interpretation problem. The anterior leaflet touches the interventricular septum during diastole with relatively normal chamber proportions. Phase S8. Normal function called abnormal (False Positive). Apical 4 chamber view. Image acquisition is adequate. Other views were also available that showed normal function.

Abbreviations
FOCUS: focused cardiac ultrasound; PEM: pediatric emergency medicine; POCUS: point of care ultrasound.

Authors' contributions
RTM designed and conducted the study, including patient recruitment, data collection, and data analysis. RTM, JSC, and CS had complete access to the study data with CS and JSC performing image review. KB provided statistical support in analyzing and representing the data. RTM and JSC prepared the manuscript draft with important intellectual input from CS. All authors were involved in the conceptualization, design of the study, and final approval of version to be published. All authors read and approved the final manuscript.

Author details
[1] Department of Emergency Medicine and Trauma Services, Children's National Medical Center, Washington, DC, USA. [2] Department of Cardiology, Children's National Medical Center, Washington, DC, USA. [3] Department of Cardiology, Children's Hospital of Pittsburgh, Pittsburgh, PA, USA. [4] Department of Cardiology, Goryeb Children's Hospital, Morristown, NJ, USA. [5] Department of Emergency Medicine, Icahn School of Medicine at Mt. Sinai, New York, NY, USA. [6] Faculty, George Washington University School of Medicine, Washington, DC, USA.

Acknowledgements
We want to thank the Pediatric Emergency Medicine Fellows at Children's National Medical Center (2014–2016) who participated in this study. Special thanks to Drs. James Chamberlain and Keith Boniface who provided feedback to the manuscript. The material presented here was presented in abstract form at the Pediatric Academic Society Meeting. San Francisco, CA, May 2017.

References
1. Labovitz AJ, Noble VE, Bierig M et al (2010) Focused cardiac ultrasound in the emergent setting: a consensus statement of the American society of echocardiography and American college of emergency physicians. J Am Soc Echocardiogr 23(12):1225–1230
2. Marin JR, Lewiss RE, American Academy of Pediatrics CmoPEM, Society for Academic Emergency Medicine AaoEU, American College of Emergency Physicians PdEMC, Ultrasound WINFoC (2015) Point-of-care ultrasonography by pediatric emergency medicine physicians. Pediatrics 135(4):e1113–1122
3. Marin JR, Abo AM, Arroyo AC et al (2016) Pediatric emergency medicine point-of-care ultrasound: summary of the evidence. Crit Ultrasound J 8(1):16
4. Gaspar HA, Morhy SS, Lianza AC et al (2014) Focused cardiac ultrasound: a training course for pediatric intensivists and emergency physicians. BMC Med Educ 14:25
5. Pershad J, Myers S, Plouman C et al (2004) Bedside limited echocardiography by the emergency physician is accurate during evaluation of the critically ill patient. Pediatrics 114(6):e667–e671
6. Longjohn M, Wan J, Joshi V, Pershad J (2011) Point-of-care echocardiography by pediatric emergency physicians. Pediatr Emerg Care 27(8):693–696
7. Costantino T, Burton J, Tayal V (2015) Ultrasound competency and practice: what's in a number? Acad Emerg Med 22(5):597–599
8. Vignon P, Mücke F, Bellec F et al (2011) Basic critical care echocardiography: validation of a curriculum dedicated to noncardiologist residents. Crit Care Med 39(4):636–642
9. Chisholm CB, Dodge WR, Balise RR, Williams SR, Gharahbaghian L, Beraud AS (2013) Focused cardiac ultrasound training: how much is enough? J Emerg Med 44(4):818–822
10. Blehar DJ, Barton B, Gaspari RJ (2015) Learning curves in emergency ultrasound education. Acad Emerg Med 22(5):574–582
11. Lewiss RE, Hoffmann B, Beaulieu Y, Phelan MB (2014) Point-of-care ultrasound education. J Ultrasound Med 33(1):27–32
12. Amini R, Stolz LA, Javedani PP et al (2016) Point-of-care echocardiography in simulation-based education and assessment. Adv Med Educ Pract 7:325–328
13. Riera A, Weeks B, Emerson BL, Chen L (2018) Evaluation of a focused cardiac ultrasound protocol in a pediatric emergency department. Pediatr Emerg Care. https://doi.org/10.1097/PEC.0000000000001495
14. Via G, Hussain A, Wells M et al (2014) International evidence-based recommendations for focused cardiac ultrasound. J Am SocEchocardiogr 27(7):683.e1–683.e33
15. Tsung JW, Blaivas M (2008) Feasibility of correlating the pulse check with focused point-of-care echocardiography during pediatric cardiac arrest: a case series. Resuscitation 77(2):264–269
16. Hu K, Gupta N, Teran F, Saul T, Nelson BP, Andrus P (2018) Variability in interpretation of cardiac standstill among physician sonographers. Ann Emerg Med 71(2):193–198

2

Lung ultrasound training: a systematic review of published literature in clinical lung ultrasound training

Pia Iben Pietersen[1,2,3*], Kristian Rørbæk Madsen[4], Ole Graumann[2,5], Lars Konge[6], Bjørn Ulrik Nielsen[4] and Christian Borbjerg Laursen[1,2]

Abstract

Background: Clinical lung ultrasound examinations are widely used in the primary assessment or monitoring of patients with dyspnoea or respiratory failure. Despite being increasingly implemented, there is no international consensus on education, assessment of competencies, and certification. Today, training is usually based on the concept of mastery learning, but is often unstructured and limited by bustle in a clinical daily life. The aim of the systematic review is to provide an overview of published learning studies in clinical lung ultrasound, and to collect evidence for future recommendations in lung ultrasound education and certification.

Methods: According to PRISMA guidelines, three databases (PubMed, Embase, Cochrane Library) were searched, and two reviewers examined the results for eligibility. Included publications were described and assessed for level of evidence and risk of bias according to guidelines from Oxford Centre for Evidence-Based Medicine and Cochrane Collaboration Tool for Risk of Bias assessment.

Results: Of 7796 studies screened, 16 studies were included. Twelve pre- and post-test studies, three descriptive studies and one randomized controlled trial were identified. Seven studies included web-based or online modalities, while remaining used didactic or classroom-based lectures. Twelve (75%) studies provided hands-on sessions, and of these, 11 assessed participants' hands-on skills. None of the studies used validated neither written nor practical assessment. The highest level of evidence score was 2 ($n = 1$), remaining scored 4 ($n = 15$). Risk of bias was assessed high in 11 of 16 studies (68.75%).

Conclusion: All educational methods proved increased theoretical and practical knowledge obtained at the ultrasound courses, but the included studies were substantial heterogeneous in setup, learning-, and assessment methods, and outcome measures. On behalf of current published studies, it was not possible to construct clear guidelines for the future education and certification in clinical lung ultrasound, but the use of different hands-on training facilities tends to contribute to different aspects of the learning process. This systematic review proves a lack of learning studies within this content, and research with validated theoretical and practical tests for assessment is desired.

Keywords: Thoracic ultrasound, Pulmonary ultrasound, Point-of-care ultrasound, Medical education, Training

*Correspondence: pia.iben.pietersen3@rsyd.dk
[1] Department of Respiratory Medicine, Odense University Hospital, Sdr. Boulevard 29, 5000 Odense C, Denmark
Full list of author information is available at the end of the article

Introduction

The clinical use of lung ultrasound (LUS) in emergency departments, critical care units as well as in respiratory departments has increased substantially. LUS has an excellent diagnostic accuracy for many of the most common causes of acute respiratory failure (e.g., cardiogenic pulmonary edema, pneumonia, pleural effusion, and pneumothorax) and increases the proportion of patients receiving a correct diagnosis and treatment [1–6]. Furthermore, LUS is a rapid, bedside, non-invasive, radiation-free diagnostic tool, which the clinician can use as an integrated part of the initial clinical assessment as well as for monitoring purposes. However, the value of LUS is dependent on competent operators performing the examination.

Several societies, e.g., the European Federation of Societies for Ultrasound in Medicine and Biology, British Thoracic Society and European Association of Cardiovascular Imaging, have clear guidelines and descriptions of logbook, number of performed supervised examinations needed, and basic knowledge curricula, which must be obtained before performing unsupervised lung ultrasound examinations [7–9]. However, no clear evidence-based guidelines or recommendations exist on the training needed to obtain adequate skills for performing an LUS examination.

Like other procedures and treatments, LUS education and certification should be based on best available evidence, and with gathered validity evidence in learning- or clinical studies. The aims of this systemic review were to provide an overview of the literature published in learning studies in clinical LUS, and to explore and collect evidence for future recommendations in lung ultrasound education and competency assessment.

Materials and methods

The systematic review was performed according to the Preferred Reporting Items for Systematic Review and Meta-Analysis (PRISMA) guidelines [10]. A systematic literature search was conducted in PubMed, Embase, and Cochrane Library in collaboration with a research librarian from the Medical Research library at Odense University Hospital, Denmark. Terms used: lung OR lungs OR pulmonal OR pulmonary OR thoracic OR thorax OR thoracal OR mediastinal OR mediastinum, ultrasound OR ultrasonic OR ultrasonography OR ultrasonics OR sonography OR sonographic, medical education OR education OR learning OR training OR clinical competences OR curriculum including MeSH terms. The search was completed on March 7, 2017. The inclusion criterion was: learning- or education studies in lung or thoracic ultrasound. No exclusion criteria were provided within languages, animal studies, etc.

After removing duplicates, all titles and abstracts were screened by two authors (PP and KRM). All articles that potentially met the broad inclusion criterion or indeterminate articles were assessed with full article reading. Abstracts regarding the following studies were excluded: ultrasound education in other organ systems or anatomical structures than lungs or thorax, cost–benefit analysis, case reports, author responses, letter to the editor, and comments. Diagnostic accuracy studies were excluded from this review, except from those, which also included a learning study or had objectives or outcomes that assessed training or development of competencies in LUS. The same two authors then subsequently read all eligible articles, and each article was discussed until consensus. In case of disagreement, a third reviewer (CBL) was conferred. Hand search was conducted on references of included full articles. Level of evidence was categorized using the Oxford Centre for Evidence-Based Medicine (OCEBM) system for Level of Evidence [11]. Bias in each included article were discussed and marked according to Cochrane Collaboration risk of bias [12].

Results

Search strategy

The initial search yielded 7796 publications. After removal of duplicates, author responses and conference abstracts, 4656 publications remained. Of these, 4622 were excluded. Most of the excluded studies did not meet the inclusion criterion at all, and comprised complete different topics, aims, and objectives than education or assessment in LUS or thoracic ultrasound. Because of the wide search strategy, the amount of publications not relevant for this systematic review was large. Figure 1 presents the eligibility process and exclusion of articles. Causes of the full-text exclusions were: diagnostic accuracy studies ($n=6$), testing the effectiveness and use of different models/phantoms or hands-on facilities for LUS ($n=7$), describing implementation, use and feasibility of LUS ($n=3$), train-the-trainer course ($n=1$), and assessment of respiratory therapists' theoretical and clinical skills in LUS ($n=1$). The reference lists of included papers were screened without leading to inclusion of further studies. Study design, participants, learning strategy, hands-on facilities, and assessment are described below. Additional information is shown in Tables 1 and 2.

Study design

In total, there were 12 pre- and post-test studies that used improvement in written test scores to evaluate the educational Cochrane [13–24]. Five of the pre- and post-test studies had a follow-up time from 1 week to 6 months, average 13 weeks ± 4.83 [14, 16, 18, 20, 25], and one recorded number of scans performed from baseline to

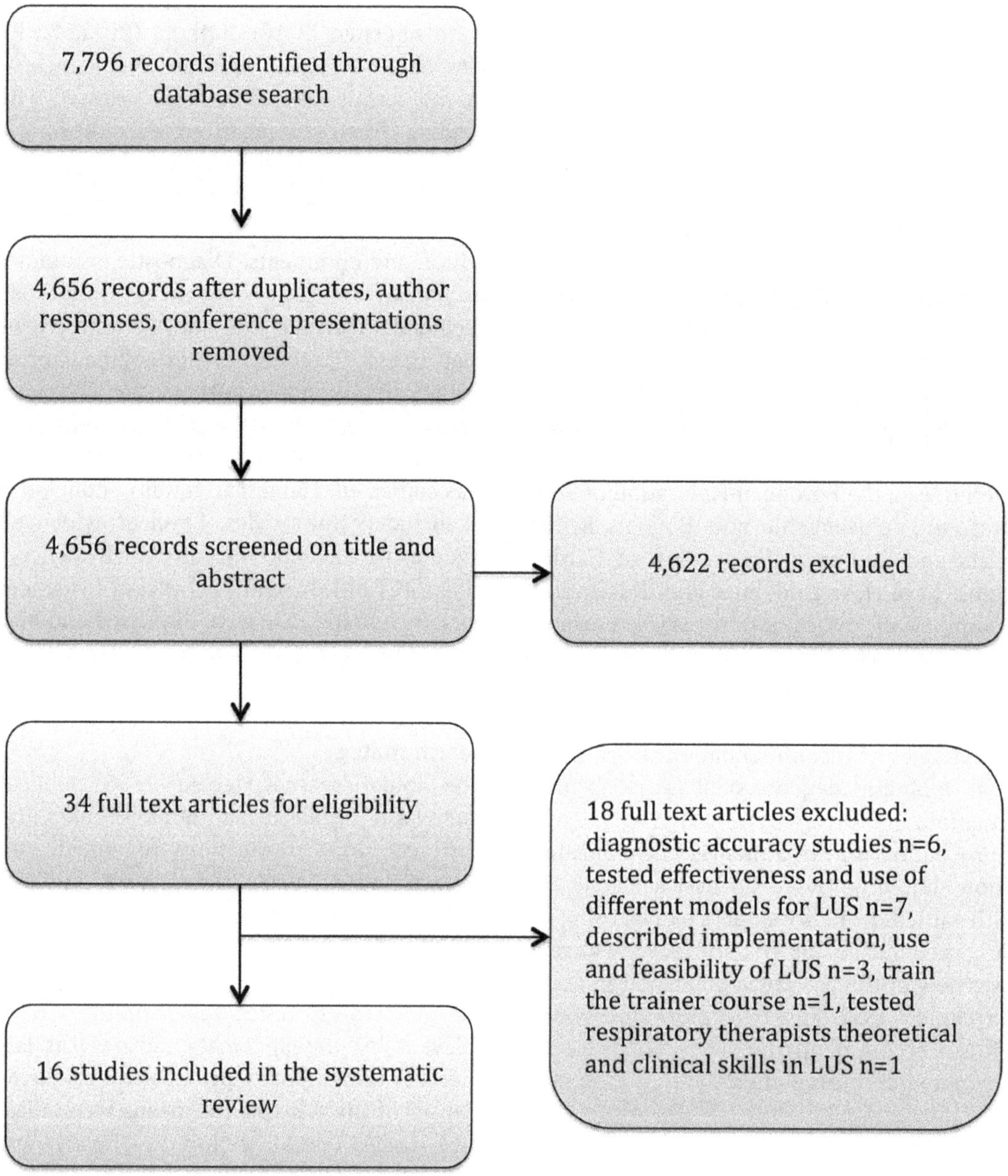

Fig. 1 Flowchart of search strategy, and selection process based on the Preferred Reporting Items for Systematic Reviews and Meta-analysis (PRISMA)

follow-up [20]. Three descriptive studies were identified [25–27] and one randomized controlled trial [28]. Five of the studies (31%) were courses in general critical care ultrasound, or basic skill ultrasound, where thoracic or lung ultrasound was a specific and independently evaluated topic [17, 19–21, 24].

Participants

Most study participants were ultrasound novices, and especially novices in clinical LUS, and varied from medical students to respiratory therapists, emergency department residents, and anesthesiologists. Three studies also included other healthcare professionals as prehospital providers, nurses, and veterinarians [18, 22, 24]. Two studies excluded participants with the previous ultrasound certification or attendance in a formal critical care ultrasound course within 12 months [20, 28], and two studies only included a study population with no experience [21, 24].

Learning strategy

Learning strategies in the studies included were heterogeneous in both time spent on lectures, theoretical presentation, and method used for assessment. The most

Table 1 Publications on education in lung ultrasound: study characteristics

	Study design	Assessment	Facility	Education tool	Participants
Pre and post-test studies					
Noble et al. [13]	Pre- and post-test	Theoretical pre- and post-test (50 video clips)	Ultrasound video clips	2 h didactic lecture (one for pneumothorax and one for pulmonary oedema)	27 physicians working for the SAMU at l'Hôpital Necker in Paris, France
Oveland et al. [14]	Pre- and post-test and 6-months follow-up	Theoretical pre- and post-test (34 MCQs, 10 US physics questions, 17 recognition pictures, 7 video clips) and hands-on practical examination (6 months follow-up	Healthy live models and porcine models	8 h attendance course including didactic (2 h), practical (2 h) and experimental (4 h) sessions	20 first-year to graduate-year medical students (11 at 6 months follow-up)
Breitkreutz et al. [15]	Pre- and post-test	Theoretical pre- and post-test (15 MCQs and 5 recognition images), post course recognition quiz (15 video clips) and practical post course examination (16 predefined sonoanatomic items)	Healthy live models, patients with chronic or malignant lung diseases or who had recently underwent thoracotomy. Custom-made gel phantoms	Two and a half hour theoretical training (six brief lectures in anatomy, physiology and pathology of thorax and four case presentations). Two and a half hour hands-on training	54 trainees. Group A: 14 medical students, Group B: 32 anaesthesiologists, Group C: 8 trauma surgeons
Cuca et al. [16]	Pre- and post-test	Theoretical pre-, post-, and sustainability test (20 MCQs, results compared with THOLUUSE-study [14])	–	E-learning module including physiological and pathological sonographic patterns (Five topics: basics and pleural effusion, pneumothorax, pulmonary oedema and consolidation, trachea, workflow of LUS) estimated time 30–50 min	29 medical students and medical doctors
Hulett et al. [17]	Pre- and post-test	Theoretical pre- and post-test (46 questions including MCQs, true/false, matching items, fill-in-the blank image and video recognition), practical pre- and post course skills	Patients located in medical ICU at the North Carolina Hospital	1 h didactic instruction, 1 h image interpretation workshop and image acquisition training, in 1 work week supervised hands-on training	Eight critical care medicine fellows
Bhat et al. [18]	Pre- and post-test and 1-week follow-up	Theoretical (16 MCQs)	Ultrasound images and video clips obtained in the Emergency Department by trained ultrasound physicians	1 h didactic lecture including basic scan technique, normal ultrasound anatomy, image interpretation of normal or pathological pattern	57 prehospital providers (19 medical technicians students, 16 paramedic students, 18 certified medical technicians and four certified paramedics
Connolly et al. [19]	Pre- and post-test	Theoretical pre- and post-test (21 MCQs) and practical examination (real-time scans saved and blinded evaluated by instructors)	Live models and phantom task trainer models and simulators	Five 1-h workshops and 4 h didactic online preparatory training. Hands-on with supervised scans	24 medical students in MCQ pre- and post-test evaluation and 16 in clinical skill assessment

Table 1 (continued)

	Study design	Assessment	Facility	Education tool	Participants
Dinh et al. [20]	Pre- and post-test and 3 months follow-up	Theoretical pre-, post-, and sustainability test (50 MCQs—12 pulmonary) (84 point checklist). Pathologic image interpretation (4 cases with each 20 questions each). Ultrasound comfort level and use of ultrasound	Healthy live models, simulators	2 days course including didactic lectures, live demonstrations, hands-on sessions on healthy models, pathologic image interpretation with cases using ultrasound simulator	Eight ICU fellows, participants with the previous ultrasound experience were excluded
Heiberg et al. [21]	Pre- and post-test	Theoretical pre- and post-test (56 MCQs) and practical three test sessions	Four healthy medical students	E-learning course including text, pictures, animations and movies (5–8 h) and hands-on session (4 h; 30 min LUS)	20 medical students
Sanchez-de-Toledo et al. [22]	Pre- and post-test	Theoretical pre-, and post-test (four written cases). Practical skill test after 60 min hands-on session (four cases)	Porcine models	One and a half hour theoretical and practice-based course	Four veterinaries, eight neonatologists, seven paediatric intensive care specialists, two intensive care nurses, three paediatric surgeons, eight paediatric anaesthesiologists, four paediatricians
See et al. [23]	Pre- and post-test	Theoretical pre- and post-test (20 MCQs) and hands-on (blinded evaluation of image acquisition and interpretation)	Mechanically ventilated patients or patients with respiratory failure, requiring at least 40% inspired oxygen fraction to maintain an oxygen saturation of 90%	30 min didactic introduction, 1 month self-study (powerpoint slides, criticalecho.com and court.net). Supervised scans with immediately feedback with focus on image acquisition, afterwards image interpretation by blinded observer	22 respiratory therapists
Greenstein et al. [24]	Pre- and post-test	Theoretical pre- and post-test (20 MCQs) and hands-on assessment	Healthy human models	3 days course including didactic lectures with real-time ultrasound scan on healthy models, image interpretation sessions and hands-on training	363 critical care physicians, hospitalists, surgeons, physician assistants, advanced practice nurses and medical residents
Descriptive studies					
Krishnan et al. [25]	Post course evaluation and sustainability test	Theoretical post- and sustainability test (20 video clips ± pneumothorax)	Ultrasound video of 53 patients before and after elective thoracic surgery. In all, 99 videos were compiled (52 without pneumothoraces and 47 with)	5-min online presentation of the use of ultrasound for detection of pneumothorax	79 (70 at 6 month follow-up) residents and faculty members from Department of anaesthesia

Table 1 (continued)

	Study design	Assessment	Facility	Education tool	Participants
Abbasi et al. [26]	Prospective cross-sectional study	Hands-on assessment (± pneumothorax)	Healthy live models and patients admitted in Emergency Department with thoracic trauma	2 h training course including 30 min didactic lecture, 30 min hands-on training on healthy volunteers, 1 h training on patients	Four emergency physicians
Gargani et al. [27]	Post course evaluation	Online assessment of uploaded LUS examinations and theoretical assessment of *b*-line interpretation (44 videos)	Patients	Part A: web-based training program; 26 min educational video with focus on *b*-line assessment. Upload of 7 self-performed lung ultrasound videos, when videos were approved by experts, trainees proceed to Part B: *b*-line interpretation	Thirty nephrologists and 14 cardiologists
Randomized controlled trial					
Edrich et al. [28]	Randomized controlled trial with 4 weeks follow-up	Theoretical pre-, post-, and sustainability test (10 MCQs and one video clip) and practical examination (blinded reviewers)	Healthy live models	Group I: web-based (powerpoint 25 min and online demonstration 5 min). Group II: Classroom-based (powerpoint) 45 min didactic lectures and 20 min hands-on training. Group III: No education or hands-on training. Blinded reviewers	138 anaesthesiologists from four academic hospitals. Participants with the previous ultrasound experience excluded

Table 2 Publications in education in lung ultrasound: study statistics and conclusion

	Statistical analysis	Outcome measures	Study conclusion	Level of evidence
Noble et al. [13]. Evaluation of thoracic ultrasound training module for the detection of pneumothorax and pulmonary edema by prehospital physician care providers. 2009	Paired *t* test compared mean score of pre- and post-test	Improvement in pre- and post-test scores	With minimal didactic and image recognition skill sessions are needed before physicians can recognize the key artifacts, which lead to the diagnosis of pulmonary edema and pneumothorax.	4
Oveland et al. [14]. Animal laboratory training improves lung ultrasound proficiency and speed. 2013	Sensitivity, specificity, positive and negative predictive value	Confidence level, scan time, improvement in theoretical score and sensitivity/specificity	Novices can quickly learn how to diagnose PTX using lung US. Training in an animal facility imparts a high level of long-term diagnostic proficiency and speed for diagnosing PTX	4
Breitkreutz et al. [15]. Thorax, trachea and lung ultrasonography in Emergency and Critical care medicine: Assessment of an Objective Structured training concept. 2013	Non-parametric Wilcoxon matched pairs (within groups), Mann–Whitney *U* test (between groups)	Improvement in pre- and post-test scores. Recognition and interpretation skill scores. Practical imaging performance scores	1-day training program like THOLUUSE significantly improves theoretical and practical skills for sonographic diagnosis of including PLE and PTX	4
Cuca et al. [16]. Assessment of a new e-learning system on thorax, trachea and lung ultrasound. 2013	Wilcoxon matched pairs test. Self-assessment survey	Improvement in pre- and post-test score and sustainability test, qualitative program evaluation score	Results of written tests from the e-learning attendance course are comparable and with same progress as attendance-based courses	4
Hulett et al. [17]. Development and Preliminary Assessment of Critical Care Ultrasound Course in an Adult Pulmonary and Critical Care Fellowship Program. 2014	Paired t-test on pre- and postcourse performances	Improvement in pre- and post-test scores, practical pre- and postcourse skill score and self-assessment score	A formal curriculum dedicated to critical care ultrasound can be developed and implemented on site in a fellowship training program. After validation studies testing longer term retention of knowledge and bedside skills on trainees at other broadly representative medical centres, the curriculum described here might form the basis of a widely applicable onsite critical care ultrasound course curriculum	4
Bhat et al. [18]. Prehospital Evaluation of Effusion, Pneumothorax and standstill (PEEPS): Point-of-care Ultrasound in emergency medical services. 2015	Two-tailed, paired *t* test	Improvement in pre-, post- and sustainability test. Level of confidence	This study showed potential promise for training prehospital EMS providers in accurate US interpretation through a 1-h didactic lecture focused on US technique and anatomy for the assessment of pericardial effusion, pneumothorax, and cardiac standstill	4
Connolly et al. [19]. Ultrafest: a novel Approach to Ultrasound in Medical Education Leads to Improvement in Written and Clinical Examinations, 2014	Paired *t* test analysis	Improvement in pre- and post-test score and practical pre- and postcourse skill score	A 1-day, 9-h, small group instruction and practice symposium improved student knowledge on trauma and pulmonary US, and improved image acquisition, but the latter fell short of significant proficiency	4

Table 2 (continued)

	Statistical analysis	Outcome measures	Study conclusion	Level of evidence
Dinh et al. [20]. Impact of a 2-day critical care ultrasound course during fellowship training: a pilot study. 2015	Students *t* test, Chi square or ANOVA	Improvement in pre-, post-, and 3 month follow-up test score, comfort level score. Number of self-reported scans	Introduction of a 2-day critical care ultrasound course has both a positive short- and long-term impact on fellows' confidence and proficiency with ultrasound use. Utilizing tools such as written tests to assess basic knowledge, live models to teach practical skills, and ultrasound simulators to teach pathological image identification can help standardize critical care ultrasound training	4
Heiberg et al. [21]. Point-of-care clinical ultrasound for medical students. 2015	Paired Students *t* test, Wilcoxon rank sum test, Chi squared test, linear regression	Improvement in pre- and post-test score and practical pre- and postcourse skill score	Medical students with no previous experience of ultrasound techniques demonstrated a significant increase in their ability to acquire and interpret an ultrasound image after completion of interactive e-learning, and this competence was further improved after 4 h of systematic hands-on training	4
Sanchez-de-Toledo et al. [22]. Teaching chest ultrasound in an porcine model. 2016	Sensitivity, specificity, positive and negative predictive values	Improvement in sensitivity and specificity after 30 and 60 min	Brief training in theory combined with animal models facilitates learning for medical professionals with no previous training in US and enables them to recognize the three most relevant thoracic US patterns. The introduction of advanced simulation with animal models can facilitate training of personnel in the recognition and management of acute lung disease	4
See et al. [23]. Lung ultrasound training: curriculum implementation and learning trajectory among respiratory therapists. 2016	Paired *t* test. Three patients block (36 images) Overall performance score with linear regression	Improvement in pre- and post-test scores and practical skill scores	We devised a pragmatic lung ultrasound curriculum, which involved building rapport, stimulating self-directed learning, and avoiding cognitive overload. Our training method allowed RTs to acquire the ability to independently perform lung ultrasound after at least ten directly supervised scans	4

Table 2 (continued)

	Statistical analysis	Outcome measures	Study conclusion	Level of evidence
Greenstein et al. [24]. Effectiveness of a Critical Care ultrasonography Course. 2016	Two-tailed student *t* test	Improvement in pre- and post-test score and practical pre- and postcourse skill score	This 3-day CHEST CCUS course is an effective method to train large groups of clinicians in the skills requisite for CCUS. The majority of learners demonstrated improved performance in both image interpretation and hands-on ultrasonography skills across all educational domains at the completion of the course	4
Krishnan et al. [25]. Efficacy of an online education program for ultrasound diagnosis of pneumothorax. 2013	Sensitivity and specificity at the time of educational program and after 6 months	Improvement in sensitivity/specificity, use of ultrasound from baseline to follow-up	After viewing a 5-min online training video, physicians can reliably rule out pneumothorax on an optimal ultrasound image. They are also able to retain this skill for up to 6 months	4
Abbasi et al. [26]. Accuracy of emergency physician-performed ultrasound in detecting traumatic pneumothorax after 2-h training course. 2012	Sensitivity and specificity, positive after 5, 10 and 20 ultrasound examinations, × 2-test for proportions and the Student *t* test for continuous variables	Improvement in sensitivity/specificity after 5, 10 and 20 examinations	By a brief learning course, the emergency physicians easily diagnosed PTX in trauma patients with a reasonable accuracy in comparison with CT scan as the gold standard	4
Gargani et al. [27]. Efficacy of a remote web-based lung ultrasound training for nephrologists and cardiologists: an LUST trial sub-project. 2016	Mean number of *b* lines ± SD. Pearsons correlation coefficient (trainer vs. trainee). Intraclass correlation coefficient and confidence interval. Interobserver agreement by Bland–Altman plot	Test-score agreement (trainee vs. trainer)	In conclusion, this study performed in the framework of the LUST trial shows that nephrologists and cardiologists can be effectively trained to measure lung congestion by an entirely web-based educational program	4
Edrich et al. [28]. A comparison of web-based with traditional classroom-based training of lung ultrasound for the exclusion of pneumothorax. 2016	Agreement of reviewers results assessed with Krippendorff test. Total score in percent. One-sided, 2-sample *t* test	Improvement in pre-, post-, and sustainability test score and practical test	When training anaesthesiologists to perform LUS for the exclusion of pneumothorax, we found that web-based training was not inferior to traditional classroom-based training and was effective, leading to test scores that were similar to a group of clinicians experienced in LUS	2

commonly used educational tool used was didactic lectures ($n = 12$, 75%), with a variation of time spent from 30 min sessions [26] to 2.5 h sessions [15]. Abbasi et al. presented a single topic course (detection of pneumothorax with LUS), and time spent on didactic lecture was 30 min. This study was the only single topic course that used didactic lecture as educational tool [26]. Remaining studies introduced classroom-based learning covering a more comprehensive introduction to full LUS, primarily with 15–30 min education in each of the main topic. Some studies had a clear overview and description of topics included in the didactic lectures, whereas other studies only stated the overall general topics (Table 1).

Four studies describe a full day to 3 days courses with alternating theoretical and hands-on sessions [14, 19, 20, 24]. Four studies incorporated live ultrasound examinations by instructors in the theoretic session to combine the theoretic and practical understanding [19, 20, 24, 26]; otherwise, images and video clips were frequently used in the lectures.

Web-based learning or online presentations were used in 7 (44%) studies [16, 19, 21, 23, 25, 27, 28]. Four of those had only online presentations or web-based learning modules without didactic lectures or hands-on sessions [16, 25, 27, 28]. Cuca et al. studied a web-based learning program evaluated by nine experts of the international lung ultrasound consensus committee [16], and used the same written tests, topics, and curriculum as the study by Breitkreutz et al. [15]. Cuca et al. compared the results from the two studies. Krishnan et al. [25] presented a 5 min online presentation in the use of ultrasound as a diagnostic tool to confirm pneumothorax. Gargani et al. had a 26 min online presentation with primary focus on *b*-line presentation, interpretation, and the possibility of real-time demonstrations or meeting with instructors on Skype. Subsequently, participants were to upload seven LUS examinations for evaluation. When the instructors had approved the seven videos, the participants could proceed to the second part of the training, including a set of 44 videos with the focus of counting *b* lines [27]. In the randomized trial by Edrich et al., one of the study groups received a web-based educational learning program and had no hands-on session, another group had a 45 min classroom-based lecture and 20 min hands-on, whereas the control group had no lectures at all. The participants were evaluated with a pretest, post-test, and 4 week retention test [28].

Hands-on training facilities

Twelve of sixteen studies included hands-on sessions in the educational program [13–15, 17, 19–24, 26, 28]. Simulators were used in three studies [19, 20, 26], and healthy live models in eight studies [14, 15, 19–21, 24, 26, 28]. In five studies, emergency department patients or patients with respiratory failure in other departments were assessed as a part of the training program [15, 17, 23, 26, 27], including three studies, where LUS video clips from patients hospitalized were obtained and used in the assessment [13, 18, 25]. Porcine models were used in two studies [14, 22]. Four studies combined the use of different models, patients and/or simulators [14, 15, 19, 20, 26].

Assessment

Thirteen studies used written examinations to assess theoretical knowledge obtained at the educational programs [13–25]. They all used multiple-choice items format covering true/false questions, one-best-answer questions, single-correct-answer questions and multiple-response questions, all included images and/or video clips in the questions. None of the studies described gathering validity evidence for neither the pre- and post-tests nor the practical skill assessment tools. One study, however, had the multiple-choice questions (MCQs) peer-reviewed by the instructors ahead of the study [20], but the vast majority of the assessment checklists, written tests, and curricula were described as based on the international consensus recommendations for point-of-care lung ultrasound by Volpicelli et al. [29].

Eleven studies assessed participants' practical skills [14, 15, 17, 19–24, 26, 28]. The most common method used for evaluation and assessment of practical skills was observer checklists but varied greatly. Participants in See et al. [23] scanned 12 zones with an instructor bedside, who was allowed to comment or help if needed, videos were stored, and participants then interpreted the clips in front of the instructor. Connolly et al. [19] assessed the participants' practical skills by letting participants scan four windows, and videos were stored and rated by blinded instructors. Breitkreutz et al. [15] had 16 predefined sonoanatomical structures that participants should present and were then rated on a standardized sheet. Respectively, 46 and 84 checklist items were to be scanned in Hulett et al. and Dinh et al. [17, 20] and were evaluated regarding image acquisition and interpretation. Furthermore, Dinh et al. presented four cases with 20 case questions each [20]. Heiberg et al. [21] performed online testing of the students' practical skills by correct/incorrect and offline evaluation of image quality and interpretation. Greenstein et al. used 20 standardized examination tasks and 20 video-based examinations [24], whereas Oveland et al. presented scans on porcine models with confirmation or validation of pneumothorax, oral feedback from instructor and yet another scan session [14].

Level of evidence of the included studies is presented in Table 2 according to OCEBM guidelines, and assessment of risk of bias in Table 3. No studies scored the highest level of evidence, one study scored 2, remaining part of the studies scored 4. Bias was assessed as high in the majority of the studies (Table 3).

Discussion

The vast majority of the currently published LUS learning studies are one-group pre- and post-tests studies with low level of evidence. This study design can just inform us that trainees learned something from the specific intervention, but does not provide any evidence on how to build a curriculum [30]. The studies are heterogeneous in choice of: educational program, teaching methods, participant assessment, and study outcome. In

Table 3 Scores of the Cochrane Collaboration risk of bias assessment tool [12]

	Selection bias		Performance bias	Detection bias	Attrition bias	Reporting bias	Other bias	Overall risk of bias
	Random sequence generation	Allocation concealment	Blinding of participants and personnel	Blinding of outcome assessment	Incomplete outcome data	Selective reporting	Other sources of bias	
Pre and post-test studies								
Noble et al. [13]. 2009	#	#	1	1	1	1	?	Low
Oveland et al. [14]. 2013	#	#	?	0	0	0	?	High
Breitkreutz et al. [15]. 2013	#	#	1	0	1	1	?	Low
Cuca et al. [16]. 2013	#	#	0	1	0	1	?	High
Hulett et al. [17]. 2014	#	#	0	0	1	0	?	High
Bhat et al. [18]. 2015	#	#	0	0	0	1	?	High
Connolly et al. [19]. 2014	#	#	1	0	0	0	?	High
Dinh et al. [20]. 2015	#	#	0	0	1	1	?	High
Heiberg et al. [21]. 2015	#	#	0	0	1	0	?	High
Sanchez-de-Toledo et al. [22]. 2016	#	#	1	1	1	1	?	Low
See et al. [23]. 2016	#	#	0	0	1	1	?	High
Greenstein et al. [24]. 2016	#	#	1	0	0	0	?	High
Descriptive studies								
Krishnan et al. [25]. 2013	#	#	0	1	1	1	?	Low
Abbasi et al. [26]. 2012	#	#	0	0	1	1	?	High
Gargani et al. [27]. 2016	#	#	0	0	1	1	?	High
Randomized controlled trial								
Edrich et al. [28]. 2016	?	0	1	1	1	1	?	Low

0 = high risk of bias, 1 = low risk of bias, ? = unclear risk of bias, # = irrelevant in this study (non-randomized trial)

addition to conventional classroom-based didactic lectures, web-based learning was often chosen as an alternative or additional method and was used in 7 of the 16 included studies [16, 19, 21, 23, 25, 27, 28], but only one study measured the effect of the two educational methods, and compared the results from the two groups in a randomized controlled trial [28].

Web-based learning strategies have been proven to have several advantages. Ruiz et al. describe increased accessibility and flexibility as important advantages. It standardizes course content and delivery independent of teacher presentation and variation. Students are in control of their learning sequence and learning pace, and web-based learning can be designed to include outcome assessment [31, 32]. Furthermore, it is possible to implement different types of multimedia such as graphics, videos, animations, and texts to increase learning ability. A meta-analysis by Cook et al. [33] proved that medical web-based learning was significantly superior to no intervention, and participants could achieve results similar to traditional learning methods like classroom-based learning in numerous diagnostic and therapeutic content areas. Edrich et al. [28] correspondingly found the same improvement. Since web-based education has similar outcome as classroom-based lectures, it would be obvious to include other parameters like maintenance of both theoretical and practical skills with follow-up assessments, time efficiency, and user satisfaction surveys. The meta-analysis, like this systematic review, suffers from considerable heterogeneity in study participants, learning methods, and outcome measures.

Web-based learning in general point-of-care ultrasound has advantageously been evaluated in several studies [34–36]. In Kang et al. [36], outcome measures were not only improvement in test score, but also hours spent on organizing the course and course costs. In both cases, web-based learning was more cost-effective. None of the studies included in this systematic review incorporated cost–benefit analysis, but one concluded that an ultrasound symposium requires a massive setup and great financial resources because of the number of ultrasound machines, phantoms, volunteers, instructors, and rooms. When building a theoretical curriculum in medical education, the teacher:student ratio can be low without affecting the learning ability significantly. However, when training practical skills, it requires a closer relation and interaction between instructor and trainee, and the most optimal trainee to instructor ratio is as close as 1:1 as possible. Oveland et al. [14] also discussed cost–benefit issues and concluded that porcine models as simulators and animal laboratory training in general, combined with ethical considerations, may be an option but have time, venue, and cost dilemmas.

The practical skill assessments of course participants in the included studies diverge in amount of checkpoints and topics. Even though the studies included used various checklists to keep the assessment as objective and standardized as possible, only two studies had blinded reviewers scoring the stored images or ultrasound sequences afterwards [19, 28], and no validity evidence was provided for any checklists.

LUS imaging and examinations differ from other point-of-care ultrasound examinations, because image interpretation and pathological recognition are based on sonographic artifacts instead of directly imaging diagnostics as, e.g., thickening of gallbladder wall, pericholecystic fluid, and sludge as a sign of acute cholecystitis. Therefore, there is a great need for a standardized and validated tool for assessing the understanding of LUS, image acquisition, and image interpretation, additionally, to demonstrate the capability to correlate the patterns and interpretations to lung pathology and physiology.

In general, when introducing a new assessment tool, validity evidence should be gathered, to ensure the reliability, and to make it possible for meaningful interpretation. Today, one of the most described and recognized frameworks for validity testing is by Messick [37]. Five distinct sources of validity evidence in scientific experimental data have been discussed; content, response process, internal structure, relationship to other variables, and consequences [38]. Some types of assessment demand a stronger emphasis on one or more sources of evidence depending on the curriculum, consequences, and properties of inferences. All sources should be researched with the highest level of evidence possible, but within this setting, an assessment tool should emphasize content-related evidence with some evidence of response quality, internal structure, and consequences.

A new study have constructed and gathered validity evidence for an instrument to assess LUS competences by obtaining international consensus by experts in multiple specialties [39]. The objective structured assessment of lung ultrasound skills (LUS-OSAUS) could form the foundation of further and more homogeneous studies in the future.

The theoretical assessment was a preferred method for measuring the degree of obtained theoretical knowledge before and after a course, but single-group pretest post-test design suffers from minimal internal and external validity. In the case of evaluating medical education through this set-up, it would be surprising if an increased post-test score was not found. This setup has been discussed and criticized for decades and is today considered obsolete [30, 40, 41]. A single topic curriculum like presented in Krishnan et al., where participants were presented for a 5 min online presentation in detection of pneumothorax with LUS, and assessed theoretical with 20 videos, proves that even a very short theoretical session leads to increased knowledge and pattern recognition. However, it does not provide any guarantee that the trainees can obtain the ultrasound images themselves, or connect the patterns to relevant differential diagnosis in a clinical setting.

One study reported that their theoretical test was validated, but did not describe how this was done [18]. Another had the questions peer reviewed by authors of the study [20]. Written tests, in general, are proven to be authoritative motivating, facilitating the learning process and cost-effective [42]. Disadvantages of using the same theoretical test as pretest, post-test, and follow-up test are recall bias or "learning the test" [43, 44]. The majority of the studies have tried to eliminate this bias by changing the order of questions as well as the order of answers. None of the participants in the included studies were blinded to the studies. Since the participants knew that they were being evaluated, they may have been more motivated to enhance their performance in the tests.

There were large differences in the use of healthy live models, patients with respiratory failure or lung diseases, phantoms/simulators, or porcine models for the hands-on training. The overall conclusion was that all models could contribute to increased hands-on competencies. Summarized, the different models could contribute to different aspects of the learning process; healthy live models were well suited for getting comfortable with the ultrasound devices, learning advantages and disadvantages of various transducers, improving image optimization, and learning hand–eye coordination. When using porcine models, it was possible to create pneumothoraces or pleural effusions allowing trainees to train the visual understanding of these diagnoses, but as discussed animal laboratory models have several other limitations. Dinh et al. [20] discuss the use of patients in an educational setting, and found it difficult to incorporate and standardize live pathology given the logistical challenges of recruiting patients with specific diseases and sonographic pattern. See et al. [23] reported problems with only a minority of the trainees scanned patients with pneumothorax due to a low prevalence of pneumothoraces. In addition, it is crucial not to delay diagnostic or initial treatment when using admitted patients in a learning study. Two studies used simulators for learning pathological patterns; both found simulators useful, and state that with the use of simulators, the students engage in both acquiring image and interpreting the abnormal finding while assimilating muscle memory with cognitive learning [20].

We acknowledge that the literature review was constrained by the quantity and quality of available evidence. Three databases were searched, decided being relevant for the topic, but a broader search strategy could potentially reveal more studies eligible for this systematic review, and we did not include data that were not published. However, all reference lists of publications eligible for full-text reading were searched with no additional findings. A minor part of the excluded publications contains education in lung ultrasound in context with ultrasound in other organ systems, e.g., abdominal ultrasound or eFAST (extended focused assessment with sonography for trauma). Different alternative expanded protocols for lung ultrasound or combined ultrasound have been developed and anchored in different specialties, and the evaluation of education of these different protocols was beyond the aim of this study. Therefore, studies were only included if the educational outcome was based on lung ultrasound separately.

The included studies failed to contribute to compelling body of evidence to support the educational evidence in LUS, and a meta-analysis was not possible to conduct because of the differences in assessment tools, and lack of comparability.

Standardized recommendations for education and certification in LUS is not possible to establish based on published studies because of heterogeneity in study design, low evidence-level, and high risk of bias among included literature. All courses showed progress in both theoretical and practical skills no matter which educational method used. If recommendations should be assigned from the current studies included in this systematic review and existing medical education literature, it would be ideal to use a three-step mastery-learning approach. First, trainees should obtain theoretical knowledge through either classroom-based education or web-based lectures with a curriculum based on experts' opinion and a validated post-test with a pass–fail standard to ensure sufficient theoretical knowledge. Second, focused hands-on sessions on simulators, pigs, or healthy subjects until competency are demonstrated in the training environment using a performance test with solid evidence of validity. Third, supervised scanning of real patients with feedback from a trained instructor who preferably uses an assessment tool to decide when the trainee is ready for independent practice. Virtual-reality simulators could play an important role in the training of LUS, especially of pathologic cases, and could also provide standardized and objective assessments of competence. As far as we know, no studies have developed valid simulator-based tests of competence in LUS, even though simulators are commonly used in other specialties and are demonstrated to have a great potential for reproducible and objective assessment and effects on skill and behavior [45–47].

In conclusion, more uniform, competency-based training programs and assessment tools are needed to ensure a higher standard of education and assessment in LUS. Furthermore, simulation training could potentially `bute to the hands-on training in a calm environment making it possible to train high-risk cases without putting patients in risk.

Abbreviations

LUS: lung ultrasound; BTS: British Thoracic Society; EFSUMB: European Federation of Societies for Ultrasound in Medicine and Biology; PRISMA: Preferred Reporting Items for Systematic Review and Meta-analysis; OCEBM: Oxford Centre for Evidence-Based Medicine; MCQ: multiple-choice question.

Authors' contributions

Conception and design: PIP, KRM, LK, and CBL. Analysis and interpretation: PIP, KRM, OG, LK, BUN, and CBL. Data collection: PIP, KRM, and CBL. Overall responsibility and guarantor: PIP, OG, LK, and CBL. All authors read and approved the final manuscript.

Author details

[1] Department of Respiratory Medicine, Odense University Hospital, Sdr. Boulevard 29, 5000 Odense C, Denmark. [2] Institute for Clinical Research, University of Southern Denmark, Odense, Denmark. [3] Regional Center for Technical Simulation, Region of Southern Denmark, Odense, Denmark. [4] Department of Anaesthesiology and Intensive Care Medicine, Odense University Hospital, Odense, Denmark. [5] Department of Radiology, Odense University Hospital, Odense, Denmark. [6] Copenhagen Academy for Medical Education and Simulation (CAMES), University of Copenhagen and the Capital Region of Denmark, Copenhagen, Denmark.

Acknowledgements

Not applicable.

References

1. Grimberg A, Shigueoka DC, Atallah AN et al (2010) Diagnostic accuracy of sonography for pleural effusion: systematic review. Sao Paulo Med J 128:90–95
2. Alrajab S, Youssef AM, Akkus NI et al (2013) Pleural ultrasonography versus chest radiography for the diagnosis of pneumothorax: review of the literature and meta-analysis. Crit Care 17:R208
3. Laursen CB, Sloth E, Lassen AT et al (2014) Point-of-care ultrasonography in patients admitted with respiratory symptoms: a single-blind, randomised controlled trial. Lancet Respir Med 2:638–646
4. Pivetta E, Goffi A, Lupia E et al (2015) Lung ultrasound-implemented diagnosis of acute decompensated heart failure in the ED: a SIMEU multicenter study. Chest 148:202–210
5. Alzahrani SA, Al-Salamah MA, Al-Madani WH et al (2017) Systematic review and meta-analysis for the use of ultrasound versus radiology in diagnosing of pneumonia. Crit Ultrasound J 9:6
6. Long L, Zhao HT, Zhang ZY et al (2017) Lung ultrasound for the diagnosis of pneumonia in adults: a meta-analysis. Medicine 96:e5713
7. Education, Practical Standards Committee EFoSfUiM, Biology (2006) Minimum training recommendations for the practice of medical ultrasound. Ultraschall Med 27:79–105
8. Havelock T, Teoh R, Laws D et al (2010) Pleural procedures and thoracic ultrasound: British Thoracic Society pleural disease guideline 2010. Thorax 65(Suppl 2):ii61–ii76
9. Neskovic AN, Hagendorff A, Lancellotti P et al (2013) Emergency echocardiography: the European association of cardiovascular imaging recommendations. Eur Heart J Cardiovasc Imaging 14:1–11
10. Moher D, Liberati A, Tetzlaff J et al (2010) Preferred reporting items for systematic reviews and meta-analyses: the PRISMA statement. Int J Surg 8:336–341
11. Medicine CfE-b (2009) Oxford Centre for evidence-based medicine 2011—level of evidence
12. Higgins JP, Altman DG, Gotzsche PC et al (2011) The Cochrane Collaboration's tool for assessing risk of bias in randomised trials. BMJ 343:d5928
13. Noble VE, Lamhaut L, Capp R et al (2009) Evaluation of a thoracic ultrasound training module for the detection of pneumothorax and pulmonary edema by prehospital physician care providers. BMC Med Educ 9:3
14. Oveland NP, Sloth E, Andersen G et al (2012) A porcine pneumothorax model for teaching ultrasound diagnostics. Acad Emerg Med 19:586–592
15. Breitkreutz R, Dutine M, Scheiermann P et al (2013) Thorax, trachea, and lung ultrasonography in emergency and critical care medicine: assessment of an objective structured training concept. Emerg Med Int 2013:312758
16. Cuca C, Scheiermann P, Hempel D et al (2013) Assessment of a new e-learning system on thorax, trachea, and lung ultrasound. Emerg Med Int 2013:145361
17. Hulett CS, Pathak V, Katz JN et al (2014) Development and preliminary assessment of a critical care ultrasound course in an adult pulmonary and critical care fellowship program. Ann Am Thorac Soc 11:784–788
18. Bhat SR, Johnson DA, Pierog JE et al (2015) Prehospital evaluation of effusion, pneumothorax, and standstill (PEEPS): point-of-care ultrasound in emergency medical services. West J Emerg Med 16:503–509
19. Connolly K, Beier L, Langdorf MI et al (2015) Ultrafest: a novel approach to ultrasound in medical education leads to improvement in written and clinical examinations. West J Emerg Med 16:143–148
20. Dinh VA, Giri PC, Rathinavel I et al (2015) Impact of a 2-day critical care ultrasound course during fellowship training: a pilot study. Crit Care Res Pract 2015:675041
21. Heiberg J, Hansen LS, Wemmelund K et al (2015) Point-of-care clinical ultrasound for medical students. Ultrasound Int Open 1:E58–E66
22. Sanchez-de-Toledo J, Renter-Valdovinos L, Esteves M et al (2016) Teaching chest ultrasound in an experimental porcine model. Pediatr Emerg Care 32:768–772
23. See KC, Ong V, Wong SH et al (2016) Lung ultrasound training: curriculum implementation and learning trajectory among respiratory therapists. Intensive Care Med 42:63–71
24. Greenstein YY, Littauer R, Narasimhan M et al (2017) Effectiveness of a critical care ultrasonography course. Chest 151:34–40
25. Krishnan S, Kuhl T, Ahmed W et al (2013) Efficacy of an online education program for ultrasound diagnosis of pneumothorax. Anesthesiology 118:715–721
26. Abbasi S, Farsi D, Hafezimoghadam P et al (2013) Accuracy of emergency physician-performed ultrasound in detecting traumatic pneumothorax after a 2-h training course. Eur J Emerg Med 20:173–177
27. Gargani L, Sicari R, Raciti M et al (2016) Efficacy of a remote web-based lung ultrasound training for nephrologists and cardiologists: a LUST trial sub-project. Nephrol Dial Transplant 31:1982–1988
28. Edrich T, Stopfkuchen-Evans M, Scheiermann P et al (2016) A comparison of web-based with traditional classroom-based training of lung ultrasound for the exclusion of pneumothorax. Anesth Analg 123:123–128
29. Volpicelli G, Elbarbary M, Blaivas M et al (2012) International evidence-based recommendations for point-of-care lung ultrasound. Intensive Care Med 38:577–591
30. Cook DA, Beckman TJ (2010) Reflections on experimental research in medical education. Adv Health Sci Educ Theory Pract 15:455–464
31. Ruiz JG, Mintzer MJ, Leipzig RM (2006) The impact of e-learning in medical education. Acad Med 81:207–212
32. Cook DAL, Levinson AJ, Garside S (2010) Time and learning efficiency in internet-based learning: a systematic review and meta-analysis. Adv Health Sci Educ 15:755–770
33. Cook DA, Levinson AJ, Garside S et al (2008) Internet-based learning in the health professions: a meta-analysis. JAMA 300:1181–1196
34. Platz E, Goldflam K, Mennicke M et al (2010) Comparison of web-versus classroom-based basic ultrasonographic and EFAST training in 2 European hospitals. Ann Emerg Med 56:660–667
35. Hempel D, Sinnathurai S, Haunhorst S et al (2016) Influence of case-based e-learning on students' performance in point-of-care ultrasound courses: a randomized trial. Eur J Emerg Med 23:298–304
36. Kang TL, Berona K, Elkhunovich MA et al (2015) Web-based teaching in point-of-care ultrasound: an alternative to the classroom? Adv Med Educ Pract 6:171–175

37. Messick S (1995) Validity of psychological assessment: validation of inferences from persons' responses and performances as scientific inquiry into score meaning. Am Psychol 50:741–749
38. Downing SM (2003) Validity: on meaningful interpretation of assessment data. Med Educ 37:830–837
39. Skaarup SH, Laursen CB, Bjerrum AS et al (2017) Objective and structured assessment of lung ultrasound competence. A multispecialty delphi consensus and construct validity study. Ann Am Thorac Soc 14:555–560
40. Campell DT, Stanley JC (1963) Experimental and quasi-experimental designs for research. Houghton Mifflin Company, Boston
41. Yarris LM, Gruppen LD, Hamstra SJ et al (2012) Overcoming barriers to addressing education problems with research design: a panel discussion. Acad Emerg Med 19:1344–1349
42. Schuwirth LWT, van der Vleuten CP (2003) ABC of learning and teaching in medicine: written assessment. BMJ 326:643–645
43. Downing SM, Yudkowsky R (2009) Assessment in health professions education. Routledge, New York
44. Haladyna TM, Downing SM, Rodriguez MC (2002) A review of multiple-choice item-writing guidelines for classroom assessment. Lawrence Erlbaum Associates, Inc., Mahwah
45. Ostergaard ML, Nielsen KR, Albrecht-Beste E et al (2017) Development of a reliable simulation-based test for diagnostic abdominal ultrasound with a pass/fail standard usable for mastery learning. Eur Radiol. https://doi.org/10.1007/s00330-017-4913-x
46. Jensen K, Bjerrum F, Hansen HJ et al (2017) Using virtual reality simulation to assess competence in video-assisted thoracoscopic surgery (VATS) lobectomy. Surg Endosc 31:2520–2528
47. Cook DA, Hatala R, Brydges R et al (2011) Technology-enhanced simulation for health professions education: a systematic review and meta-analysis. JAMA 306:978–988

3

Combined ultrasound–CT approach to monitor acute exacerbation of interstitial lung disease

Silvia Mongodi[1*], Andrea Colombo[2], Anita Orlando[1], Lorenzo Cavagna[3], Bélaid Bouhemad[4,5], Giorgio Antonio Iotti[1,2] and Francesco Mojoli[1,2]

Abstract

Background: Lung ultrasound is a bedside non-irradiating tool for assessment and monitoring of lung diseases. A lung ultrasound score based on visualized artefacts allows reliable quantification of lung aeration, and is useful to monitor mechanical ventilation setting, fluid resuscitation and antibiotic response in critical care. In the context of interstitial lung diseases associated to connective tissue disorders, lung ultrasound has been integrated to computed tomography for diagnosis and follow-up monitoring of chronic lung disease progression.

Case presentation: This case describes a severe acute exacerbation of interstitial lung disease associated to dermatomyositis–polymyositis requiring prolonged extra-corporeal life support. Lung ultrasound score was performed daily and allowed monitoring and guiding both the need of advanced imaging as computed tomography and immunosuppressive therapy.

Conclusions: This case suggests lung ultrasound may be a useful monitoring tool for the response to immunosuppressive therapy in acute severe rheumatic interstitial lung disease, where chest X-ray is poorly informative, and transportation is at high risk.

Keywords: Interstitial lung disease, Lung ultrasound, High-resolution CT, ECMO, Lung monitoring

Introduction

Lung ultrasound is increasingly used to assess and monitor pulmonary diseases in critically ill patients [1]. Although computed tomography scan (CT) represents the gold standard for the majority of lung pathologies, it is burdened with several limitations as exposure to ionizing radiations and need of transportation to radiology department. Lung ultrasound helps in the differential diagnosis of acute respiratory failure [2], reducing ionizing radiation and relative medical costs [3]. In particular, ultrasound-aided diagnostic criteria for ARDS have been proposed [4]. Moreover, a lung ultrasound score can be computed to quantify lung loss of aeration, with strong association with quantitative CT assessment [5]. In ARDS patients, lung ultrasound score may guide positive end-expiratory pressure titration [6] and fluid resuscitation [7] and can be used for daily monitoring of lung recovery [8]. In critically ill patients with ventilator-associated pneumonia, it has been applied to monitor the response to antibiotics [9].

In the context of interstitial lung disease (ILD) associated to connective tissue diseases, lung ultrasound has been proposed as an integration to CT for diagnosis [10] and follow-up monitoring [11]; in this chronic setting, different quantitative approaches based on the total number of visualized B-lines in all the intercostal spaces have been applied to monitor ILD progression [12] and evaluate timing of radiological follow-up [13]. However, how to use lung ultrasound to monitor the response to

*Correspondence: silvia.mongodi@libero.it
[1] Anaesthesia and Intensive Care, San Matteo Hospital, Viale Golgi 19, Pavia, Italy
Full list of author information is available at the end of the article

treatment in acute respiratory failure associated to rheumatic diseases is still unclear. We describe a prolonged ultrasound monitoring in acute exacerbation of ILD associated to connective tissue disease.

Case presentation

A 28-year-old man affected by dermatomyositis–polymyositis was admitted to our general intensive care unit for hypoxemic respiratory failure. He had been diagnosed with dermatomyositis–polymyositis 1 year before after muscular and cutaneous symptoms, had been treated with cyclophosphamide and was under chronic corticosteroid therapy. In intensive care unit, he was first supported with high-flow nasal cannula (HFNC) oxygen therapy. Infectious aetiology was ruled out by negative microbiological specimens (bronchoalveolar lavage for virus, bacteria and parasites, haemocultures, uroculture, serology for *Chlamydia*, *Legionella* and *Mycoplasma Pneumoniae*, urinary antigens for *Legionella* and *Streptococcus Pneumoniae*). A transthoracic echocardiogram was performed but no alterations of the left ventricular systolic and diastolic function were found (ejection fraction > 55%). Patient was also negative for acute or chronic valvular diseases. Autoimmune analyses showed antinuclear antibody positivity (speckled pattern 1:160) and weak reactivity of anti-melanoma differentiation-associated protein 5 antibodies. Immunosuppressive therapy with high-dose intravenous immunoglobulin (2 g/kg/day for 5 days, then 0.4 g/kg/day) and methylprednisolone (1 g daily for 3 days, then 40 mg twice daily) was then started. Nevertheless, he rapidly deteriorated and required intubation for refractory hypoxemia [partial arterial oxygen pressure (PaO_2) 63.4 mmHg with fraction of inspired oxygen (FiO_2) 0.8 by HFNC, pH 7.45, $PaCO_2$ 45.3 mmHg]. A second-line immunosuppressive treatment was introduced, with rituximab (375 mg/m^2 once a week for five cycles) and plasma exchange. Veno-venous femoro-jugular extracorporeal membrane oxygenation (ECMO) was also placed percutaneously to extubate the patient and reduce the risk of overinfection whilst immunosuppressed. Once the ECMO started and the patient extubated, non-invasive respiratory support was provided by HFNC associated to 2–3 daily cycles of mask non-invasive ventilation. Initial CT showed multiple parenchymal consolidations and diffuse ground-glass pattern affecting all lobes, bilateral architectural distortion and nodular-pattern blurred opacities with partial sparing of inferior right lobe. Lung ultrasound score was performed daily to monitor ILD response to immunosuppressive therapy, being chest X-ray poorly informative in an almost completely white lung and being transportation to CT at particularly high risk for both immunosuppression and extra-corporeal support. 12 standard thoracic regions were examined in supine position with thorax elevation around 45°, using in transversal scan a 10-MHz linear probe or a 2.5-MHz phased-array probe when a tissue-like pattern was visualized. Four steps of progressive loss of aeration were distinguished; each region was scored from 0 (normal aeration) to 3 (complete aeration loss), according to the visualized pattern, as previously described [5–9, 14]. The sum of each region's score gives the global lung ultrasound score [1, 5–8], therefore ranging from 0 to 36. Lung ultrasound score, HFNC FiO_2, ECMO settings and patient's PaO_2 are shown in Fig. 1. Initial lung ultrasound score was 28; a progressive reduction of the score from 28 to 17 was observed in the first 5 weeks, confirming the positive response to immunosuppressive therapy, as also supported by the CT performed after 15 days. Gas exchanges also improved with reduced ECMO and inspired FiO_2. However, a complete lung recovery was not observed; the lung ultrasound score ranged between 17 and 22 for days and the patient failed two tests of ECMO discontinuation. A third CT was then performed, where evolution to fibrosis was described. Once overinfection was ruled out again, a third-line immunosuppressive therapy with a second cycle of intravenous immunoglobulin and intravenous cyclosporine (100 mg twice daily) was introduced. Non-invasive respiratory approach was also changed, pursuing with HFNC only. After an initial worsening, a second slower reduction in lung ultrasound score was observed, corresponding to better lung aeration at CT. The patient was finally weaned from ECMO after 93 days with a lung ultrasound score of 15 and good gas exchanges in HFNC (PaO_2 96.1 mmHg with FiO_2 0.3, pH 7.38, $PaCO_2$ 51.2 mmHg).

Conclusions

Lung ultrasound score and CT were here combined to assess and monitor lung aeration of acute exacerbation of dermatomyositis–polymyositis. CT provides the best assessment of ILD and optimal quantification of lung aeration loss; however, for its costs, irradiation and risk related to transportation of critical patients it cannot be considered a monitoring tool. Lung ultrasound score is a reliable alternative for quantification of lung aeration [5]; it can reduce the radiation exposure in critically ill patients, can be performed bedside and requires few minutes for a complete examination in expert hands. In this case of prolonged extra-corporeal support, the need of advanced imaging was triggered by lung ultrasound findings; this led to a very limited number of CTs. Whilst the absolute value of lung ultrasound score does not provide clear information, it can be useful if compared to initial CT and to monitor lung aeration variations in response to treatments finalized at pulmonary

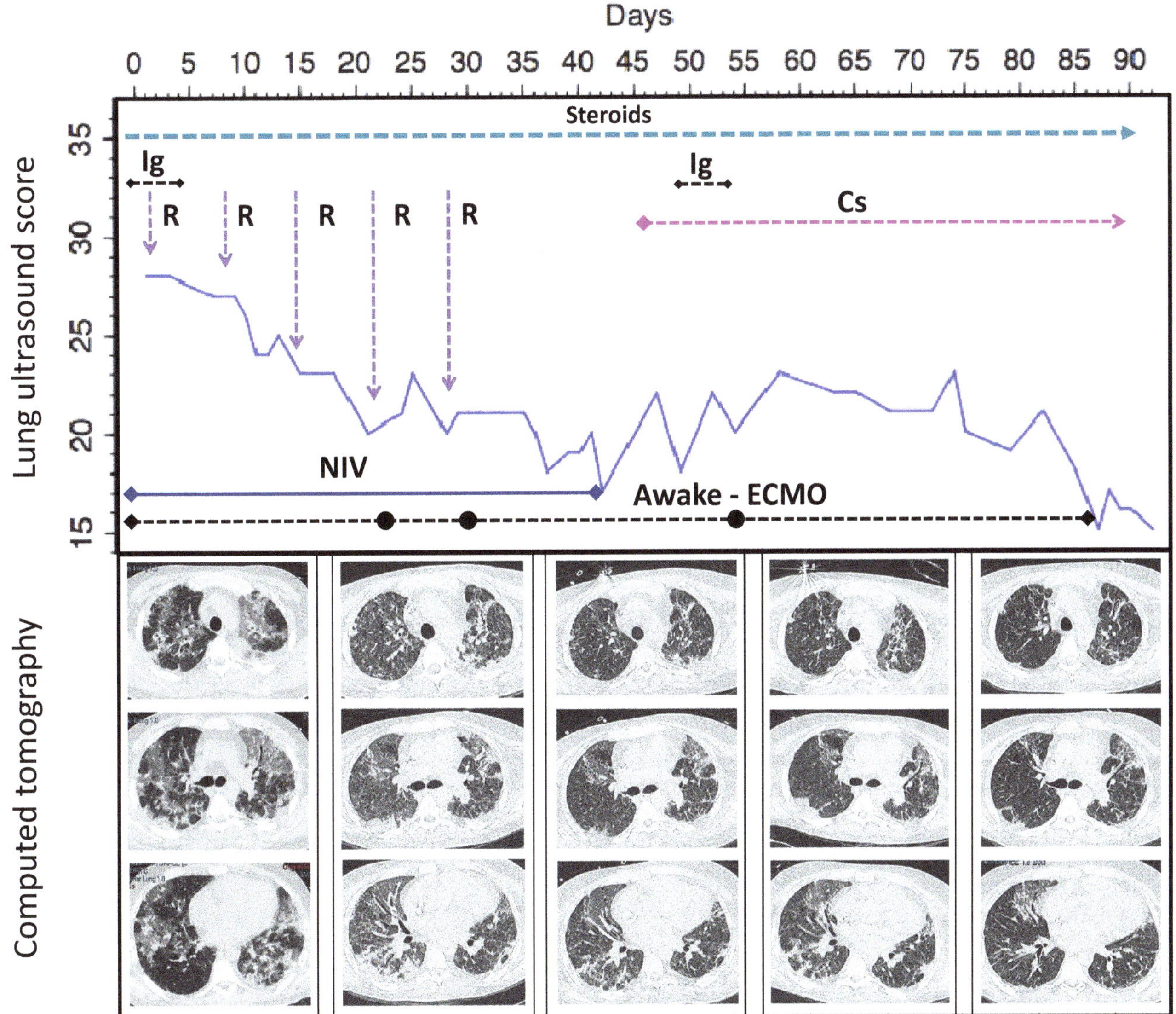

HFNC-FiO_2	100 [100-100]	60 [70-90]	45 [45-50]	45 [45-50]	40 [40-45]	35 [35-40]	35 [35-35]	50 [35-50]	40 [40-40]	30 [30-40]	30 [30-30]	30 [30-30]	30 [30-30]	30
ML-FiO_2	100 [100-100]	100 [100-100]	70 [70-80]	60 [50-70]	40 [30-45]	21 [21-21]	35 [35-35]	50 [35-50]	40 [40-40]	40 [40-40]	40 [40-45]	40 [40-40]	21 [21-21]	
BF (L/min)	3.5 [3.5-3.6]	3.6 [3.6-3.6]	3.0 [3.0-3.1]	3.5 [3.1-3.5]	3.0 [2.9-3.2]	3.1 [2.8-3.5]	3.2 [3.0-3.3]	3.5 [3.2-3.5]	3.0 [3.0-3.1]	3.0 [3.0-3.0]	3.0 [3.0-3.1]	2.9 [2.9-2.9]	3.3 [3.0-3.5]	
SGF (L/min)	7.0 [6.5-8.0]	8.0 [6.0-8.5]	4.0 [3.5-4.5]	5.5 [4.5-5.4]	4.0 [3.0-4.0]	1.0 [0.7-1.5]	3.0 [3.0-3.0]	5.0 [4.0-6.0]	3.0 [3.0-3.0]	3.0 [2.5-3.0]	2.5 [2.5-2.5]	2.5 [2.5-2.5]	1.3 [0.5-2.0]	
PaO_2 (mmHg)	57.5 [56.5-62.2]	66.0 [63.8-79.7]	73.0 [71.5-87.9]	97.5 [82.3-103.6]	85.8 [85.1-91.0]	86.6 [84.9-101.7]	100.1 [99.7-105.2]	93.7 [88.9-102.6]	98.1 [87.3-99.9]	83.0 [82.3-97.8]	88.6 [86.0-92.9]	88.1 [85.1-92.6]	88.0 [82.8-90.1]	87.7

Fig. 1 Lung ultrasound score trend, computed tomography and clinical parameters during 93 days of extra-corporeal life support for acute exacerbation of interstitial lung disease in dermatomyositis–polymyositis (*R* rituximab, *Ig* immunoglobuline, *Cs* cyclosporine, *NIV* non-invasive ventilation, *ECMO* extra-corporeal membrane oxygenation—red dot: membrane lung replacement, *HFNC-*FiO_2 fraction of inspired oxygen delivered by high flow nasal cannula, *ML-*FiO_2 fraction of inspired oxygen delivered by the membrane lung, *SGF* sweep gas flow, PaO_2 patient's partial arterial oxygen pressure)

aeration improvement, as mechanical ventilation setting [6], antibiotics [9] or, in case of rheumatic diseases, immunosuppressive therapy. Whilst more and more used for many common respiratory diseases in critical care [1], lung ultrasound in acute ILD associated to connective tissue diseases has been less investigated. In particular, the interest of lung ultrasound score for aeration monitoring in response to immunosuppressive therapy has not been explored yet in this context. This case suggests lung ultrasound may integrate the classical imaging and clinical management of acute exacerbations of ILD, providing useful daily information on lung aeration and on its response to immunosuppressive treatment, whilst integrating and eventually guiding the need of advanced imaging as CT.

Abbreviations

CT: Computed tomography; ECMO: Extra-corporeal membrane oxygenation; FiO_2: Fraction of inspired oxygen; HFNC: High-flow nasal cannula; ICU: Intensive care unit; ILD: Interstitial lung disease; LUS: Lung ultrasound; PaO_2: Partial arterial oxygen pressure.

Acknowledgements

None.

Authors' contributions

All the authors gave substantial contribution to the conception and design of the work, drafted the work and revised it critically before submission. SM, AO, AC and FM acquired, analysed and interpreted data. All authors read and approved the final manuscript.

Author details

[1] Anaesthesia and Intensive Care, San Matteo Hospital, Viale Golgi 19, Pavia, Italy. [2] Department of Clinical-Surgical, Diagnostic and Paediatric Sciences, Unit of Anaesthesia and Intensive Care, University of Pavia, Pavia, Italy. [3] Division of Rheumatology, University of Pavia, San Matteo Hospital, Pavia, Italy. [4] Dijon and Université Bourgogne Franche-Comté LNC UMR866, F-21000 Dijon, BP 77908, Dijon Cedex 21709, France. [5] Department of Anesthesiology and Intensive Care, C.H.U. Dijon, Dijon Cedex, France.

References

1. Mojoli F, Bouhemad B, Mongodi S, Lichtenstein D (2019) Lung ultrasound in the critically ill. Am J Resp Crit Care Med 199:701–714
2. Laursen CB, Sloth E, Lassen AT, Christensen Rd, Lambrechtsen J, Madsen PH, Henriksen DP, Davidsen JR, Rasmussen F (2014) Point-of-care ultrasonography in patients admitted with respiratory symptoms: a single-blind, randomised controlled trial. Lancet Respir Med 2:638–646
3. Brogi E, Bignami E, Sidoti A, Shawar M, Gargani L, Vetrugno L, Volpicelli G, Forfori F (2017) Could the use of bedside lung ultrasound reduce the number of chest x-rays in the intensive care unit? Cardiovasc Ultrasound 15(1):23
4. Riviello ED, Kiviri W, Twagirumugabe T, Mueller A, Banner-Goodspeed VM, Officer L, Novack V, Mutumwinka M, Talmor DS, Fowler RA (2016) Hospital incidence and outcomes of the acute respiratory distress syndrome using the Kigali modification of the Berlin definition. Am J Respir Crit Care Med 193:52–59
5. Chiumello D, Mongodi S, Algieri I, Vergani GL, Orlando A, Via G, Crimella F, Cressoni M, Mojoli F (2018) Assessment of lung aeration and recruitment by CT scan and ultrasound in ARDS patients. Crit Care Med 46:1761–1768
6. Bouhemad B, Brisson H, Le-Guen M, Arbelot C, Lu Q, Rouby JJ (2011) Bedside ultrasound assessment of positive end-expiratory pressure-induced lung recruitment. Am J Respir Crit Care Med 183:341–347
7. Caltabeloti F, Monsel A, Arbelot C, Brisson H, Lu Q, Gu WJ, Zhou GJ, Auler JO, Rouby JJ (2014) Early fluid loading in acute respiratory distress syndrome with septic shock deteriorates lung aeration without impairing arterial oxygenation: a lung ultrasound observational study. Crit Care 18:R91
8. Mongodi S, Pozzi M, Orlando A, Bouhemad B, Stella A, Tavazzi G, Via G, Iotti GA, Mojoli F (2018) Lung ultrasound for daily monitoring of ARDS patients on extracorporeal membrane oxygenation: preliminary experience. Intensive Care Med 44:123–124
9. Bouhemad B, Liu ZH, Arbelot C, Zhang M, Ferarri F, Le-Guen M, Lu Q, Rouby JJ (2010) Ultrasound assessment of antibiotic-induced pulmonary reaeration in ventilator-associated pneumonia. Crit Care Med 38:84–92
10. Song G, Bae SC, Lee YH (2016) Diagnostic accuracy of lung ultrasound for interstitial lung disease in patients with connective tissue diseases: a meta-analysis. Clin Exp Rheumatol 34:11–16
11. Gargani L, Doveri M, D'Errico L, Frassi F, Bazzichi ML, Delle Sedie A, Scali MC, Monti S, Mondillo S, Bombardieri S, Caramella D, Picano E (2009) Ultrasound lung comets in systemic sclerosis: a chest sonography hallmark of pulmonary interstitial fibrosis. Rheumatology (Oxford) 48:1382–1387
12. Wang Y, Gargani L, Barskova T, Furst DE, Cerinic MM (2017) Usefulness of lung ultrasound B-lines in connective tissue disease-associated interstitial lung disease: a literature review. Arthritis Res Ther 18(19):206
13. Gasperini ML, Gigante A, Iacolare A, Pellicano C, Lucci S, Rosato E (2020) The predictive role of lung ultrasound in progression of scleroderma interstitial lung disease. Clin Rheumatol 39(1):119–123
14. Mongodi S, Bouhemad B, Orlando A, Stella A, Tavazzi G, Via G, Iotti GA, Braschi A, Mojoli F (2017) Modified lung ultrasound score for assessing and monitoring pulmonary aeration. Ultraschall Med 38:530–537

4

The "pandemic" increase in lung ultrasound use in response to Covid-19: can we complement computed tomography findings? A narrative review

Luigi Vetrugno[1], Marco Baciarello[2*], Elena Bignami[2], Andrea Bonetti[2], Francesco Saturno[2], Daniele Orso[1], Rossano Girometti[3], Lorenzo Cereser[3] and Tiziana Bove[1]

Abstract

Coronavirus disease of 2019 (COVID-19) is a highly infectious disease caused by severe acute respiratory syndrome coronavirus 2 (SARS-CoV-2), which has rapidly spread to a global pandemic in March 2020. This emergency condition has been putting a severe strain on healthcare systems worldwide, and a prompt, dynamic response is instrumental in its management. While a definite diagnosis is based on microbiological evidence, the relationship between lung ultrasound (LU) and high-resolution computed tomography (HRCT) in the diagnosis and management of COVID-19 is less clear. Lung ultrasound is a point-of-care imaging tool that proved to be useful in the identification and severity assessment of different pulmonary conditions, particularly in the setting of emergency and critical care patients in intensive care units; HRCT of the thorax is regarded as the mainstay of imaging evaluation of lung disorders, enabling characterization and quantification of pulmonary involvement. Aims of this review are to describe LU and chest HRCT main imaging features of COVID-19 pneumonia, and to provide state-of-the-art insights regarding the integrated role of these techniques in the clinical decision-making process of patients affected by this infectious disease.

Keywords: COVID-19, SARS-CoV-2, Ultrasonography, Lung, Pneumonia, Respiratory distress syndrome, adult, Severe acute respiratory syndrome, Multidetector computed tomography

Introduction

In the ongoing battle against the disease caused by SARS-CoV-2 (COVID-19), which first broke out in the city of Wuhan, China, in December 2019, lung ultrasound (LU) [1] has quickly been recognized as a useful tool in the diagnosis and monitoring of the disease [2]. Ultrasound cannot replace lung computed tomography (CT) when examining the whole lung to choose a ventilator strategy [3], but point-of-care ultrasound (POCUS) may complement CT thanks to ease of access and general safety.

In this review, we summarize the main LU findings in COVID-19 pneumonia next to the equivalent CT signs [4], in the hopes that a correlation can be established to facilitate patient care. In clinical practice, the two imaging modalities can be integrated with great benefits for both patients and clinicians. Although limited in the extent of lung tissue it can explore, LU is particularly advantageous when confronting a COVID-19 outbreak: for one, ventilated patients need to be transferred to a CT suite, which can be outright dangerous in the face of severely impaired gas exchange commonly seen in COVID-19 intensive care unit (ICU) patients. We are not yet aware of LU signs specific for COVID-19, but signs of interstitial pneumonia are well recognized and have been found to be applicable in these cases, with some exhibiting high

*Correspondence: marco.baciarello@unipr.it
[2] Anesthesia, Critical Care and Pain Medicine Unit, Department of Medicine and Surgery, University of Parma, Viale Gramsci, 14, 431236 Parma, Italy
Full list of author information is available at the end of the article

sensitivity [5, 6]. Additionally, it is now sufficiently clear that LU outperforms plain chest radiography in terms of sensitivity for acute respiratory symptoms in critical illness [7, 8].

A reasonable approach may be to perform CT scans on ICU admission to finalize diagnosis and to better inform the choice of ventilation (lung phenotyping) [3]; in order to reduce radiation and viral exposure, it could be repeated after a reasonable interval of time for prognostic information, whereas POCUS could be used to reduce ionizing radiation load and device contamination in many situations where it has been shown to be superior to chest x-ray and (in selected cases) as useful as CT [9]. Another setting in which LU is becoming essential is that of community outreach by specialized teams screening residents of nursing homes and long-term care facilities, which may have acted as a reservoir for SARS-CoV-2 [10]. Conversely, LU may not explore the entirety of the organ, and one should always consider CT when point-of-care monitoring fails to explain the current clinical respiratory status, especially in COVID-19, where thrombotic complications are increasingly found to be pivotal in the disease [11]. The aim of this review is thus to help physicians become familiar with LU and CT imaging in COVID-19.

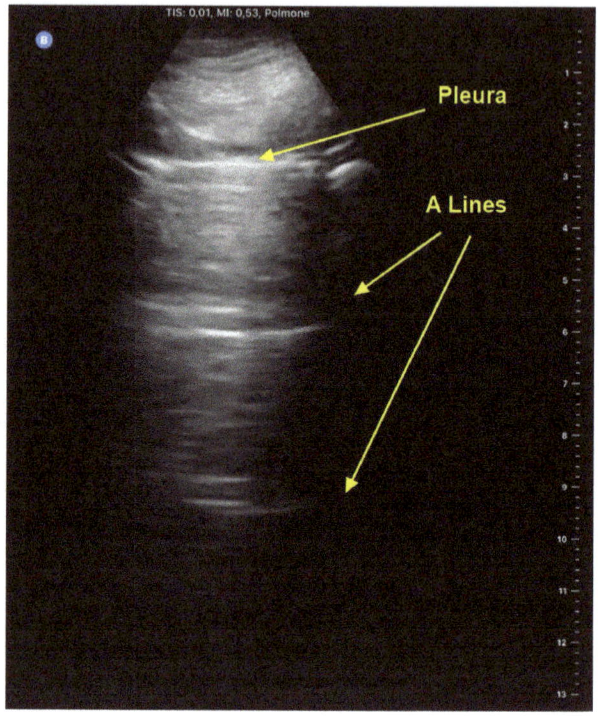

Fig. 1 Anterior parasagittal lung ultrasound scan of the thorax. The parietal and visceral pleura appear as a hyperechoic line with sliding movements (also see Additional file 1: Clip S1). A lines are thought to be mirror artifacts from the near-total ultrasound reflection by the pleura-alveolar gas interface

Lung ultrasound and COVID-19

Patients with interstitial syndromes usually display two types of artifacts. A-lines are the 'default' artifacts in healthy lung tissue, caused by soundwaves reverberating between pleura and the transducer, as the air-tissue interface reflects almost all the ultrasound packets. The sliding motion of the hyperechoic line in the near field depicts the movement of visceral over parietal pleural. The presence of A-lines and lung sliding signifies normal lung aeration (Fig. 1 and Additional file 1: Clip S1) [12].

B-lines are hyperechoic artifacts arising from single points along the pleural line and projecting to the bottom of the screen. They are thought to originate from locally increased tissue density which enhances reverberation from alveoli and distal airways [9] (Fig. 2 and Additional file 2: Clip S2).

The clinical significance of B-lines depends mostly on quality and quantity: ≤ 2 B-lines per intercostal space, interspersing A-line, and a sliding pleural line rule out pneumothorax and are considered normal variation. Three or more well-spaced B-lines (a "B-profile") are associated with interstitial syndromes [12, 13].

The pleural line is normally thin and bright but, when inflamed, it can become thickened and less mobile, with B-lines arising from it and arcing slowly. The pleural line can also be interrupted by lung consolidation and loss of aeration (the "shred sign") [14]. At the beginning of lung

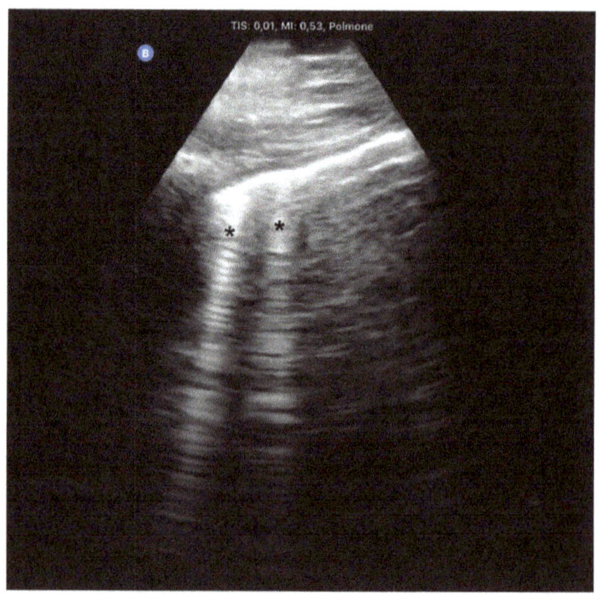

Fig. 2 B-lines. Hyperechoic artifacts descending from the pleural line to the bottom of the screen are called "B lines" (black asterisks); by definition, a B line obscures any A line along its path. Two B lines per scan field are considered normal; ≥ 3 lines are associated with varying degrees of interstitial syndrome

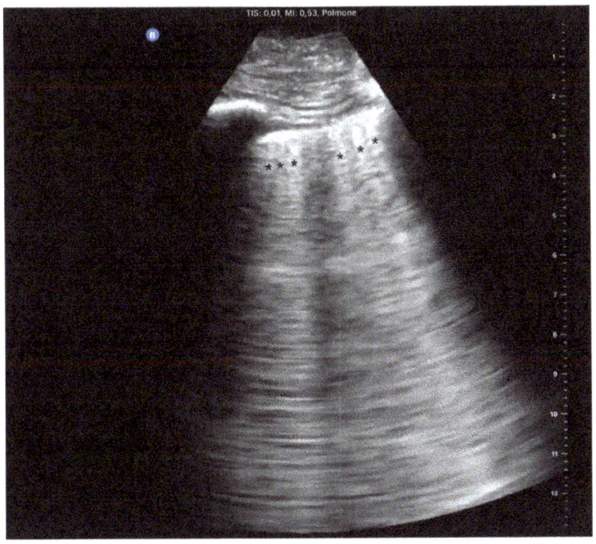

Fig. 3 Confluent B-lines. Multiple confluent B-lines (asterisks) and occupying ≥ 50% of the field of view define the “rocket launch” sign or “glass rockets.” This is associated with more overt interstitial syndrome. Additional file 1: Clip S1: Anterior parasagittal scan of the thorax. The parietal and visceral pleura appear as a hyperechoic line. Pleural sheaths are seen sliding with respiration

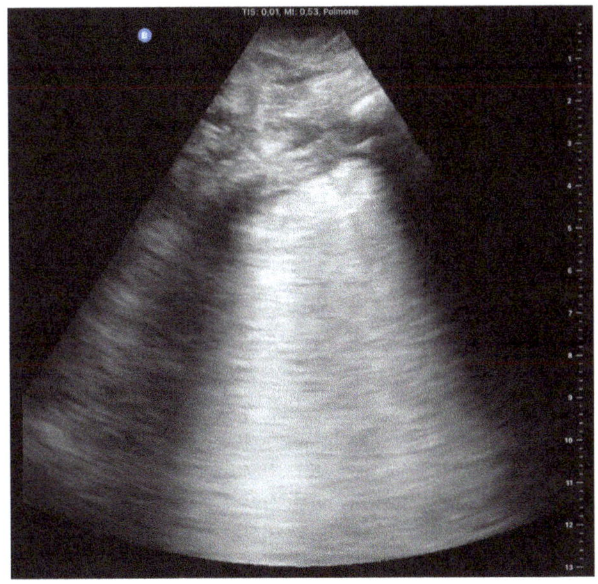

Fig. 4 White lung. In this parasagittal scan, the whole intercostal space is occupied by continuous hyperechoic artifact commonly referred to as “white lung.” The pleural line also appears coarser and thicker than normal. This image is associated with advanced interstitial syndrome and may precede complete loss of aeration (consolidation)

involvement in COVID-19, B-lines (with lung sliding) are distributed heterogeneously between spared regions of A-lines (Fig. 3). As the disease progresses, lung density increases, as does the amount of B-lines, leading to coalescence of the artifacts into “glass-rockets” and then “white lung” (Figs. 3 and 4, respectively; see also Additional file 3: Clip S3 and Additional file 4: Clip S4), equivalent ground-glass opacities (GGO) in CT scans [1]. Amid a pandemic with a very high prevalence of the disease, high density of B-lines with spared areas and lung sliding plus fever and cough is high suspicious for COVID-19 infection, and these patients should be managed accordingly [15, 16]. Glass rockets or white lung are typically associated with impaired oxygenation requiring supplemental oxygen.

Finally, in advanced disease, lung density further increases as alveoli fill up with inflammatory cells and Lung ultrasound findings in patients with COVID-19 pneumonia byproducts, with loss of aeration and a corresponding LU aspect called “tissue-like” (Fig. 5). This is equivalent to consolidation as seen in CT scans. The appearance of consolidations in LU is similar to that of liver tissue, with hyperechoic inclusions corresponding to distal bronchi which may or may not be filled with secretions [14].

What is new in this context?

Recently, Volpicelli et al. have described some aspects of B-lines that seem to increase the diagnostic probability

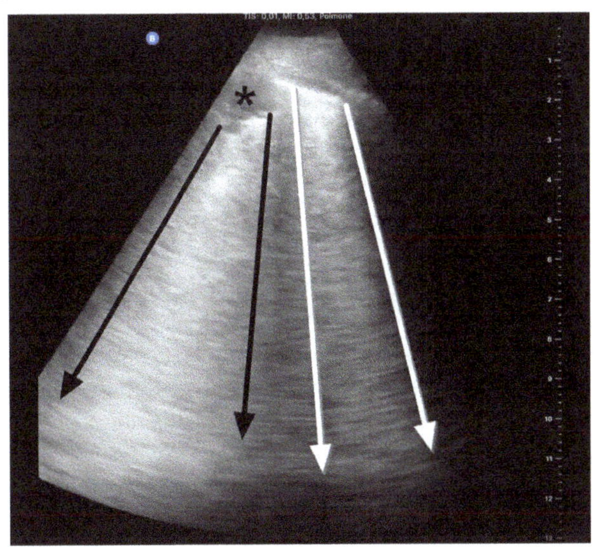

Fig. 5 Subpleural consolidations and “light beam”. Two artifacts frequently seen in COVID-19 with significant respiratory symptoms: small subpleural consolidation (asterisk), with white lung-like artifact projecting from its interface with aerated lung (between black arrows); and a “light beam”, a hyperechoic artifact (between white arrows), also similar in quality to white lung, but arising from a discrete region of normal pleura. The light beam is so called also because it is “turned off and on” (i.e., disappears and reappears) repeatedly, even in a single respiratory cycle

in patients suspected of COVID-19 pneumonia [5], in combination with clinical phenotype, blood tests and nasal-pharyngeal swab. They report on a sonographic sign named "light beam" and described as a shining vertical band artifact arising from a wide portion of a regular pleura, as opposed to the discrete points of origin of B-lines. The artifact is thought to be present in the earlier phase of viral spread in the peripheral lung and associated with the early GGO alterations visible at CT scan. This sign has also been described by Huang et al. in patients with COVID-19 infection as a "waterfall" sign [17]. In COVID-19, the light beam artifact is typically interspersed among areas of normal lung aeration or discrete B-lines, often alternating with areas of pleural line irregularity and peripheral consolidations. These signs identify affected regions, with patchy distribution in the two lungs [17–19] (Additional file 5: Clip S5).

In COVID-19, two pathological phenotypes have been described. One is the L-type, with normal or minimally reduced respiratory system compliance; these patients have been dubbed by some Authors as "happy hypoxic", and a prospective multicenter study is currently investigating whether the light beam sign could be an early sign of disease in these cases. On CT, they show diffuse infiltrates but a low margin of recruitability (hence the name), defined as a relatively minor volume of de-aerated lung tissue [3]. The H-phenotype is characterized by low- to very low respiratory system compliance with high potential for recruitment with higher mean airway pressures; CT of these patients typically shows extensive consolidation with or without superimposed bacterial pneumonia. While L-type COVID-19 is intuitively characterized by the presence of LU signs such as those we described above (a multicenter study is ongoing to confirm this hypothesis), LU of H-type COVID-19 might have more in common with bacterial pneumonia and atelectasis. On CT, up to three different profiles can be described according to the distribution of consolidations [20].

From their characteristics, it has been proposed that different phenotypes require distinct respiratory management strategies, based on recruitment potential [3]. However, not all experts concur with this view, promoting instead the concept of a continuous disease which may worsen with mechanical ventilation itself and/or opportunistic infection [21].

What is known about LU?

Certain characteristics of B-lines can help rule out COVID-19 infection, for example when B-lines are unilateral, which is more typical of initial pneumonia of likely bacterial origin, although underlying COVID-19 pneumonia cannot be ruled out [12]: theoretically, H-type COVID-19 pneumonia might share these features on LU. A unilateral consolidation within a large pleural effusion suggests bacterial pneumonia rather than COVID-19 pneumonia [22]. Pleural effusion is a well-known sign that appears as a hypo- or anechoic space in LU, distributed in gravity-dependent fashion [23, 24]. Pleural effusion is easy to see, and it may be possible to be estimate its volume with simple calculations (Balik formula) [22]. Sometimes septa can be seen floating in effusions, which is more typical of bacterial or fungal infection. However, in COVID-19, we have observed that large pleural effusions are rarely present and an alternative diagnosis, or superimposed infection, should be considered when confronted with such sign.

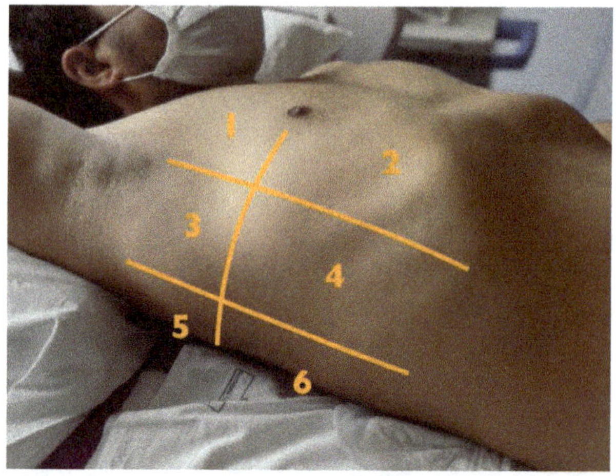

Fig. 6 Representation of the 6-zone model for lung ultrasound score (see Ref. [21]). The parasagittal lines are the midclavicular, anterior and posterior axillary lines; the transverse line is at the 4th intercostal space, roughly equivalent to hilar lines

Lung ultrasound score (LUS)

When performing LU, it is customary to divide the chest into 8 to 16 regions. We will describe an approach where the chest is divided into 12, defined by the intersections of the anterior and posterior axillary lines with a transverse plane passing through both nipples (Fig. 6). These regions can be scanned with different probes, depending on personal experience and preference, the most common being convex low-frequency and phased array (echocardiography) transducers [25].

Lung ultrasound score is a system in which each of 12 lung zones is assigned points, which are then added up [26]. One point is assigned to zones with A-lines and pleural sliding, or ≤ 2 B-lines; 1 point is for ≥ 3 well-spaced B-lines (interstitial syndrome); and 2 points are calculated for coalescent B-lines or "glass-rockets"—equivalent to GGO in CT; finally, consolidation with "tissue like-sign" has a score of 3. Therefore, the total score may range between 0 (normal lungs) and 36, in the worst-case scenario of completely de-aerated lungs [25]. We do not know how the "light beam" sign or small superficial lung consolidations may affect this score.

Diagnostic performance of LU

Ultrasound distinction between acute cardiogenic pulmonary edema and acute respiratory distress syndrome (ARDS) in a critically ill patient can be difficult [27]. As is the case in every interstitial syndrome, non-infectious causes of pulmonary edema are always a differential diagnosis [28, 29].

The presence of bilateral B lines is associated with an interstitial syndrome, as previously reported [30], but it is poorly specific (while sensitivity is close to 100%). On the one hand, the presence of some ultrasound signs such as abnormalities of the pleural line, the reduction of pleural sliding, interspersed sparing areas, and the presence of consolidations can suggests ARDS over cardiogenic pulmonary edema (sensitivity 83–100% and specificity 45–100%) [29]. On the other hand, evidence on the diagnostic value of LU in ARDS is still very discordant. Diagnostic accuracy of LU for interstitial syndrome suffers considerably from variability between different research groups [area under the curve (AUC) of the receiver operating characteristic curve (ROC) from 85 to 95%] [31, 32]. The diagnosis of pneumonia by detection of lung consolidations (typical of bacterial pneumonia) was found to have sensitivity and specificity approaching those of CT (up to 95% and 91%, respectively). Ultimately, the diagnostic accuracy of LU seems to be greater than 90% [24, 25]. In viral pneumonia, LU has shown good sensitivity (94.1%) but inferior specificity (84.8%), with positive and negative predictive values of 86.5% and 93.3%, respectively [33]. Again, signs of interstitial syndromes can be present in a host of different conditions. [34], and at the time of this writing only anecdotal reports have been published for LU diagnosis of COVID-19.

Chest CT and COVID-19

Imaging features

The spectrum of chest CT findings encountered in viral pneumonias reflects variable combinations of a few histopathologic features (i.e., diffuse alveolar damage, intra-alveolar hemorrhage, and interstitial inflammatory cell infiltration), and include: (i) mosaic attenuation pattern (caused by hypoventilation of alveoli distal to bronchiolar obstruction and secondary vasoconstriction of the same areas); (ii) ground-glass opacity (GGO) and consolidation (related to the coexistence of airspaces partial filling and thickening of interstitial tissue); (iii) nodules, micronodules, and tree-in-bud opacities (indicative of centrilobular bronchioles that are dilated and impacted with mucus or fluid, along with peribronchiolar interstitial

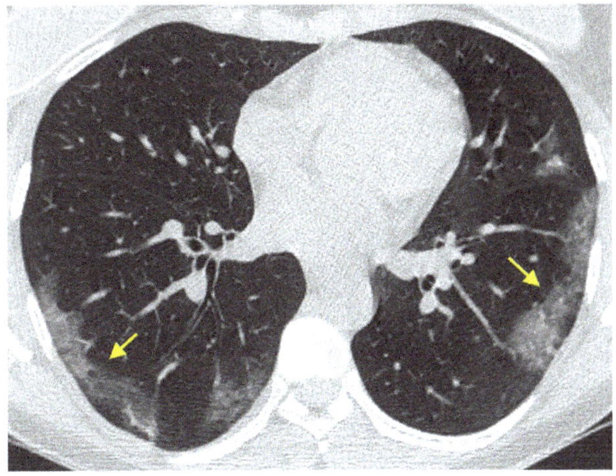

Fig. 7 Typical chest CT imaging appearance of COVID-19 pneumonia. High-resolution CT image of a female COVID-19 patient presenting fever with cough for 5 days shows bilateral, multifocal, and peripheral areas of pure ground-glass opacity (GGO) (arrows)

inflammation, infiltration, or fibrosis); (iv) interlobular septal thickening (due to the presence of interstitial fluid, cellular infiltration, or fibrosis); and (v) bronchial and/or bronchiolar wall thickening (due to inflammation or fibrosis) [35].

As a general rule, all the viruses of the same family causing pneumonia share the main pathological changes and, consequently, show similar CT findings [36]. For this reason, pneumonias due to SARS-CoV-2 show HRCT features that resemble SARS-CoV and MERS-CoV pneumonias (all viruses belonging to Coronaviridae family), caused by injury to pulmonary epithelial cells with hyaline membrane formation in the alveoli, along with proliferative fibrous tissue blocking alveoli and small airways, and interstitial inflammatory infiltrates (mainly lymphocytes) [36, 37]. These pathologic alterations are supposed to be the causes of most typical CT findings of COVID-19 pneumonia, namely GGO and consolidation, with a prevalence range of 36–86% for GGO alone, and of 36–64% for the combination of GGO and consolidation. Their distribution is usually bilateral (87%), peripheral (in 56–97% of cases) and multifocal (76%), often with lower lung predominance (54%) [38–41] (Fig. 7). GGO may have round morphology and, in up to 5–36% of cases, configures a "crazy-paving" pattern (defined as thickened interlobular septa and intralobular lines superimposed on a background of GGO, resembling irregularly shaped paving stones; see Fig. 8) [42–44]. The prevalence of consolidation tends to increase later in the course of the disease, possibly reflecting an inflammatory reaction of the lung tissue (Fig. 9) [40, 43].

The presence of GGO and/or consolidation with a typical pattern of distribution in patients with high clinical

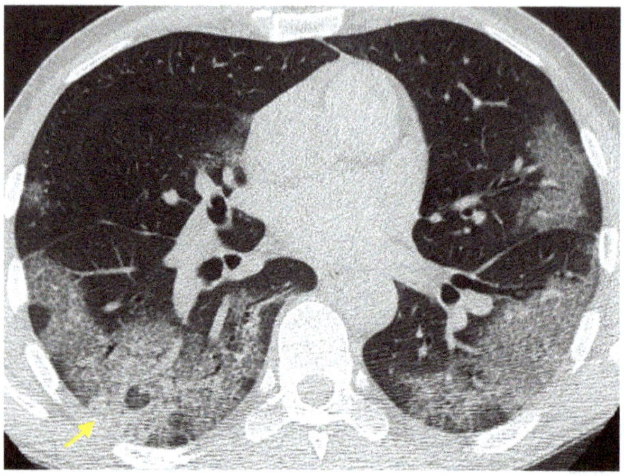

Fig. 8 Typical chest CT imaging appearance of COVID-19 pneumonia. High-resolution CT image of a COVID-19 patient presenting fever with dry cough and myalgia for 10 days shows bilateral, multifocal, peripheral, and confluent areas of ground-glass opacity (GGO) with "crazy-paving" pattern, along with perilobular consolidation in the right lower lobe (arrow)

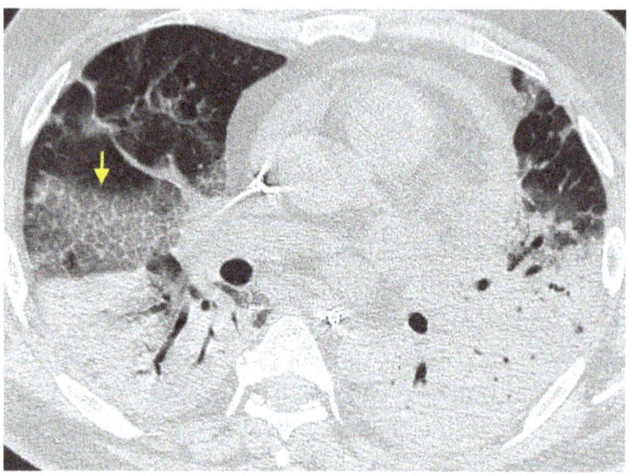

Fig. 9 Chest CT imaging appearance of severe COVID-19 pneumonia and acute respiratory distress syndrome (ARDS). High-resolution CT image of a COVID-19 patient admitted to intensive care unit shows bilateral areas of consolidation predominantly affecting the dependent areas of both lungs, along with ground-glass opacity (GGO) with "crazy-paving" pattern in the right middle lobe (arrow)

likelihood of disease helps consolidating the suspicion of COVID-19 pneumonia in clinically borderline cases (e.g., when the results of RT-PCR are still unavailable on initially negative) [45].

Other CT findings have been reported in COVID-19 pneumonia, including: air bronchogram (in up to 90%), bronchial wall thickening (in up to 30%), bronchus deformation (in up to 32%), pulmonary nodules (in up to 23%, mainly centrilobular, with or without tree-in-bud pattern), bubble-like air-containing spaces (in 80% of advanced-stage disease cases), and dilatation of pulmonary vessels around and/or within the lesions (in almost half cases) (Fig. 10) [38, 40, 46].

Those findings are of limited significance in patients with confirmed diagnosis and presence of GGO and consolidation. When presenting alone in less defined clinical situations (e.g., patients with negative RT-PCR results), they can act as confounders in imaging interpretation, or suggest alternate diagnosis.

Of note, GGO and consolidation in COVID-19 pneumonia can reflect an organizing pneumonia (OP) pattern [47]; OP is usually part of the normal repair process of an acute or subacute lung injury [e.g., diffuse alveolar damage, (DAD)], mainly infectious in origin, displaying characteristic plugs of fibroblasts and myofibroblasts that organize both in airspaces and interstitial tissue [48]. In COVID-19 pneumonia chest CT may show certain features that, albeit nonspecific, may suggest coexistence of DAD in its fibrotic phase and OP pattern of lung injury (e.g., reverse halo sign, consolidation with perilobular pattern, peribronchial or peribronchiolar nodules) (Fig. 11). It has been supposed that the pathological pathway of COVID-19 pneumonia is sustained by two consecutive and overlapping stages, triggered by the virus itself in the earlier phase, and by the host response in the second phase [49]. Consequently, when chest CT is performed in patients with clinical signs of viral pneumonia, pulmonary findings presumably reflect a combination of concurrent viral and host inflammatory response. One may argue that, in case of predominant OP features, chest CT may hint at a self-reinforcing systemic inflammatory process, thus potentially suggesting the use of immunosuppressant drugs.

In order to aid radiologists in recognizing CT findings of COVID-19 pneumonia and improving their communication with referring clinicians, the Radiological Society of North America (RSNA) has grouped the above-described CT findings into four categories (typical, indeterminate, atypical or negative), according to their reported incidence in COVID-19 pneumonia [50]. However, radiologists should always keep in mind that patients who have underlying lung pathologies (e.g., extensive emphysema, lung fibrosis), or are immunocompromised might present with atypical chest CT pattern, thus reducing the diagnostic confidence [51, 52].

Diagnostic performance and role in clinical practice

The role of imaging in the clinical decision-making of COVID-19 should be tailored depending on locally available resources, with the aim of assisting referring physicians in clinical decision-making, while guaranteeing the safety of healthcare professionals performing examinations, and minimizing the risk that themselves become vectors of infection [51, 53, 54].

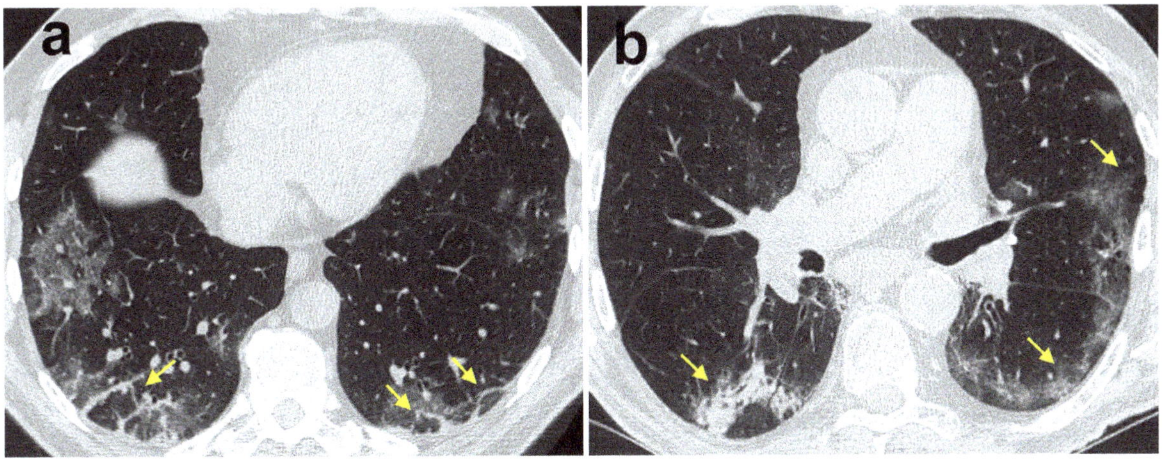

Fig. 10 Organizing pneumonia pattern of lung injury in COVID-19 pneumonia. High-resolution CT images of a male COVID-19 patient presenting fever with cough and dyspnea for 15 days (**a**) and of a different male COVID-19 patient 14 days after the clinical onset (**b**) show perilobular thickening and parenchymal opacities (both ground-glass opacity and consolidation), along with superimposed signs of distortion, in the posterior subpleural regions of both lower lobes (arrows)

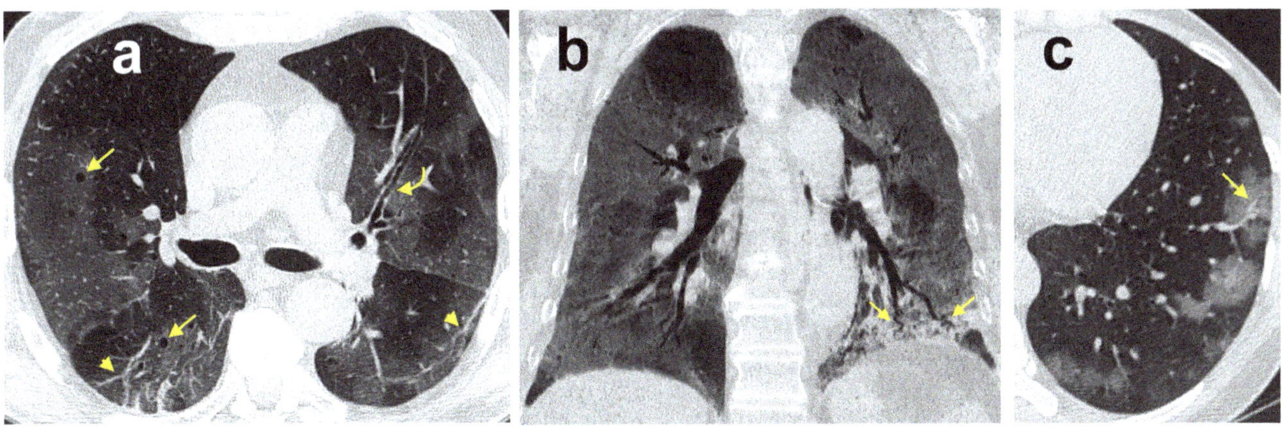

Fig. 11 Ancillary chest CT imaging findings in COVID-19 pneumonia. **a** High-resolution CT image of a 73-year-old male COVID-19 patient presenting fever with dry cough for 5 days shows bilateral, multifocal, peripheral areas of ground-glass opacity (GGO) with mosaic appearance, along with superimposed fibrous stripes in the lower lobes (arrowheads), bronchial wall thickening (curved arrow) and bubble-like air-containing spaces (straight arrows). **b** 8-mm Min-IP coronal CT image of a 73-year-old female COVID-19 patient presenting fever for 5 days shows bilateral, multifocal, peripheral GGO, along with consolidation in the left lower lobe presenting with air bronchogram and bronchus deformation (arrows). **c** High-resolution CT image of the same patient as inset (**a**) shows dilatation of pulmonary vessels within one of the multiple GGO in the left lower lobe (arrow)

A Multinational Consensus Statement from the Fleischner Society, involving a panel of experts in different fields (e.g., thoracic radiologists, pulmonologists, and anesthesiologists), stated that radiological imaging (plain x-ray or CT, depending on local resources and expertise): (i) has generally no role in patients with no symptoms or mild features of COVID-19; (ii) is advised when a patient present with moderate-to-severe features suggesting COVID-19 infection (regardless of COVID-19 testing results), since it can establish baseline pulmonary status, help in risk stratification for clinical worsening, assess complications (e.g., pulmonary embolism, superimposed bacterial pneumonia, or heart failure due to myocardial injury), or reveal alternative diagnoses explaining patient's clinical features; (iii) can provide a presumptive diagnosis of COVID-19 for rapid triage and consequent decisions about clinical management and measures of epidemic control, when the pre-test probability of COVID-19 is high and the healthcare setting is resource-constrained (with potential limited availability of viral testing kits) [45].

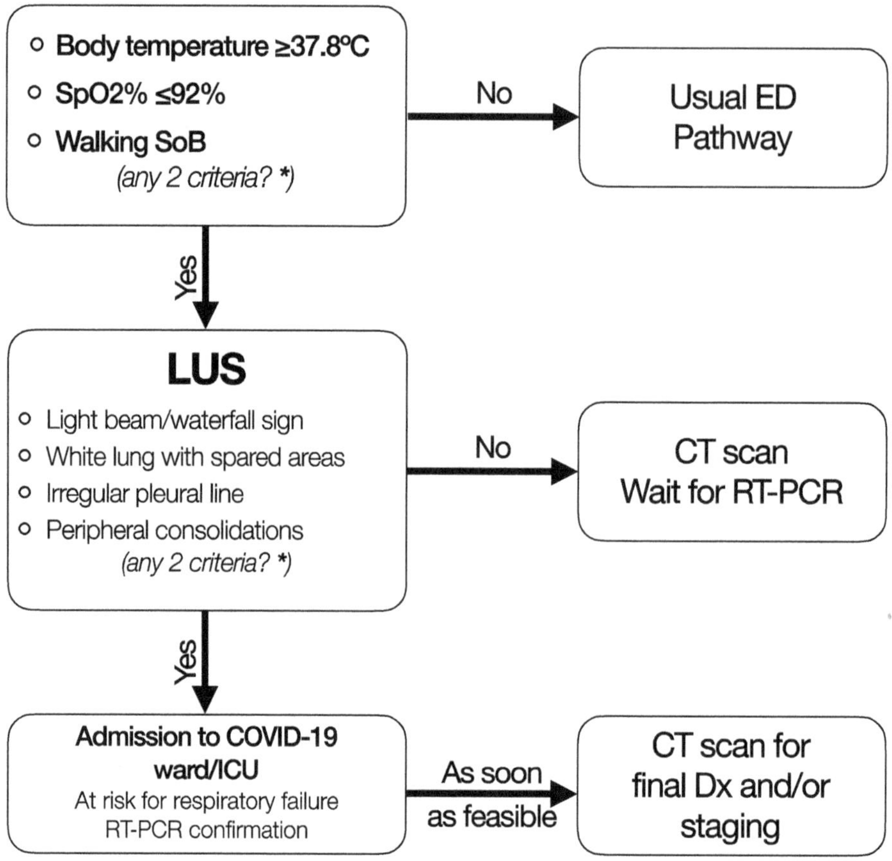

* There is currently no scientific evidence that this is the appropriate criteria. Please consider this as a proposal, to be validated.

Fig. 12 A proposal for a LU-based approach to triage and admission during outbreaks with high-volume influx of patients. There is not enough evidence, yet, to recommend specific LU criteria over others, but we hypothesize these may be the most useful ones. During resource constraint phases, feasibility and throughput volume can be maximized by the use of LU, followed by CT when appropriate. *LU* lung ultrasound, *CT* computed tomography, *ICU* intensive care unit, *RT-PCR* real-time polymerase chain reaction, *Dx* diagnosis

Concerning the latter scenario, a valuable complementary role for CT has been reported by Ai et al. [4] in a cohort of 1014 COVID-19 patients in Wuhan, Hubei, China. With RT-PCR as reference standard, sensitivity, specificity, positive predictive value (PPV), negative predictive value (NPV), and accuracy of chest CT in diagnosing COVID-19 were 97%, 25%, 65%, 83%, and 68%, respectively [4]. At the beginning of February 2020, the National Health Committee of China (NHC) established for Hubei Province the equivalence between COVID-19 RT-PCR-confirmed cases and clinically diagnosed cases, the latter identified only by means of clinical history, physical and laboratory findings, and "chest imaging revealing abnormalities", preferably CT [55]. Nevertheless, such an approach may be less suitable in other scenarios, especially with lower prevalence of disease (i.e., lower pretest probability) [56]. According the Royal College of Radiologists "the CT appearances alone will not obviate the need for viral testing and should not be viewed as equivalent to or replacing this" [57]. Reconsidering the data expressed by Ai et al. [4], we may expect a PPV lower than 65%, implying that even more than 35% of patients with positive CT are actually *false* positive. Such an image-centric approach poses serious decision-making problems, since non-COVID patients hospitalized in a COVID-dedicated healthcare floor are at high risk to become infected soon, as highlighted in a communication by the Italian Society of Radiology to the members on March 26, 2020 (Sardanelli F, personal communication). In addition, chest CT can be negative for pneumonia in symptomatic patients with RT-PCR-confirmed COVID-19. As an example, in a cohort of cruise ship passengers and crewmembers, Inui et al. reported a 20% of symptomatic cases having no CT findings consistent with viral pneumonia [39]. Of note, according to the American College of Radiology (ACR) recommendations, "a normal CT should not dissuade a patient from being quarantined or provided other clinically indicated treatment when otherwise medically appropriate" [58]. Conversely, RT-PCR should be repeated whenever initially negative in the face of a chest CT suggestive of COVID-19 (Fig. 12) [59].

Conclusion

In conclusion, chest CT in patients with COVID-19 has a high potential to give valuable help to clinicians, as long as it is used in accordance with existing guidelines and recommendations. Further studies, particularly on a radio-pathological correlation basis, are warranted in order to tailor the CT to different clinical scenarios.

In a recent interview, Dr. Roberto Cosentini, the head of the Emergency Department at the main hospital the Bergamo province of Italy (one of the most stricken by the epidemic), mentioned up to 60–80 COVID-19 admissions, mostly concentrated in afternoon hours. Such circumstances may force even major hospitals into resource constraints,[1] and when that happens, it may be conceivable to sacrifice diagnostic specificity in exchange for increased sensitivity and patient throughput through triage units; experience at one of our institutions led to the proposal of a LU-based algorithm for faster admission of patients with pneumonia during a possible future COVID-19 outbreak (Fig. 12). In such emergency contexts, LU may temporarily be the most feasible imaging modality, by allowing high-throughput patient assessment without transportation throughout the hospital; its high sensitivity when screening patients in the admission area may avert the risk of inappropriate discharges (i.e., compensating but sick patients). In the ICU, daily monitoring including LU allows for early detection of deterioration and/or improvement, which may influence the decision to transfer patients to lower-intensity units, although a correlation between LU findings and disease evolution over time has not been established [60]. LU is an interdisciplinary tool that can be used throughout the acute care hospital, with a common language when treating (COVID-19) lung pathology. However, for this to happen, definitions and skills need to be shared, diffused and consolidated in prospective evidence.

Supplementary information

Additional file 1: Clip S1. Anterior parasagittal scan of the thorax. From top to bottom, the first (most superficial) hyperechoic line is the pleural line, characterized by its sliding layers. Further down, multiple A lines "mirror" the pleural shape and move together with it as the transducer is slightly tilted and rocked.

Additional file 2: Clip S2. Anterior parasagittal scan of the thorax. Up to 3 B lines appear on screen throughout respiratory cycles (white asterisks). A lines are erased where B lines appear.

[1] "Like an earthquake." Interview with Dr. Roberto Cosentini. The Italian Society of Emergency Medicine Official Website. https://www.simeu.it/w/articoli/leggiArticolo/3977/leggi [in Italian]. Last accessed June 16, 2020.

Additional file 3: Clip S3. Coalescing B-lines with distinct points of origin in the pleural line and moving with it, while filling ≥ 50% of the field of the view. This artifact can be described as a "rocket launch" or "glass rocket". Note how A lines become visible again as B lines slide out of view with respiratory cycles (spared areas).

Additional file 4: Clip S4. White lung artifact arising from an irregular ("shredded") pleural line, just next to a spared area of the lung. No single B line is detectable. Also note how the visceral pleura appears detached from the chest wall: a millimetric effusion (shown as a thin hypoechoic line just above the visceral pleura) is quite common in severe interstitial syndrome.

Additional file 5: Clip S5. Two artifacts frequently seen in COVID-19 with significant respiratory symptoms. A small subpleural consolidation, indicated by the white caret ('^') projects a white-lung artifact from its interface with deeper aerated tissue. To the right, a similar artifact arising instead from normal pleura disappears an reappears multiple times: a "light beam".

Abbreviations

ARDS: Acute (or adult) respiratory distress syndrome; AUC: Area under the curve; CT: Computed tomography; DAD: Diffuse alveolar damage; GGO: Ground-glass opacity; HRCT: High-resolution computed tomography; ICU: Intensive care unit; LU: Lung ultrasound; NPV: Negative predictive value; OP: Organizing pneumonia; PPV: Positive predictive value; RT-PCR: Reverse-transcription polymerase chain reaction.

Acknowledgements

The authors would like to thank Katia Zatorri, MS, for her technical help annotating images and videoclips.

Authors' contributions

LV and DO conceived the paper and wrote the first draft; MB finalized the manuscript and annotated ultrasound pictures; RG and LC wrote about computed tomography, collected and analyzed relevant pictures; AB and FS made ultrasound recordings; EB and TB revised the manuscript and oversaw the work. All authors read and approved the final manuscript.

Author details

[1] Anesthesia and Intensive Care Clinic, Department of Medicine, University of Udine, University Hospital S. Maria della Misericordia, Udine, Italy. [2] Anesthesia, Critical Care and Pain Medicine Unit, Department of Medicine and Surgery, University of Parma, Viale Gramsci, 14, 431236 Parma, Italy. [3] Institute of Radiology, Department of Medicine, University of Udine, University Hospital S. Maria della Misericordia, Udine, Italy.

References

1. Lichtenstein DA (2019) Current misconceptions in lung ultrasound. A short guide for experts. Chest 156:21–25. https://doi.org/10.1016/j.chest.2019.02.332
2. Vetrugno L, Bove T, Orso D, Barbariol F, Bassi F, Boero E, Ferrari G, Kong R (2020) Our Italian experience using lung ultrasound for identification, grading and serial follow-up of severity of lung involvement for management of patients with COVID-19. Echocardiography 37:625–627. https://doi.org/10.1111/echo.14664
3. Gattinoni L, Chiumello D, Caironi P, Busana M, Romitti F, Brazzi L, Camporota L (2020) COVID-19 pneumonia: different respiratory treatments for different phenotypes? Intensive Care Med. https://doi.org/10.1007/s00134-020-06033-2
4. Ai T, Yang Z, Hou H, Zhan C, Chen C, Lv W, Tao Q, Sun Z, Xia L (2020) Correlation of chest CT and RT-PCR testing in coronavirus disease 2019 (COVID-19) in China: a report of 1014 cases. Radiology. https://doi.org/10.1148/radiol.2020200642

5. Volpicelli G, Gargani L (2020) Sonographic signs and patterns of COVID-19 pneumonia. Ultrasound J 12:22. https://doi.org/10.1186/s13089-020-00171-w
6. Vetrugno L, Bove T, Orso D, Bassi F, Boero E, Ferrari G (2020) Lung ultrasound and the COVID-19 "Pattern": not all that glitters today is gold tomorrow. J Ultrasound Med. https://doi.org/10.1002/jum.15327
7. Maw AM, Hassanin A, Ho PM, McInnes MDF, Moss A, Juarez-Colunga E, Soni NJ, Miglioranza MH, Platz E, DeSanto K, Sertich AP, Salame G, Daugherty SL (2019) Diagnostic accuracy of point-of-care lung ultrasonography and chest radiography in adults with symptoms suggestive of acute decompensated heart failure: a systematic review and meta-analysis. JAMA Netw Open 2:e190703. https://doi.org/10.1001/jamanetworkopen.2019.0703
8. Alzahrani SA, Al-Salamah MA, Al-Madani WH, Elbarbary MA (2017) Systematic review and meta-analysis for the use of ultrasound versus radiology in diagnosing of pneumonia. Crit Ultrasound J 9:6. https://doi.org/10.1186/s13089-017-0059-y
9. Brogi E, Bignami E, Sidoti A, Shawar M, Gargani L, Vetrugno L, Volpicelli G, Forfori F (2017) Could the use of bedside lung ultrasound reduce the number of chest x-rays in the intensive care unit? Cardiovasc Ultrasound 15:23. https://doi.org/10.1186/s12947-017-0113-8
10. Nouvenne A, Zani MD, Milanese G, Parises A, Baciarello M, Bignami E, Odone A, Sverzellati N, Meschi T, Ticinesi A (2020) Lung ultrasound in COVID-19 pneumonia: correlations with chest CT at hospital admission. Respiration. https://doi.org/10.1159/000509223
11. Klok FA, Kruip MJHA, van der Meer NJM, Arbous MS, Gommers DAMPJ, Kant KM, Kaptein FHJ, van Paassen J, Stals MAM, Huisman MV, Endeman H (2020) Incidence of thrombotic complications in critically ill ICU patients with COVID-19. Thromb Res. https://doi.org/10.1016/j.thromres.2020.04.013
12. Lichtenstein DA, Mezière GA (2008) Relevance of lung ultrasound in the diagnosis of acute respiratory failure: the BLUE protocol. Chest 134:117–125. https://doi.org/10.1378/chest.07-2800
13. Lichtenstein DA (2014) Lung ultrasound in the critically ill. Ann Intensive Care 4:1. https://doi.org/10.1186/2110-5820-4-1
14. Lichtenstein DA, Lascols N, Mezière G, Gepner A (2004) Ultrasound diagnosis of alveolar consolidation in the critically ill. Intensive Care Med 30:276–281. https://doi.org/10.1007/s00134-003-2075-6
15. Lu W, Zhang S, Chen B, Chen J, Xian J, Lin Y, Shan H (2020) A clinical study of noninvasive assessment of lung lesions in patients with coronavirus disease-19 (COVID-19) by bedside ultrasound. Ultraschall Der Medizin Stuttgart Ger 41:300–307. https://doi.org/10.1055/a-1154-8795
16. Xing C, Li Q, Du H, Kang W, Lian J, Yuan L (2020) Lung ultrasound findings in patients with COVID-19 pneumonia. Crit Care 24:174. https://doi.org/10.1186/s13054-020-02876-9
17. Huang Y, Wang S, Liu Y, Zhang Y, Zheng C, Zheng Y, Zhang C, Min W, Zhou H, Yu M, Hu M (2020) A preliminary study on the ultrasonic manifestations of peripulmonary lesions of non-critical novel coronavirus pneumonia (COVID-19). SSRN Electron J. https://doi.org/10.2139/ssrn.3544750
18. Nazerian P, Volpicelli G, Vanni S, Gigli C, Betti L, Bartolucci M, Zanobetti M, Ermini FR, Iannello C, Grifoni S (2015) Accuracy of lung ultrasound for the diagnosis of consolidations when compared to chest computed tomography. Am J Emerg Med 33:620–625. https://doi.org/10.1016/j.ajem.2015.01.035
19. Volpicelli G, Lamorte A, Villén T (2020) What's new in lung ultrasound during the COVID-19 pandemic. Intensive Care Med. https://doi.org/10.1007/s00134-020-06048-9
20. Robba C, Robba C, Battaglini D, Ball L, Patroniti N, Loconte M, Brunetti I, Vena A, Giacobbe D, Bassetti M, Rocco PRM, Pelosi P (2020) Distinct phenotypes require distinct respiratory management strategies in severe COVID-19. Respir Physiol Neurobiol. https://doi.org/10.1016/j.resp.2020.103455
21. Tobin MJ, Laghi F, Jubran A (2020) Caution about early intubation and mechanical ventilation in COVID-19. Ann Intensive Care 10:78. https://doi.org/10.1186/s13613-020-00692-6
22. Brogi E, Gargani L, Bignami E, Barbariol F, Marra A, Forfori F, Vetrugno L (2017) Thoracic ultrasound for pleural effusion in the intensive care unit: a narrative review from diagnosis to treatment. Crit Care 21:325. https://doi.org/10.1186/s13054-017-1897-5
23. Vetrugno L, Guadagnin GM, Barbariol F, D'Incà S, Delrio S, Orso D, Girometti R, Volpicelli G, Bove T (2019) Assessment of pleural effusion and small pleural drain insertion by resident doctors in an intensive care unit: an observational study. Clin Med Insights Circul Respir Pulm Med 13:117954841987152. https://doi.org/10.1177/1179548419871527
24. Vetrugno L, Brogi E, Barbariol F, Forfori F, Bignami E (2018) A message in the bottle. Anesthesiology 128:677. https://doi.org/10.1097/aln.0000000000002039
25. Bouhemad B, Mongodi S, Via G, Rouquette I (2015) Ultrasound for "lung monitoring" of ventilated patients. Anesthesiology 122:437–447. https://doi.org/10.1097/aln.0000000000000558
26. Bouhemad B, Liu Z-H, Arbelot C, Zhang M, Ferarri F, Le-Guen M, Girard M, Lu Q, Rouby J-J (2010) Ultrasound assessment of antibiotic-induced pulmonary reaeration in ventilator-associated pneumonia. Crit Care Med 38:84–92. https://doi.org/10.1097/ccm.0b013e3181b08cdb
27. Pesenti A, Musch G, Lichtenstein D, Mojoli F, Amato MBP, Cinnella G, Gattinoni L, Quintel M (2016) Imaging in acute respiratory distress syndrome. Intensive Care Med 42:686–698. https://doi.org/10.1007/s00134-016-4328-1
28. Soldati G, Copetti R, Sher S (2009) Sonographic interstitial syndrome: the sound of lung water. J Ultrasound Med 28:163–174. https://doi.org/10.7863/jum.2009.28.2.163
29. Copetti R, Soldati G, Copetti P (2008) Chest sonography: a useful tool to differentiate acute cardiogenic pulmonary edema from acute respiratory distress syndrome. Cardiovasc Ultrasound 6:16. https://doi.org/10.1186/1476-7120-6-16
30. Mayo PH, Copetti R, Feller-Kopman D, Mathis G, Maury E, Mongodi S, Mojoli F, Volpicelli G, Zanobetti M (2019) Thoracic ultrasonography: a narrative review. Intensive Care Med 45:1200–1211. https://doi.org/10.1007/s00134-019-05725-8
31. Pisani L, Vercesi V, van Tongeren PSI, Lagrand WK, Leopold SJ, Huson MAM, Henwood PC, Walden A, Smit MR, Riviello ED, Pelosi P, Dondorp AM, Schultz MJ, Consortium LU (2019) The diagnostic accuracy for ARDS of global versus regional lung ultrasound scores—a post hoc analysis of an observational study in invasively ventilated ICU patients. Intensive Care Med Exp 7:44. https://doi.org/10.1186/s40635-019-0241-6
32. Huang D, Ma H, Xiao Z, Blaivas M, Chen Y, Wen J, Guo W, Liang J, Liao X, Wang Z, Li H, Li J, Chao Y, Wang XT, Wu Y, Qin T, Su K, Wang S, Tan N (2018) Diagnostic value of cardiopulmonary ultrasound in elderly patients with acute respiratory distress syndrome. BMC Pulm Med 18:136. https://doi.org/10.1186/s12890-018-0666-9
33. Ye X, Xiao H, Chen B, Zhang S (2015) Accuracy of lung ultrasonography versus chest radiography for the diagnosis of adult community-acquired pneumonia: review of the literature and meta-analysis. PLoS ONE 10:e0130066. https://doi.org/10.1371/journal.pone.0130066
34. Testa A, Soldati G, Copetti R, Giannuzzi R, Portale G, Gentiloni-Silveri N (2012) Early recognition of the 2009 pandemic influenza A (H1N1) pneumonia by chest ultrasound. Crit Care 16:R30. https://doi.org/10.1186/cc11201
35. Franquet T (2011) Imaging of pulmonary viral pneumonia. Radiology 260:18–39. https://doi.org/10.1148/radiol.11092149
36. Koo HJ, Lim S, Choe J, Choi S-H, Sung H, Do K-H (2018) Radiographic and CT features of viral pneumonia. Radiographics 38:719–739. https://doi.org/10.1148/rg.2018170048
37. Xu Z, Shi L, Wang Y, Zhang J, Huang L, Zhang C, Liu S, Zhao P, Liu H, Zhu L, Tai Y, Bai C, Gao T, Song J, Xia P, Dong J, Zhao J, Wang F-S (2020) Pathological findings of COVID-19 associated with acute respiratory distress syndrome. Lancet Respir Med 8:420–422. https://doi.org/10.1016/s2213-2600(20)30076-x
38. Zhao W, Zhong Z, Xie X, Yu Q, Liu J (2020) Relation between chest CT findings and clinical conditions of coronavirus disease (COVID-19) pneumonia: a multicenter study. AJR Am J Roentgenol 214:1–6. https://doi.org/10.2214/ajr.20.22976
39. Inui S, Fujikawa A, Jitsu M, Kunishima N, Watanabe S, Suzuki Y, Umeda S, Uwabe Y (2020) Chest CT findings in cases from the cruise ship "Diamond Princess" with coronavirus disease 2019 (COVID-19). Radiol Cardiothorac Imaging 2:e200110. https://doi.org/10.1148/ryct.2020200110
40. Zhou Z, Guo D, Li C, Fang Z, Chen L, Yang R, Li X, Zeng W (2020) Coronavirus disease 2019: initial chest CT findings. Eur Radiol. https://doi.org/10.1007/s00330-020-06816-7

41. Salehi S, Abedi A, Balakrishnan S, Gholamrezanezhad A (2020) Coronavirus disease 2019 (COVID-19): a systematic review of imaging findings in 919 patients. AJR Am J Roentgenol. https://doi.org/10.2214/ajr.20.23034
42. Hansell DM, Bankier AA, MacMahon H, McLoud TC, Müller NL, Remy J (2008) Fleischner society: glossary of terms for thoracic imaging. Radiology 246:697–722. https://doi.org/10.1148/radiol.2462070712
43. Bernheim A, Mei X, Huang M, Yang Y, Fayad ZA, Zhang N, Diao K, Lin B, Zhu X, Li K, Li S, Shan H, Jacobi A, Chung M (2020) Chest CT findings in coronavirus disease-19 (COVID-19): relationship to duration of infection. Radiology. https://doi.org/10.1148/radiol.2020200463
44. Pan Y, Guan H, Zhou S, Wang Y, Li Q, Zhu T, Hu Q, Xia L (2020) Initial CT findings and temporal changes in patients with the novel coronavirus pneumonia (2019-nCoV): a study of 63 patients in Wuhan, China. Eur Radiol. https://doi.org/10.1007/s00330-020-06731-x
45. Rubin GD, Haramati LB, Kanne JP, Schluger NW, Yim J-J, Anderson DJ, Altes T, Desai SR, Goo JM, Inoue Y, Luo F, Prokop M, Richeldi L, Tomiyama N, Leung AN, Ryerson CJ, Sverzellati N, Raoof S, Volpi A, Martin IBK, Kong C, Bush A, Goldin J, Humbert M, Kauczor H-U, Mazzone PJ, Remy-Jardin M, Schaefer-Prokop CM, Wells AU (2020) The role of chest imaging in patient management during the COVID-19 pandemic: a multinational consensus statement from the Fleischner Society. Radiology. https://doi.org/10.1148/radiol.2020201365
46. Ye Z, Zhang Y, Wang Y, Huang Z, Song B (2020) Chest CT manifestations of new coronavirus disease 2019 (COVID-19): a pictorial review. Eur Radiol. https://doi.org/10.1007/s00330-020-06801-0
47. Kong W, Agarwal PP (2020) Chest imaging appearance of COVID-19 infection. Radiol Cardiothorac Imaging 2:e200028. https://doi.org/10.1148/ryct.2020200028
48. Kligerman SJ, Franks TJ, Galvin JR (2013) From the radiologic pathology archives: organization and fibrosis as a response to lung injury in diffuse alveolar damage, organizing pneumonia, and acute fibrinous and organizing pneumonia. Radiographics 33:1951–1975. https://doi.org/10.1148/rg.337130057
49. Siddiqi HK, Mehra MR (2020) COVID-19 illness in native and immunosuppressed states: a clinical-therapeutic staging proposal. J Heart Lung Transplant. https://doi.org/10.1016/j.healun.2020.03.012
50. Simpson S, Kay FU, Abbara S, Bhalla S, Chung JH, Chung M, Henry TS, Kanne JP, Kligerman S, Ko JP, Litt H (2020) Radiological Society of North America Expert Consensus Statement on Reporting Chest CT findings related to COVID-19. Endorsed by the Society of Thoracic Radiology, the American College of Radiology, and RSNA. Radiol Cardiothorac Imaging 2:e200152. https://doi.org/10.1148/ryct.2020200152
51. Sverzellati N, Milone F, Balbi M (2020) How imaging should properly be used in COVID-19 outbreak: an Italian experience. Diagn Interv Radiol 26:204–206. https://doi.org/10.5152/dir.2020.30320
52. Jin Y-H, Cai L, Cheng Z-S, Cheng H, Deng T, Fan Y-P, Fang C, Huang D, Huang L-Q, Huang Q, Han Y, Hu B, Hu F, Li B-H, Li Y-R, Liang K, Lin L-K, Luo L-S, Ma J, Ma L-L, Peng Z-Y, Pan Y-B, Pan Z-Y, Ren X-Q, Sun H-M, Wang Y, Wang Y-Y, Weng H, Wei C-J, Wu D-F, Xia J, Xiong Y, Xu H-B, Yao X-M, Yuan Y-F, Ye T-S, Zhang X-C, Zhang Y-W, Zhang Y-G, Zhang H-M, Zhao Y, Zhao M-J, Zi H, Zeng X-T, Wang Y-Y, Wang X-H, (CPAM) for the Zhongnan Hospital of Wuhan University Novel Coronavirus Management and Research Team, Evidence-Based Medicine Chapter of China International Exchange and Promotive Association for Medical and Health Care (2020) A rapid advice guideline for the diagnosis and treatment of 2019 novel coronavirus (2019-nCoV) infected pneumonia (standard version). Mil Med Res 7:4. https://doi.org/10.1186/s40779-020-0233-6
53. Hope MD, Raptis CA, Shah A, Hammer MM, Henry TS, Signatories on Behalf of Six (2020) A role for CT in COVID-19? What data really tell us so far. Lancet 395:1189–1190. https://doi.org/10.1016/s0140-6736(20)30728-5
54. Raptis CA, Hammer MM, Short RG, Shah A, Bhalla S, Bierhals AJ, Filev PD, Hope MD, Jeudy J, Kligerman SJ, Henry TS (2020) Chest CT and coronavirus disease (COVID-19): a critical review of the literature to date. Am J Roentgenol. https://doi.org/10.2214/ajr.20.23202
55. Li R, Liu G, Zhang X, Li H (2020) Letter to the Editor: Chest CT and RT-PCR: radiologists' experience in the diagnosis of COVID-19 in China. https://www.european-radiology.org/opinions/chest-ct-and-rt-pcr-radiologists-experience-in-the-diagnosis-of-covid-19-in-china/. Accessed 28 Apr 2020
56. Sardanelli F, Leo GD (2020) Assessing the value of diagnostic tests in the new world of COVID-19 pandemic. Radiology. https://doi.org/10.1148/radiol.2020201845
57. The Royal College of Radiologists (2020) RCR position on the role of CT in patients suspected with COVID-19 infection. https://www.rcr.ac.uk/college/coronavirus-covid-19-what-rcr-doing/clinical-information/rcr-position-role-ct-patients. Accessed 28 Apr 2020
58. American College of Radiography (2020) ACR recommendations for the use of chest radiography and computed tomography (CT) for suspected COVID-19 infection. https://www.acr.org/Advocacy-and-Economics/ACR-Position-Statements/Recommendations-for-Chest-Radiograph y-and-CT-for-Suspected-COVID19-Infection. Accessed 28 Apr 2020
59. Winkler M, Touw H, Pm Ven, Twisk J, Tuinman P (2018) Diagnostic accuracy of chest radiograph, and when concomitantly studied lung ultrasound, in critically ill patients with respiratory symptoms. Crit Care Med 46:e707–e714. https://doi.org/10.1097/ccm.0000000000003129
60. Guarracino F, Vetrugno L, Forfori F et al (2020) Lung, heart, vascular, and diaphragm ultrasound examination of COVID-19 patients: a comprehensive approach. J Cardiothorac Vasc Anesth. https://doi.org/10.1053/j.jvca.2020.06.013 **(published online ahead of print, 2020 Jun 1)**

5

Success rate to complete optimal 20 + 2 ISUOG planes for foetal ultrasonographic structural screening during early second trimester pregnancy in Thailand

Ravita Chaichanalap and Tharangrut Hanprasertpong*

Abstract

Objective: To compare the success rates of obtaining optimal 20 + 2 (2 overview + 20 planes) International Society of Ultrasound in Obstetrics and Gynaecology (ISUOG) planes for foetal ultrasound structural screening between pregnant women at gestational age (GA) 18–20 weeks and 20–22 weeks 6 days

Methods: A prospective descriptive study was conducted. Singleton pregnant women at GA 18–22 weeks + 6 days attending antenatal clinic between December 2019 and March 2020 were invited to participate in the study. Women whose foetuses had obvious structural anomalies were excluded. The ultrasound screening using 20 + 2 ISUOG protocol was performed by 21 operators who had completed the online ISUOG basic training programme with an experience of ultrasound scanning of at least 30 cases. The success rates of achieving optimal planes between GA 18–20 weeks and 20–22 weeks 6 days were compared using Chi-square test. Common suboptimal planes in the ultrasound scan were also presented.

Results: Optimal 20 + 2 ISUOG planes were successfully assessed in 97/126 (77%) and 112/126 (88.9%) patients in the group with a GA < 20 weeks and in the group with a GA ≥ 20 weeks, respectively. Overall success rate was 82.9%. The success rate for the GA < 20 weeks group was significantly lower than that for the GA ≥ 20 weeks group. The group with a GA ≥ 20 weeks had a 1.2 times higher success rate than the group with a GA < 20 weeks. The most common suboptimal planes were the facial planes, especially the median facial profile, and foetal thoracic planes.

Conclusions: We prefer to perform foetal structural screening using US with the 20 + 2 ISUOG protocol at a GA 20 to 22 weeks and 6 days with the aim reducing the need for repeat scans.

Keywords: Foetal structural screening, Success rate, Ultrasonographic

Introduction

Ultrasonography (US) is a standard investigation for detecting foetal structural abnormalities. There are many reports that have evaluated the detection rate, accuracy, and cost-effectiveness of US in detecting routine foetal structural abnormalities in low-risk pregnancies [1–3]. Most experts suggest performing routine US investigations for foetal structural abnormalities at 18–22 weeks of gestation, although this may be performed earlier to evaluate such abnormalities during the first trimester aneuploidy screening [4]. For a foetal anatomical survey, the evaluation should be systematically examined. International Society of Ultrasound in Obstetrics and Gynaecology (ISUOG) launched the good guidance (the 20 + 2 approach) for obstetricians to perform an effective foetal evaluation since 2018. The protocol consisted

*Correspondence: tharangrut@hotmail.com; tharangrut@gmail.com
Department of Obstetrics and Gynecology, Faculty of Medicine, Srinakharinwirot University, Ongkharak 26120, Nakornnayok, Thailand

of a combination of 2 overview sweeps with 20 planes (divided into 7 anatomical areas: head, thorax, abdomen, pelvis, limbs, spine and face) of the foetus. It also has been backed up by ISUOG online education and training. Each plane relates to a specific foetal section or view that enables the potential exclusion of 50 abnormal foetal appearances.

In Thailand, there is no recommendation about when to perform routine US foetal structural screening. Consequently, the practice varies depending on the location and availability of a suitably qualified physician and US instrument, but US may be performed in certain cases such as genetic Down syndrome screening for high-risk pregnancies [5]. The Antenatal Outpatient Unit, Department of Obstetrics and Gynaecology, Faculty of Medicine, Srinakharinwirot University, serves as a maternal foetal medicine centre for general obstetrics, and for other hospitals in eastern Thailand. We arrange routine US foetal structural screening for all pregnant women who attend the antenatal care (ANC) clinic at our hospital and for pregnant women who visit ANC units at other hospitals or clinics nearby. Generally, we prefer a gestational age (GA) of 18 to 22 weeks and 6 days for screening. Unfortunately, suboptimal screening results are occasionally obtained and lead to the need for a repeat scan during the next visit. A suboptimal screening result and the need for a repeat scan are not ideal for pregnant women or physicians. We postulated that the GA may affect the chance of obtaining suboptimal screening results. Thus, we conducted this study to investigate this hypothesis. The primary objective was to compare the success rates of the complete optimal 20 + 2 (2 overviews + 20 planes) International Society of Ultrasound in Obstetrics and Gynaecology (ISUOG) protocol for foetal US structural screening between women with pregnancies at a GA < 20 weeks and those with a GA ≥ 20 weeks. The secondary objective was to identify the planes that most commonly resulted in suboptimal results. Finally, we also aimed to determine the possible factors that influence the chance of obtaining a suboptimal result.

Methods

A prospective descriptive study was conducted between December 2019 and March 2020. Singleton pregnant women who visited our ANC clinic during 18 to 22 weeks and 6 days of gestation who were scheduled for routine US foetal structural screening at the Antenatal Outpatient Unit, Department of Obstetrics and Gynaecology, Faculty of Medicine, Srinakharinwirot University, Thailand, were enrolled in our study. The exclusion criteria were refusal to participate or detection of foetal abnormality during US screening.

The study was approved by the institutional ethics committee (SWUEC/E-294/62) and was registered with the Thai Clinical Trials Registry (TCTR 20200107005). After routine ANC was performed, all singleton pregnant women with a GA between 18 and 22 weeks and 6 days were routinely requested to undergo US foetal structural screening. Before the US examination, we explained our study to the women and if they agreed to participate in our study, we asked each woman to give signed informed consent. The participants' demographic data and possible factors influencing the success rate of the complete optimal 20 + 2 ISUOG protocol were collected, including history of an abdominal surgery. Then, the participants were asked to undergo an US examination performed by the doctor on duty that day. If there was more than one service doctor working that day, the doctor with the greatest availability was asked to do the examination. US screening in our study was performed by 21 operators, classified as 6, 3 or 12 doctors who were qualified to practise maternal foetal medicine by The Royal Thai College of Obstetricians and Gynaecologists (RTCOG), the residents attending of maternal foetal medicine fellowship training programme or obstetrics and gynaecologic training programme, respectively, at the Department of Obstetrics and Gynaecology, Faculty of Medicine, Srinakharinwirot University, under the RTCOG curriculum. The 20 + 2 ISUOG protocol was applied for the screening [6]. We set the qualifications of the operators before taking part in this study, including: (1) completion of the online ISUOG basic training programme, and (2) experience in US scanning of at least 30 cases. For maternal foetal medicine fellowship training doctors, they independently performed US scan without confirmation. For obstetrics and gynaecologic training doctors, all US images were audited by maternal foetal medicine staffs.

All retrieved images of cases and controls were assessed offline by two independent examiners (R.C., T.H.) who were unaware of the final diagnosis.

The US information sought included the 20 + 2 ISUOG foetal anatomical area planes, amniotic fluid deepest vertical pocket (DVP), placental location and thickness, presence of pelvic mass, and maternal anterior abdominal wall thickness. The maternal anterior abdominal wall thickness was measured along the linea nigra at the midportion between the umbilicus and the pubic symphysis. The results of the US examination were recorded in the hospital-based system and reported to the primary doctor for antenatal management planning. Each scan took approximately 15 to 20 min. Suboptimal scan defined by operator when the scan took more than 30 min and changing position of pregnant women on the examination bed was tried. If the examination results were suboptimal, the remarks of concerning failure such as foetal position or maternal habitus and suboptimal anatomical area was recorded and the pregnant women were asked to make another appointment for a second scan as per the hospital protocol.

The required sample size was estimated on the basis of sufficiency to compare two independent proportions. Based on a previous study [7], the proportion of successfully completed optimal examinations were 90% and 70% for women with a GA ≥ 20 weeks and GA < 20 weeks, respectively. To achieve a power of at least 80% to detect significant differences at an alpha error of 0.05, beta error of 0.2, and for a sample ratio between two groups of 1:1, the sample size required for each group was determined to be approximately 126 subjects, or 252 in total. The statistical analysis was performed with R2.10.0 software (freeware distributed by the R Development Care Team). The patients' basic characteristics were collected and the data distribution was analysed by the Kolmogorov–Smirnov test and presented as the number, percentage, median, range, mean, and standard deviation (SD). The differences in the patients' basic characteristics between the two groups were analysed using the Chi-square test and Fisher's exact test. The success rates of obtaining complete 20 + 2 ISUOG planes for foetal US screening in each group are presented herein as the number and percentage. The difference in success rates between the two groups was compared using Chi-square test. Other possible factors that may affect the success rate were analysed using the bivariate, co-linearity and multiple logistic regression. Finally, the common foetal structural system when complete 20 + 2 ISUOG planes were successfully obtained for foetal US screening is presented as the number and percentage and was correlated to a GA < 20 weeks or GA ≥ 20 weeks as analysed by Fisher exact test. A probability value of $p < 0.05$ is considered significant in all cases.

Results

In total, 252 participants were enrolled in the study, with 126 in each group. The patients' basic characteristics are shown in Table 1. Maternal age, race, body mass index (BMI), gravidity, parity, history of abdominal surgery, type of previous abdominal scar incision, abdominal wall thickness, DVP, placental location, and the presence of myoma uteri showed no statistically significant differences between the two groups. Information about the operator who performed the foetal US screening is presented in Table 2. The median US durations were 15 (12–21), 24 (15–30), and 19 (15–30) minutes for the GA < 20 weeks group, the GA ≥ 20 weeks group, and overall, respectively. The time needed to perform the US was significantly longer for the pregnant women with a GA ≥ 20 weeks than for those with a GA < 20 weeks ($p < 0.001$).

Overall, 209 of the 252 pregnant women (82.9%) had 20 + 2 ISUOG planes completed for foetal US screening in our study. The success rates were 97/126 (77%) and 112/126 (88.9%) for participants with GA < 20 weeks and GA ≥ 20 weeks, respectively. The success rate for the group with a GA < 20 weeks was significantly lower than the success rate for the group with a GA ≥ 20 weeks. The GA ≥ 20 weeks group had a 1.2 times higher success rate for obtaining complete optimal 20 + 2 ISUOG planes for foetal US screening than the GA < 20 weeks group (Table 3). Other variables, including BMI, history of abdominal surgery, type of previous abdominal scar, presence of myoma uteri, placental location, experience of the operators and maternal abdominal wall thickness, were not statistically significant factors for the success rate of obtaining a complete and optimal scan. The means ± SDs of DVP were 3.98 ± 0.95 cm and 3.95 ± 0.99 cm in the optimal scan and suboptimal scan groups, respectively, which was not a significant difference ($p = 0.87$). The median (interquartile range) maternal abdominal wall thicknesses were 1.66 (1.34–2.10) cm and 1.78 (1.31–2.56) cm in the optimal scan and suboptimal scan groups, respectively, which was not a significant difference ($p = 0.39$). Subgroup analysis of US screening performed by maternal foetal medicine fellows showed that the suboptimal rate of the GA < 20 weeks group was 3 times significantly higher than that of GA ≥ 20 weeks group (25.0% VS 8.2%, p-value = 0.003).

Table 4 presents the most common foetal suboptimal planes, which were the facial (especially median facial profile) and foetal thoracic planes. The common failure in foetal thoracic planes was presented. The most common suboptimal planes were not significantly different between the two groups. All suboptimal examinations were optimal scan in the next subsequent appointment. No structural anomalies were reported in postnatal examination by routine neonatal evaluation in all participants. The common reasons for suboptimal scan were foetal position (86%) and maternal habitus (9.3%). The detail of foetal position did not record in our study.

Discussion

Our present study is the first to evaluate the success rate of obtaining complete and optimal 20 + 2 ISUOG planes for foetal US structural screening during the early second trimester in a developing country, namely Thailand. In low-resource developing countries, the number of qualified and trained US physicians and the availability of US equipment is limited compared to the number of pregnant women. Thus, effective medical resource management is necessary. Our study chose to implement

Table 1 Patients' characteristics ($n = 252$)

	GA < 20 weeks ($n = 126$)	GA ≥ 20 weeks ($n = 126$)	Overall (252)	*P*-value
Age (years)				0.892
Median (interquartile range)	29 (23–33)	28.5 (23–32.5)	29 (23–33)	
Race, n (%)				0.593
Thai	106 (49.3%)	109 (50.7%)	215	
Other	20 (54.1%)	17 (45.9%)	37	
BMI (kg/m^2)				0.656
Median (interquartile range)	23.8 (21.4–26.7)	23.7 (20.8–27.1)	23.8 (21–26.9)	
Gravid, n (%)				0.240
Nulligravida ($G = 1$)	51 (54.8%)	42 (45.2%)	93	
Multigravida ($G \geq 2$)	75 (47.2%)	84 (52.8%)	159	
Parity, n (%)				0.253
Nulliparous ($P = 0$)	60 (54.1%)	51 (45.9%)	111	
Multiparous ($P \geq 1$)	66 (46.8%)	75 (53.2%)	141	
History of abdominal surgery, n (%)				0.357
Presence	24 (44.4%)	30 (55.6%)	54	
Absence	102 (51.5%)	96 (48.5%)	198	
Type of previous abdominal scar incision, n (%)				0.694
Midline	5 (50%)	5 (50%)	10	
Transverse	16 (41%)	23 (59%)	39	
Laparoscopic	1 (100%)	0	1	
Other	2 (50%)	2 (50%)	4	
Abdominal wall thickness (cm)				0.889
Median (interquartile range)	1.7 (1.3-2.2)	1.7 (1.3-2.1)	1.7 (1.3-2.1)	
Deep vertical pocket (cm)				0.135
Mean ± SD	3.9 ± 0.9	4.1 ± 1.0	4.0 ± 1.0	
Placental location n (%)				0.130
Anterior	72 (54.5%)	60 (45.5%)	132	
Posterior	54 (45.0%)	66 (55.0%)	120	
Myoma uteri *n* (%)				0.175
Presence	1 (20%)	4 (80%)	5	
Absence	**125 (50.6%)**	**122 (49.4%)**	**247**	

Table 2 Information about the operator ($n = 252$)

	GA < 20 weeks ($n = 126$)	GA ≥ 20 weeks ($n = 126$)	Overall (252)	*P*-value
Operator, *n* (%)				0.070
Obstetrics and gynaecology residents	17 (37.8%)	28 (62.2%)	45	
MFM fellows	84 (49.7%)	85 (50.3%)	169	
MFM staff with < 5-year experience	14 (60.9%)	9 (39.1%)	23	
MFM staff with ≥ 5-year experience	**11 (73.3%)**	**4 (26.7%)**	**15**	

MFM maternal foetal medicine

the 20 + 2 ISUOG protocol because foetal structural US screening using such a standard protocol improves the sensitivity of screening for all anomalies and major anomalies in populations of varying risk [8]. The application of a standard protocol is an advantage of our study. Moreover, attending the ISUOG basic training online course improves the practitioners' theoretical knowledge and

Table 3 Factors affecting the chance of success of obtaining complete 2 + 20 ISUOG planes for foetal ultrasonographic screening

Variables	Result		Prevalence rate ratio	95% CI	*P*-value*
	Incomplete	Complete			
GA					0.012
≥20 weeks (%)	14 (11.1)	112 (88.9)	1.2	1.031–1.294	
< 20 weeks (%)	29 (23)	97 (77)			
BMI					
≤25 kg/m^2 (%)	22 (14.2)	133 (85.8)	1.1	0.969–1.238	0.126
> 25 kg/m^2 (%)	21 (21.6)	6 (78.4)			
History of abdominal scar			1.1	0.974–1.227	0.190
Yes (%)	6 (11.1)	48 (88.9)			
No (%)	37 (18.7)	161 (81.3)			
Myoma uteri			1.2	1.143–1.282	0.306
Yes (%)	0	5 (100)			
No (%)	43 (17.4)	204 (82.6)			
Placenta			1.0	0.920–1.152	0.609
Anterior (%)	21 (15.9)	111 (84.1)			
Posterior (%)	22 (18.3)	98 (81.7)			
Presentation			1.0	0.912–1.144	0.716
Non-cephalic (%)	16 (16)	84 (84)			
Cephalic (%)	27 (17.8)	125 (82.2)			
Sonographer					
Staff (%)	10 (26.3)	28 (73.7)	0.871	0.714-1.062	0.100
Resident and fellow (%)	33 (15.4)	181 (84.6)			

*The univariate, co-linearity and multiple logistic regression analysis

Table 4 Details about the foetal suboptimal scanning plane

Suboptimal planes	GA < 20 weeks (*N* = 126)	GA > = 20 weeks (*N* = 126)	Overall (*N* = 256)	*P* value
Face (*n*, %)	13 (10.3)	9 (7.1)	22 (8.6)	0.240
Coronal view if upper lip, nose and nostrils (n. %)	3	0	3	
Both orbits,,both lens (n, %)	1	0	1	
Median facial profile (n, %)	9	9	9	
Thorax (*n*, %)	4 (3.2)	4 (3.2)	8 (3.1)	0.086
Lung, 4CB (n, %)	0	0	0	
LVOT (n, %)	0	0	0	
RVOT and crossover of LVOT (*n*, %)	1	0	1	
3VT (*n*, %)	1	0	1	
RVOT and crossover of LVOT and 3VT (*n*, %)	0	1	1	
LVOT, RVOT and crossover of LVOT and 3VT (*n*, %)	2	0	2	
Lungs, 4CB, LVOT, RVOT and crossover of LVOT and 3VT (*n*, %)	0	3	3	
Face and thorax (*n*, %)	11 (8.7)	1 (0.8)	12 (4.7)	
Face and abdomen (*n*, %)	1 (0.8)	0 (0)	1 (0.4)	

4CB 4 chamber view of heart, *LVOT* Left ventricular outflow tract, *RVOT* Right ventricular outflow tract, *3VT* 3 vessel trachea view of heart

* Fisher exact test

practical skills [9]. Thus, all physicians should attend such a course before performing US.

The overall success rate of obtaining optimal 20+2 ISUOG planes in our study was 82.9%. The success rates were 97/126 (77%) and 112/126 (88.9%) for participants with a GA < 20 weeks and GA ≥ 20 weeks, respectively. In previous studies, the success rates were reported to be approximately 86–94% when the examinations were performed during a GA = 18–20 weeks [10–13]. The success rate in our study is slightly lower than that in previous studies. We hypothesized that the lower rate resulted from the variation in physician experience. All previous studies concerned developed countries, where US examinations are performed by maternal foetal medicine-specialized obstetricians, while the examinations in our present study were performed by physicians with different experience levels, including maternal foetal medicine practitioners who had qualified as doctors of obstetrics or maternal foetal medicine fellowship-residents and residents in training. However, the success rates among operators with similar experience level were not different either in GA ≥ 20 weeks or GA < 20 weeks groups. Regarding the success rate of obtaining optimal 20+2 ISUOG planes between pregnant women with a GA ≥ 20 weeks and GA < 20 weeks, we found that those with a GA ≥ 20 weeks had a 1.2 times higher success rate for foetal US screening than women with a GA < 20 weeks. This is similar to previous studies, which found that a lower GA decreases the success rate of achieving optimal visualization [11–13]. We postulated that the smaller foetus and relatively smaller foetal size to amniotic fluid ratio may affect the possibility of achieving success, and hence the success rate. Moreover, the operator's confidence in making a conclusion about a normal foetal finding may be decreased when the US is performed for women with a lower GA. Furthermore, the confidence of the operator may be more affected in procedures performed by a less experienced doctor than in those performed by a more highly experienced doctor. Importantly, there is a greater risk that a diagnosis or suspicion of some malformations may be reported as a false positive when the assessment is performed in early pregnancy, such as the case for mild pyelectasis [13].

In addition to a GA ≥ 20 weeks or GA < 20 weeks, other factors did not significantly affect the success rate of obtaining optimal 20+2 ISUOG planes, including BMI, history of abdominal surgery, abdominal wall thickness, DVP, placental location, and the presence of myoma uteri. This finding is different from a previous study, which reported that foetal position, oligohydramnios, prior abdominal surgery, and maternal obesity may account for suboptimal US visualization. We hypothesized that our different result may be caused by the definition of each variable, number of sample size calculation which based on GA only and small proportion of some maternal characters such as presence of myoma, obese or abdominal scar, etc [11, 14–16]. The most common suboptimal planes in our study were the facial profile and thoracic planes. These results were similar to those another previous study [17]. We hypothesized that the success of getting both facial profile and thoracic planes depends on foetal position. Finally, the limitation of the study should be addressed. We excluded foetuses with obvious anomaly and evaluated only the success rates of achieving optimal planes of ultrasound scanning in normal foetuses. Therefore, a diagnostic performance of the 20+2 ISUOG protocol to detect foetal anomalies could not be assessed. Future research should be performed focusing on this issue. Re-schedule for US scan on the same day and waiting for foetal position changing may be optioned.

Conclusion

Based on the results of our study, we prefer to perform foetal structural screening using US with the 20+2 ISUOG protocol at a GA 20 to 22 weeks and 6 days with the aim of reducing the chance that the patient will need a repeat scan. We recommend this as a preferred foetal US structural screening practice during the early second trimester of pregnancy in Thailand, and in other developing countries (resource-limited areas). Anyway, delaying foetal abnormal diagnosis should be cautioned.

Acknowledgements
The authors would like to thank Assistant Professor Dr. Kittipong Kongsomboon MD, MBA, PhD**, Department of Preventive and Social Medicine, Faculty of Medicine, Srinakharinwirot University, Ongkharak, Nakornnayok 26120, Thailand, for support with the statistical analysis .

Authors' contributions
RC: data collection, data analysis, manuscript writing. TH: protocol development, data analysis, manuscript writing/editing. All authors read and approved the final manuscript.

References

1. Onyambu CK, Tharamba NM (2018) Screening for congenital fetal anomalies in low risk pregnancy: the Kenyatta National Hospital experience. BMC Pregn Childbirth 18:180. https://doi.org/10.1186/s12884-01801824-z
2. Romosan G, Henriksson E, Rylander A, Valentin L (2009) Diagnostic performance of routine ultrasound screening for fetal abnormalities in an unselected Swedish population in 2000–2005. Ultrasound Obstet Gynecol 34:526–533
3. Rydberg C, Tunon K (2017) Detection of fetal abnormalities by second-trimester ultrasound screening in a non-selected population. Acta Obstet Gynecol Scand 96:176–182
4. Salomon LJ, Alfirevic Z, Berghella V, Bilardo C, Hernandez-Andrade E, Johnsen SL et al (2011) Practice guidelines for performance of the routine mid-trimester fetal ultrasound scan. Ultrasound Obstet Gynecol 37:116–126
5. Benchamanon R, Suwanrath C, Pranpanus S (2020) Fetal tricuspid regurgitation in second trimester of pregnancies at risk for fetal chromosomal defects. J Clin Ultrasound 48:97–101

6. isuog.org [homepage on the Internet]. New York: International Society of Ultrasound in Obstetrics and Gynecology; [updated 2018 Oct 20; Cited 2020 July 20]. http://www.isuog.org.
7. Schwarzler P, Senat MV, Holden D, Bernard JP, Masroor T, Ville Y (1999) Feasibility of the second-trimester fetal ultrasound examination in and unselected population at 18, 20, 22 weeks of pregnancy: a randomized trial. Ultrasound Obstet Gynecol 14:92–97
8. Karim JN, Roberts NW, Salomon LJ, Papageonghiou AT (2017) Systematic review of first-trimester ultrasound screening for detection of fetal structural anomalies and factors that affect screening performance. Ultrasound Obstet Gynecol 50:429–441
9. Vrachnis N, Papageorghiou AT, Bilardo CM, Abuhamad A, Tabor A, Cohen-Overbeek TE et al (2019) International Society of Ultrasound in Obstetrics and Gynecology (ISUOG) – the propagation of knowledge in ultrasound for the improvement of OB/GYN care worldwide: experience of basic ultrasound training in Oman. BMC Med Educ 19:434–440
10. Silver MT, Pettker CM, Raney JH, Xu X, Ross JS (2016) Frequency and importance of incomplete screening fetal anatomic sonography in pregnancy. J Ultrasound Med 35:2665–2673
11. Wood SL, Owen J, Jenkins SM, Harper LM (2018) The utility of repeat midtrimester anatomy ultrasound for anomaly detection. Am J Perinatol 35:1346–1351
12. Yagel S, Cohen SM, Porat S, Daum H, Lipschuetz M, Amsalem H et al (2015) Detailed transabdominal fetal anatomic scanning in the late first trimester versus the early second trimester of pregnancy. J Ultrasound Med 34:143–149
13. Saltvedt S, Almstrom H, Kublickas M, Valentin L, Grunewald C (2006) Detection of malformations in chromosomally normal fetuses by routine ultrasound at 12 or 18 weeks of gestation-a randomized controlled trial in 39572 pregnancies. BJOG 113:664–674
14. Thornburg LL, Miles K, Ho M, Pressman EK (2009) Fetal anatomic evaluation in the overweight and obese gravida. Ultrasound Obstet Gynecol 33:670–675
15. Hendler I, Blackwell SC, Bujold E, Threadwell MC, Mittal P, Sokol RJ et al (2005) Suboptimal second-trimester ultrasonographic visualization of the fetal heart in obese women: should we repeat the examination? J Ultrasound Med 24:1205–1209
16. Edwards L, Hui L (2018) First and second trimester screening for fetal structural anomalies. Semin Fetal Neonatal Med 23:102–111
17. Silverstri MT, Pettker CM, Raney JH, Xu X, Ross JS (2016) Frequency and importance of incomplete screening fetal anatomic sonography in pregnancy. J Ultrasound Med 35:2665–2673

6

Comparing accuracy of bedside ultrasound examination with physical examination for detection of pleural effusion

Michael H. Walsh[1], Kang X. Zhang[2], Emily J. Cox[3], Justin M. Chen[2], Nicholas G. Cowley[2], Christopher J. Oleynick[1], Leo M. Smyth[4] and Irene W. Y. Ma[1,5,6*]

Abstract

Background: In detecting pleural effusion, bedside ultrasound (US) has been shown to be more accurate than auscultation. However, US has not been previously compared to the comprehensive physical examination. This study seeks to compare the accuracy of physical examination with bedside US in detecting pleural effusion.

Methods: This study included a convenience sample of 34 medical inpatients from Calgary, Canada and Spokane, USA, with chest imaging performed within 24 h of recruitment. Imaging results served as the reference standard for pleural effusion. All patients underwent a comprehensive lung physical examination and a bedside US examination by two researchers blinded to the imaging results.

Results: Physical examination was less accurate than US (sensitivity of 44.0% [95% confidence interval (CI) 30.0–58.8%], specificity 88.9% (95% CI 65.3–98.6%), positive likelihood (LR) 3.96 (95% CI 1.03–15.18), negative LR 0.63 (95% CI 0.47–0.85) for physical examination; sensitivity 98% (95% CI 89.4–100%), specificity 94.4% (95% CI 72.7–99.9%), positive LR 17.6 (95% CI 2.6–118.6), negative LR 0.02 (95% CI 0.00–0.15) for US). The percentage of examinations rated with a confidence level of 4 or higher (out of 5) was higher for US (85% of the seated US examination and 94% of the supine US examination, compared to 35% of the PE, $P < 0.001$), and took less time to perform ($P < 0.0001$).

Conclusions: US examination for pleural effusion was more accurate than the physical examination, conferred higher confidence, and required less time to complete.

Keywords: Ultrasound, Point-of-care ultrasound, Pleural effusion, Physical examination

Introduction

Pleural effusions are common in general medical patients and may be caused by pathological states such as congestive heart failure, infections, cirrhosis, and malignancy [1, 2]. Detection of pleural effusions is important because their presence may signal a need for diagnostic and/or therapeutic interventions [2, 3]. Traditionally in internal medicine, bedside identification of pleural effusions involves performing a physical examination (PE), followed by imaging studies [4]. PE includes a number of maneuvers, with dullness to percussion and asymmetric chest expansion considered the most accurate signs [5, 6].

One study found that with minimal training, novice residents were able to reliably detect pleural effusions using bedside ultrasound (US) [7]. In contrast, only 60% of medical residents accurately detected bronchial breath sounds [8], such as those that might occur above the level of a pleural effusion [9], with no appreciable increase in auscultation accuracy between 1st year and 3rd year residents [8]. While studies suggest that US outperforms PE

*Correspondence: ima@ucalgary.ca
[5] Department of Medicine, W21C, University of Calgary, 3330 Hospital Dr NW, Calgary, AB T2N 4N1, Canada
Full list of author information is available at the end of the article

for detecting pleural effusion [10–14], many studies used only auscultation as the comparator, rather than a comprehensive PE. Thus, the superior performance of US in these studies may be exaggerated. To address this gap, our study seeks to compare the diagnostic accuracy of a multi-component PE with that of bedside US in detecting pleural effusions in medical patients.

Methods

The Conjoint Health Research Ethics Board at the University of Calgary and the Providence St. Joseph Health Institutional Review Board approved this study. This study is reported to conform to STARD guidelines for reporting studies of diagnostic accuracy [15].

Aim

This study seeks to compare the diagnostic accuracy of a PE with that of bedside US in medical inpatients.

Design and setting

A convenience sample of consenting patients were prospectively recruited from the Foothills Medical Centre (Calgary, AB, Canada) between August 2019 and March 2020 and Providence Sacred Heart Medical Center (Spokane, WA, USA) between September 2019 and June 2020. Patients admitted to the general medical ward who had chest computed tomography (CT) or chest radiography (CXR) performed within 24 h of the study period were eligible. Exclusion criteria were hemodynamic instability, inability to comply with the study protocol, or presence of pain/dressings that would preclude an US scan. Recruitment occurred when patient permission to approach the patient was provided by the admission team and when at least two researchers were available.

Consenting patients underwent both a PE and a bedside US examination independently by two researchers. The order of the examinations and the researcher performing each examination were randomized.

Physical examination (PE) protocol

With the patient in a sitting position, the researcher inspected the posterior thorax for asymmetry, and performed percussion, tactile fremitus, auscultation, and egophony. Based on these findings, the researcher recorded the PE diagnosis and rated their confidence in the diagnosis using a 5-point Likert scale, where 1 = not at all confident and 5 = very confident. This procedure was then repeated on the other side by the same researcher, and time to complete the examination was recorded.

Ultrasound examination protocol

A different researcher, blinded to the PE results, performed the US exam. With the patient in the seated position, a low-frequency transducer (2–5 MHz curvilinear array, Edge II, in Calgary; 1–5 MHz phased array, M-Turbo, Sonosite Inc., in Spokane) was used to longitudinally scan the posterior thorax inferiorly from the lung apices (Fig. 1A). The diagnosis was noted and the procedure was repeated on the other side.

Next, with the patient in a supine position, the same researcher performed coronal views of the lower lung zones (Fig. 1B). The presence of the spine sign and free fluid was used to determine the presence of pleural effusion. Time taken to complete the US examination in the seated and supine position and self-reported confidence were recorded.

Reference standard

Chest imaging findings reported by radiologists at each institution on chart review served as the reference standard for the diagnosis of pleural effusion. All researchers were blinded to the imaging study results at the time of the PE and US examinations.

Researcher training

Three researchers performed the study protocol in Calgary. Two were certified in Internal Medicine by the Royal College of Physicians and Surgeons of Canada and completing their point-of-care ultrasound fellowships (MW, LS). The third (CO) was a post-graduate year (PGY-3) medical resident who underwent a 1-h didactic session on US pleural effusion, and 6 h of supervised lung US scanning prior to patient enrollment. Of the PEs, five were completed by researcher MW, eight by CO, and four by LS. Of the US examinations, 11 were performed by MW, three by CO, and three by LS.

At the Spokane site, two researchers conducted the study protocol: one was a PGY-3 medical resident (NC), who completed eight PEs and nine US examinations for this study protocol, and the other was a PGY-4 clinical teaching fellow (JC), who completed nine PEs and eight US examinations for this study. Both completed a 4-h didactic session on bedside US and 12 h of supervised lung US scanning during a 2-week bedside US elective prior to patient enrollment.

Study outcomes

The primary outcomes were the diagnostic accuracies of PE and US. Secondary outcomes included time required to perform the examinations and overall confidence.

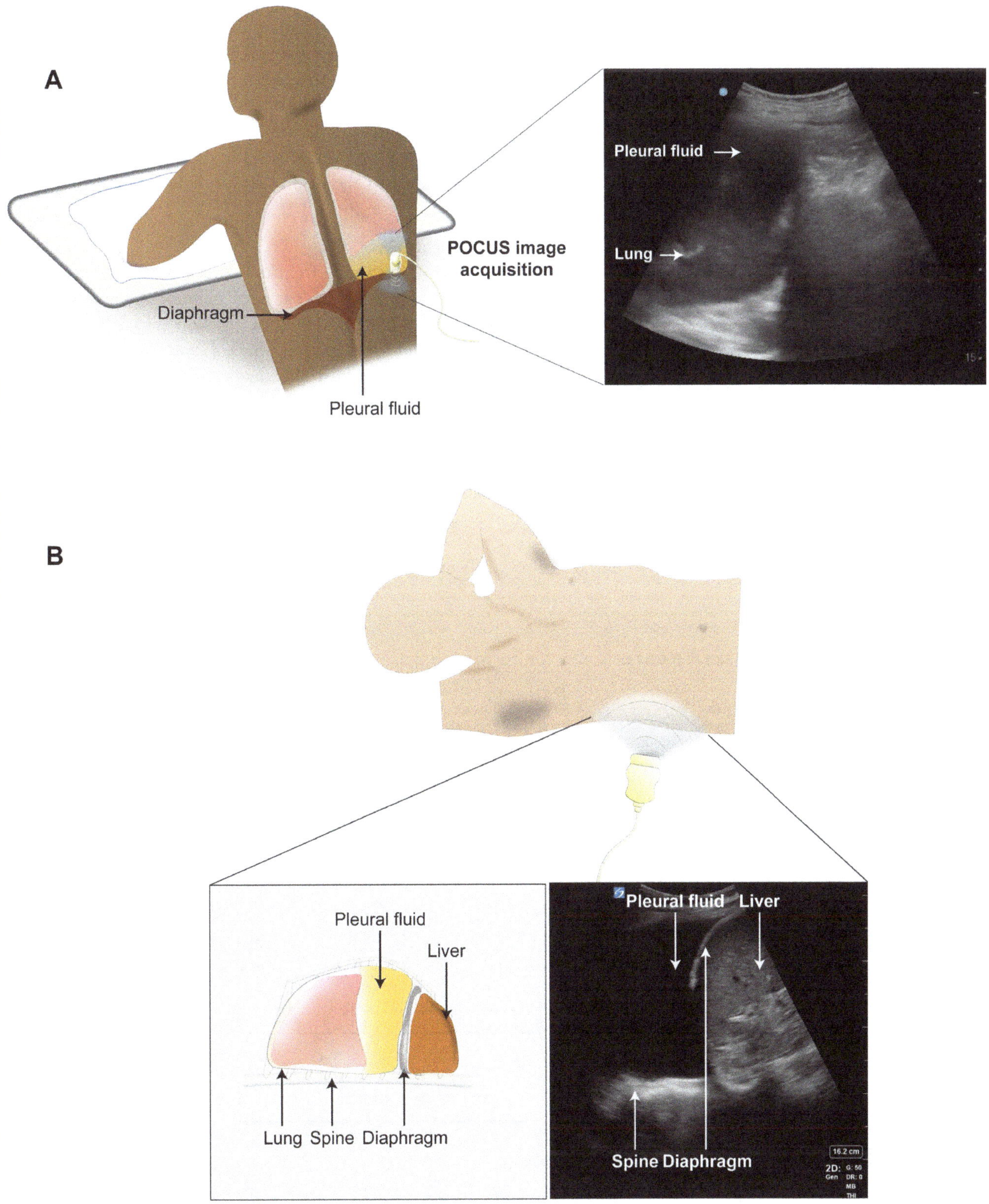

Fig. 1 Procedure for detecting pleural effusion with ultrasound. To detect the presence or absence of pleural effusion with ultrasound, the patient is evaluated in the seated position (**A**) and the supine position (**B**). With the patient in the seated position (**A**), the researcher slides the longitudinally oriented transducer inferiorly from the lung apices. With the patient in the supine position (**B**), the researcher obtains a coronal view of the lung base. A pleural effusion is detected if the researcher identifies both a positive spine sign and free fluid

Statistical analyses

Based on the previously reported pooled sensitivity of 0.93 for US [16], assuming an alpha of 0.5, and a prevalence of 0.94, a sample size of 28 would be required for our study [17, 18]. We used Wilcoxon rank-sum tests, Fisher exact tests, analysis of variance, and post hoc Tukey tests (where appropriate) to compare differences between groups. The diagnostic accuracy of the examinations was compared to the reference standard using sensitivity, specificity, positive likelihood ratio (LR) and negative LR. LRs greater than 10 or less than 0.1 were considered large effects; LRs of 5 to 10 and 0.1 to 0.2 moderate; 2 to 5 and 0.5 to 0.2 small; 1 to 2 and 0.5 to 1 negligible [19]. Confidence between groups was compared using Kruskal–Wallis tests and Fisher's exact tests adjusted for multiple comparisons using Bonferroni corrections. All analyses were performed using SAS version 9.4 (SAS Institute Inc., Cary, NC).

Results

A convenience sample of 34 patients ($n=17$ from Calgary and $n=17$ from Spokane) consented to participate (Table 1). Based on chest imaging, 22 (65%) had bilateral pleural effusions, six (27%) had unilateral, and six (27%) had no effusions. Twenty patients had a CXR performed, two had a CT performed, and 12 had both CT and CXRs performed. For those with both imaging studies performed, there was complete concordance in the pleural effusion diagnosis. There was no missing data nor known adverse events from either the reference imaging studies nor the physical examination or bedside US studies.

Physical exam

Decreased tactile fremitus and egophony were more commonly noted in cases of pleural effusion (Table 2). The overall PE for pleural effusion had a sensitivity of 44.0% and specificity of 88.9% (Table 3). Chest asymmetry had the highest specificity (94.4%) while dullness to percussion had the highest sensitivity (94.0%).

US exam

Both the seated and supine US examination had high diagnostic accuracies, (sensitivity 92% and 98%, specificity 94.4% and 94.4%, respectively for seated and supine US exam, Table 3).

Table 1 Baseline patient characteristics of the 34 patients included in the study

Characteristics	Patients with bilateral pleural effusion ($N=22$)	Patients with unilateral pleural effusion ($N=6$)	Patients with no pleural effusion ($N=6$)	*P*-value
Gender				
Male no. (%)	10 (45)	4 (67)	2 (33)	0.56
Female no. (%)	12 (55)	2 (33)	4 (67)	
Mean age (years) ± standard deviation (SD)	70 ± 10	57 ± 18	58 ± 12	0.03
Mean body mass index (kg/m^2) ± SD	24.7± 5.1	32.1 ± 7.9	32.7 ± 6.7	0.004
History of				
Coronary artery disease	13 (59)	2 (33)	1 (17)	0.20
Congestive heart failure	14 (64)	2 (33)	2 (33)	0.29
Chronic obstructive pulmonary disease	6 (27)	1 (17)	1 (17)	1.00
Diabetes mellitus	9 (41)	3 (50)	1 (17)	0.60
Hypertension	9 (41)	1 (17)	4 (67)	0.21

Square brackets indicate subgroups that are statistically different from each other ($P<0.05$) in post hoc analyses

Table 2 Physical examination and bedside ultrasound findings in 34 patients

	All lungs ($N=68$ lungs)	Lungs with pleural effusion ($N=50$ lungs)	Lungs with no pleural effusion ($N=18$ lungs)	*P*-value
Physical examination findings				
Decreased tactile fremitus—No. (%)	37 (54)	34 (68)	3 (17)	0.0002
Crackles—No (%)	30 (44)	23 (46)	7 (39)	0.78
Bronchial breath sounds—No. (%)	53 (78)	39 (78)	14 (78)	1.00
Dullness to percussion—No. (%)	62 (91)	47 (94)	15 (83)	0.33
Asymmetric chest wall expansion—No. (%)	10 (15)	9 (18)	1 (6)	0.27
Egophony—No. (%)	21 (31)	19 (38)	2 (11)	0.04
PE diagnosis—No. (%)				
Normal/diaphragm	41 (60)	25 (50)	16 (89)	0.005
Pleural effusion	24 (35)	22 (44)	2 (11)	0.02
Other (consolidation/atelectasis)	10 (15)	8 (16)	2 (11)	1.00
Median level of confidence (interquartile range) out of 5	3 (2–4)	3 (1–4)	3.5 (2–4)	0.04
Not at all confident—No. (%)	14 (21)	13 (26)	1 (6)	0.09
Somewhat not confident—No. (%)	14 (21)	10 (20)	4 (22)	
Neutral—No. (%)	16 (24)	12 (24)	4 (22)	
Somewhat confident—No. (%)	22 (32)	15 (30)	7 (39)	
Very confident—No. (%)	2 (3)	0	2 (11)	
Bedside ultrasound (US) findings				
Seated, posterior US exam				
Ultrasound diagnosis as pleural effusion	47 (69%)	46 (92)	1 (6)	<0.0001
Median level of confidence of seated, posterior US exam (interquartile range) out of 5	5 (4–5)	5 (5–5)	5 (4–5)	0.10
Not at all confident—No. (%)	5 (7)	4 (8)	1 (6)	0.15
Somewhat not confident—No. (%)	0	0	0	
Neutral—No. (%)	0	0	0	
Somewhat confident—No. (%)	10 (15)	5 (1)	5 (28)	
Very confident—No. (%)	48 (71)	38 (76)	10 (56)	
Missing responses	5 (7)	3 (6)	2 (11)	
Supine, coronal view US exam				
Ultrasound diagnosis as pleural effusion (positive spine sign)	50 (74%)	49 (98)	1 (6)	<0.0001
Median level of confidence of supine US exam (interquartile range) out of 5	5 (5–5)	5 (5–5)	5 (4–5)	0.09
Not at all confident—No. (%)	0	0	0	0.12
Somewhat not confident—No. (%)	1 (1)	0	1 (6)	
Neutral—No. (%)	1 (1)	1 (2)	0	
Somewhat confident—No. (%)	11 (17)	6 (12)	5 (28)	
Very confident—No. (%)	53 (78)	41 (82)	12 (67)	
Missing responses—No. (%)	2 (3)	2 (4)	0	

Findings are presented in terms of the individual count of lungs included in the study ($N=68$ lungs from 34 patients)

Secondary outcome measures

Mean duration of the PE [2 min 53 s ± standard deviation (SD) 39 s] was longer than the US exam in the seated and supine position (2 min 6 s ± SD 38 s and 1 min 37 s ± 43 s, respectively, $P<0.05$ for each comparison, Table 2). For confidence in the PE diagnosis, 24 (35%) of the 68 examinations were rated with a score of four or higher (out of five), while 58 (85%) of the US seated examination and 64 (94%) of the US supine examinations were rated as four or higher (Table 2). After accounting for multiple comparisons, where a $P<0.017$ is needed for statistical significance, post hoc analyses revealed that confidence in the PE was significantly lower than either of the US examinations ($P<0.001$ for both), while the confidence between the two US examinations was not significantly different ($P=0.27$).

Table 3 Diagnostic performance of physical examination and lung ultrasound for detection of pleural effusion

	Sensitivity (95% CI)	Specificity (95% CI)	Positive likelihood ratio (95% CI)	Negative likelihood ratio (95% CI)	Accuracy (95% CI)
Overall physical examination	44.0% (30.0–58.8%)	88.9% (65.3–98.6%)	3.96 (1.03–15.18)	0.63 (0.47–0.85)	55.9% (44.3–67.9%)
Individual physical examination findings					
Decreased tactile fremitus	68.0% (53.3–80.5%)	83.3% (58.6–96.2%)	4.08 (1.43–11.7)	0.38 (0.24–0.60)	72.1% (59–9-82.3%)
Dullness to percussion	94.0% (83.5–98.8%)	16.7% (3.6–41.4%)	1.13 (0.91–1.40)	0.36 (0.08–1.62)	73.5% (61.4–83.5%)
Asymmetric chest wall expansion	18% (8.6–31.4%)	94.4% (72.7–99.9%)	3.24 (0.44–23.81)	0.87 (0.73–1.03)	38.2% (26.7–50.8%)
Egophony	38.8% (25.2–53.8%)	88.9 (65.3–98.6%)	3.49 (0.90–13.50)	0.69 (0.52–0.91)	52.2% (39.7–64.6%)
Bedside ultrasound examination					
Seated (posterior exam)	92% (80.8–97.8%)	94.4% (72.7–99.9%)	16.6 (2.5–111.4)	0.08 (0.03–0.22)	92.7% (83.7–97.6%)
Supine (coronal views)	98% (89.4–100%)	94.4 (72.7–99.9%)	17.6 (2.6–118.6)	0.02 (0.00–0.15)	97.1% (89.8–99.6%)

Diagnostic parameters and their 95% confidence intervals (CI) of physical examination and sonographic findings for pleural effusion

Discussion

In our study of general medical inpatients, bedside US examination demonstrated higher accuracy than the PE. Sitting and supine US examinations resulted in diagnostic LRs that are considered large in magnitude, while LRs associated with PE were small [19]. Additionally, US examinations resulted in higher confidence and took less time to perform. While asymmetric chest wall expansion and dullness to percussion demonstrated high specificity and high sensitivity, respectively, the associated LRs were negligible to small [19].

Our supine US examination results (sensitivity of 98%, specificity 94.4%, a diagnostic accuracy of 97.1%) are consistent with existing literature. A pooled sensitivity of 93% and specificity of 96% were noted in a prior systematic review [16], while a diagnostic accuracy of 95.1% was previously reported [20]. In contrast, for dullness to percussion, our positive LR 1.13 is lower than the previously reported LR of 8.7, although a wide 95% CI (2.2–33.8) was noted [5]. Pooled negative LR of 0.31 in that review was similar to ours (0.36) [5]. Also consistent with existing literature was the finding that asymmetric chest expansion demonstrated a favorable specificity of over 90% [5, 21]. However, our positive LR was 3.24, while theirs was 8.1 [5], which may be a function of protocol differences, such as having trainees perform PE in our study, rather than experienced clinicians [5, 21]. However, even with experienced clinicians, their positive LR of 8.1 was only moderate in strength.

Few studies directly compared PE with bedside US for pleural effusion. Five prior studies reported that US was superior [10–14]. However, in at least four of these studies, only auscultation was performed [11–14], and auscultation is known to be less accurate than other PE maneuvers [5, 6]. In another study, added to PE, US resulted in significantly higher odds of identifying pleural effusion compared to PE alone [22]. Our present study adds to existing literature by directly comparing US with a comprehensive PE. Our results demonstrate that, despite the high specificity associated with asymmetric chest wall expansion and high sensitivity for dullness to percussion, the small likelihood ratios associated with these PE maneuvers suggest that US should be the preferred approach. Further, the associated large likelihood ratios for US suggest that, in the hands of a trained POCUS practitioner, the presence of pleural effusion can likely be ruled in or ruled out, with reasonably high accuracy, especially if the supine examination was used, evaluating for the presence or absence of the spine sign.

Our study has some limitations. First, our study sample had very few controls; only 6% did not have a pleural effusion. Although patients were not selected based upon the results of chest imaging studies, we cannot rule out the possibility that permission by the admitting team to approach patients for the study was more likely when the patient had pleural effusion, thereby introducing a potential selection bias. The resultant high prevalence of pleural effusions in our study sample is important to note for two reasons. First, representativeness of our conclusions may be limited, thereby limiting generalizability of our study conclusions [19]. Secondly, a high prevalence may also influence our resultant diagnostic accuracies, given the restriction in range seen as well as high reader expectations [23]. However, prior studies have reported that lower specificity may be reported in studies with higher prevalence [23]. Second, because of the multiple examinations required of our volunteer patients for this study protocol and the need for two clinician researchers present per patient, we were not able to perform an additional examination by an independent researcher. Thus, we do not have inter-rater reliability data for our study. Prior studies suggest that inter-rater reliability for

US examination is at least moderate or higher for pleural effusions [7, 24]. Third, our reported US duration did not include the time required for the machine to be located, transported to the bedside, and subsequently turned on. Thus, the actual time required may vary in the real-world setting. Fourth, resident-performed examinations may be less accurate than those performed by board-certified internists. However, senior trainees at both institutions commonly perform PEs on admission. Fifth, we did not collect information on subsequent patient management decisions, any ensuing procedures, or patient preferences regarding PE vs. US. In addition, we did not collect information on the admission diagnosis. At the Calgary site, the most common medical admission diagnoses were: congestive heart failure, alcohol withdrawal, type 1 diabetes mellitus with ketoacidosis, pneumonia, and fluid/electrolyte/acid base disorders. At the Spokane site, the most common admission diagnoses were: sepsis, acute respiratory failure, cerebral infarction, hypertensive heart and kidney disease, and alcoholic liver disease. Finally, the majority of our reference standards were based on CXR results. CT would be a preferred gold standard. However, sensitivity analysis of our diagnostic parameters did not result in significant changes to our conclusions when limiting our analyses to only those with CT results (*data not shown*). In detecting pleural effusion, US may be more sensitive than CXR [16, 25, 26], and could be identifying clinically insignificant effusions. However, US can directly visualize septations and complex effusions, and in that regard, has a theoretical advantage over CXR and CTs [27]. Neither of these outcomes were examined in our study, but should be considered in future studies.

Conclusions

In conclusion, US examination for pleural effusion is more accurate, confers greater confidence, and may be quicker to complete than PE. Thus, in situations where the device is readily accessible and practitioner is trained to scan and interpret, US examination for pleural effusion would be preferred.

Abbreviations

CXR: Chest radiography; CT: Computed tomography; CI: Confidence interval; IQR: Interquartile range; LR: Likelihood ratio; PE: Physical examination; PGY: Post-graduate year; SD: Standard deviation; US: Ultrasound.

Acknowledgements

The authors wish to thank the patients who participated in this study.

Authors' contributions

MHW, KXZ contributed to the conception and design of the work; acquisition and interpretation of data; and drafted and substantively revised the work. EJC contributed to the analysis and interpretation of data; drafted and substantively revised the work, and creation of the figures. JMC, NGC, CJO contributed to the acquisition and interpretation of data and substantively revised the work. IWYM contributed to the conception and design of the work; acquisition, analysis, and interpretation of data; and drafted and substantively revised the work. All authors read and approved the final manuscript.

Author details

[1]Division of General Internal Medicine, University of Calgary, Calgary, AB, Canada. [2]Providence Health Care, Providence Internal Medicine Residency Spokane, Spokane, WA, USA. [3]Providence Health Care, Providence Medical Research Center, Spokane, WA, USA. [4]Division of General Internal Medicine, University of Alberta, Edmonton, AB, Canada. [5]Department of Medicine, W21C, University of Calgary, 3330 Hospital Dr NW, Calgary, AB T2N 4N1, Canada. [6]Department of Community Health Sciences, W21C, University of Calgary, Calgary, AB, Canada.

References

1. Beaudoin S, Gonzalez AV (2018) Evaluation of the patient with pleural effusion. CMAJ 190(10):E291–E295
2. Hooper C, Lee YCG, Maskell N (2010) Investigation of a unilateral pleural effusion in adults: British Thoracic Society Pleural Disease guideline 2010. Thorax 65(Suppl2):Ii4–Ii17
3. Light RW (2011) Pleural effusions. Med Clin N Am 95(6):1055–1070
4. Saguil A, Wyrick K, Hallgren J (2014) Diagnostic approach to pleural effusion. Am Fam Physician 90(2):99–104
5. Wong CL, Holroyd-Leduc J, Straus SE (2009) Does this patient have a pleural effusion? JAMA 301(3):309–317
6. Mcgee S (2018) Evidence-based physical diagnosis, 4th edn. Elsevier Inc, Philadelphia
7. Begot E, Grumann A, Duvoid T et al (2014) Ultrasonographic identification and semiquantitative assessment of unloculated pleural effusions in critically ill patients by residents after a focused training. Intensive Care Med 40(10):1475–1480
8. Mangione S, Nieman LZ (1999) Pulmonary auscultatory skills during training in internal medicine and family practice. Am J Respir Crit Care Med 159(4 Pt 1):1119–1124
9. Sarkar M, Madabhavi I, Niranjan N, Dogra M (2015) Auscultation of the respiratory system. Ann Thorac Med 10(3):158–168
10. Patterson LA, Costantino TG, Satz WA (2004) Diagnosing pleural effusion: a prospective comparison of physical examination with bedside thoracic ultrasonography. Ann Emerg Med 44(4, Supplement):S112
11. Lichtenstein D, Goldstein I, Mourgeon E, Cluzel P, Grenier P, Roubyj J (2004) Comparative diagnostic performances of auscultation, chest radiography, and lung ultrasonography in acute respiratory distress syndrome. Anesthesiology 100(1):9–15
12. Vezzani A, Manca T, Brusasco C et al (2014) Diagnostic value of chest ultrasound after cardiac surgery: a comparison with chest x-ray and auscultation. J Cardiothorac Vasc Anesth 28(6):1527–1532
13. Tasci O, Hatipoglu ON, Cagli B, Ermis V (2016) Sonography of the chest using linear-array versus sector transducers: correlation with auscultation, chest radiography, and computed tomography. J Clin Ultrasound 44(6):83–89
14. Inglis AJ, Nalos M, Sue KH et al (2016) Bedside lung ultrasound, mobile radiography and physical examination: a comparative analysis of diagnostic tools in the critically ill. Crit Care Resusc 18(2):124
15. Cohen JF, Korevaar DA, Altman DG et al (2016) Stard 2015 guidelines for reporting diagnostic accuracy studies: explanation and elaboration. BMJ Open 6(11):E012799
16. Grimberg A, Shigueoka DC, Atallah AN, Ajzen S, Iared W (2010) Diagnostic accuracy of sonography for pleural effusion: systematic review. Sao Paulo Med J 128(2):90–95
17. Truc TT (2020) Statistics and sample size pro. https://Play.Google.Com/Store/Apps/Details?Id=Thaithanhtruc.Info.Sass&Hl=En_Us&Gl=Us. Accessed 21 July 2021.
18. Negida A, Fahim NK, Negida Y (2019) Sample size calculation guide—part 4: how to calculate the sample size for a diagnostic test accuracy study based on sensitivity, specificity, and the area under the roc curve. Adv J Emerg Med 3(3):E33

19. Guyatt G, Rennie D, Meade M, Cook D (2015) Users' guides to the medical literature: a manual for evidence-based clinical practice, 3rd edn. Mcgraw-Hill Education, New York
20. Xie C, Sun K, You Y et al (2020) Feasibility and efficacy of lung ultrasound to investigate pulmonary complications in patients who developed postoperative hypoxaemia-a prospective study. BMC Anesthesiol 20(1):220
21. Kalantri S, Joshi R, Lokhande T et al (2007) Accuracy and reliability of physical signs in the diagnosis of pleural effusion. Respir Med 101(3):431–438
22. Steinmetz P, Oleskevich S, Dyachenko A, Mccusker J, Lewis J (2018) Accuracy of medical students in detecting pleural effusion using lung ultrasound as an adjunct to the physical examination. J Ultrasound Med 37(11):2545–2552
23. Leeflang MMG, Rutjes AWS, Reitsma JB, Hooft L, Bossuyt PMM (2013) Variation of a test's sensitivity and specificity with disease prevalence. CMAJ 185(11):E537-544
24. Kumar A, Weng Y, Graglia S et al (2021) Interobserver agreement of lung ultrasound findings of Covid-19. J Ultrasound Med. https://doi.org/10.1002/Jum.15620
25. Hansell L, Milross M, Delaney A, Tian DH, Ntoumenopoulos G (2021) Lung ultrasound has greater accuracy than conventional respiratory assessment tools for the diagnosis of pleural effusion, lung consolidation and collapse: a systematic review. J Physiother 67(1):41–48
26. Yousefifard M, Baikpour M, Ghelichkhani P et al (2016) Screening performance characteristic of ultrasonography and radiography in detection of pleural effusion: a meta-analysis. Emergency (Tehran) 4(1):1–10
27. Svigals PZ, Chopra A, Ravenel JG, Nietert PJ, Huggins JT (2017) The accuracy of pleural ultrasonography in diagnosing complicated parapneumonic pleural effusions. Thorax 72(1):94

7

A rare ultrasound case report: intramuscular tear of the sartorius muscle

Kathryn Malherbe*

Abstract

We report a case of a 65-year-old male patient who presented with localized swelling and lump in the proximal third of the upper thigh. Most common upper thigh injuries involve the quadriceps muscle group associated with football injuries; however, in rare incidents certain forceful intrinsic injuries can cause intramuscular tear of the sartorius muscle. This is a rare case of spontaneous muscle rupture in an elderly patient with no history of recent sporting activity. Ultrasound provides a cost-effective, dynamic evaluation of the anterior upper thigh muscles to differentiate between chronic and acute phases of injury.

Keywords: Ultrasound, Sartorius muscle, Intramuscular tear, Intrinsic muscle injury

Introduction

Muscle fibres are grouped into fascicles and separated by septa of fibro-adipose tissue, the perimysium. The muscle is enclosed by a fascial sheath, the epimysium. The perimysium is seen on transverse imaging as dot echoes throughout a hypoechoic background, representing the bulk of the muscle fibres. Intramuscular septa produce a reticular pattern, and intermuscular septa appear brightly echogenic [1].

The sartorius muscle (Latin-sator, meaning tailor) is the longest muscle in the body, with its origin insertion at the level of the anterior superior iliac spine (ASIS), running obliquely across the upper anterior third of the thigh in an inferomedial direction, with its distal insertion onto the anteromedial proximal tibia [2].

The sartorius muscle assists in flexion, abduction and lateral rotation of the hip [2, 3].

Muscle injuries occur in 31–46% athlete injuries, in comparison with ligament injuries, contusion, haematomas which constitute 18% of all injuries. Most upper thigh injuries include the adductor (23%), hamstring (12–37%) or quadriceps (19%) injuries, with the incidence of injuries increasing over the age of 30 years [4].

*Correspondence: katmandukathryn@gmail.com
Diagnostic Imaging Solutions, Pretoria 0001, South Africa

The pathogenesis of muscle injuries is divided into extrinsic and intrinsic injuries.

Extrinsic injuries include factors such as contusions and penetrating wounds, whereas intrinsic injuries are caused by contraction of elongation of the muscle, leading to destruction of the internal muscle fibre. Extrinsic injuries can involve all type of muscle fibres, whereas intrinsic injuries mainly involve type II muscle fibres which rapidly contract, extended between two joints, contract eccentrically and have a fusiform muscle fibre arrangement.

Intrinsic injuries are categorized into three grades based on the extent of the lesion: grade I involves a few muscle fibres within a bundle; grade 2 involves up to ¾ of the affected muscle portion; and grade 3 involves more than ¾, and the lesion may then involve the entire muscle belly [5].

The role of US is to assess the longitudinal extent of the lesion, calculate the volume of the haematoma and detect possible compression of surrounding anatomical structures [5].

Ultrasound examination of acute muscle injuries should be preceded by accurate reporting of the medical history, mechanism of injury as well as any other symptoms.

High-frequency ultrasound is an excellent method to assess both acute and chronic type muscle injuries. Sonographic assessment in real time along with correlation of clinical findings helps with diagnosis of muscle tears and the extent thereof.

Real-time palpation of the point of tenderness during sonographic evaluation enables a complimentary assessment during clinical evaluation. Dynamic evaluation of the muscle groups can also be useful [4].

Case report

A 65-year-old male patient was referred to our department due to a suspected intrinsic muscular injury following extensive forceful traction of a heavy object along a short distance. No previous injury or trauma to the upper thigh was recorded nor any history of extraneous sporting event prior to the incident. He presented with a painful, palpable lump of the proximal third of the anterior upper thigh. Range of motion was limited with flexion, and lateral rotation of the hip. No visible ecchymosis was noted on the skin surface. The patient reported no use of oral anticoagulant therapy as well as no history of previous spontaneous bleeding.

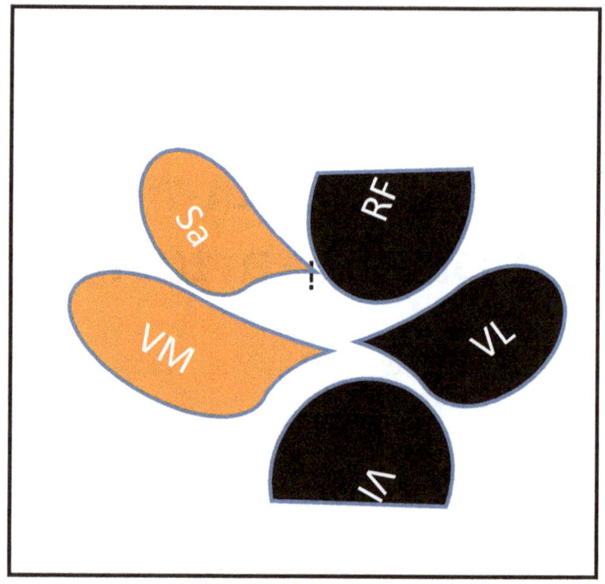

Fig. 1 Schematic drawing of the anterior upper thigh. *Sa* Sartorius muscle, *RF* rectus femoris muscle, *VM* vastus medialis muscle, *VL* vastus lateral muscle, *VI*: vastus intermedius muscle

Ultrasound image evaluation

Ultrasound evaluation was an important tool to differentiate the various upper thigh muscle groups as well as to pinpoint to clinically evident lump on the anterior surface of the thigh. Longitudinal and transverse imaging was initiated from the upper knee joint to assess distal insertion of the quadriceps tendon. Transverse imaging during upward sweep along the thigh surface enabled viewing the vastus lateralis, medialis, intermedius as well as rectus femoris muscle bellies. The full extent of the quadriceps muscle was evaluated to exclude any secondary involvement. The proximal insertion of the quadriceps tendon was also evaluated by ultrasound and was confirmed intact.

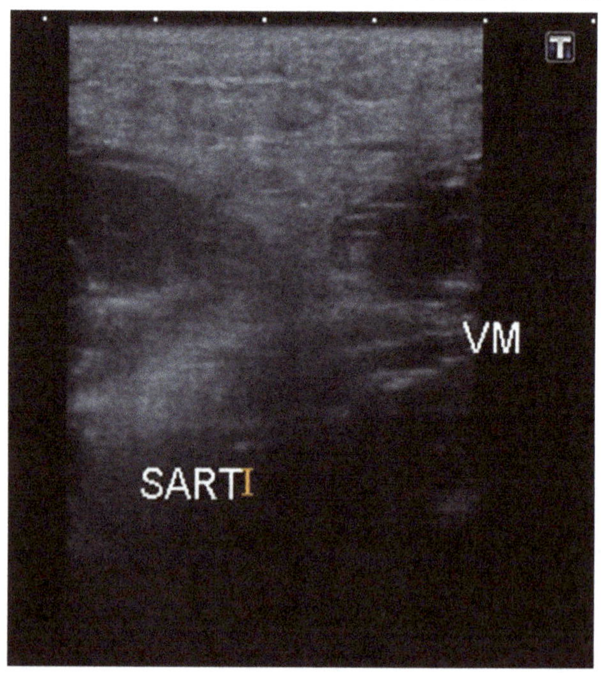

Fig. 2 Transverse ultrasound image of sartorius muscle

The lump on the anterior surface of the thigh was confirmed as medial and superficial to the vastus medialis muscle group, which coincides with the anatomical position of the sartorius muscle along its inferomedial extent towards the medial tibial surface (see Figs. 1, 2).

Increased hyperechoic, oedematous appearance of the sartorius muscle belly coincided with the palpable lump. Central to the oedematous swelling, there was a well-circumscribed hypoechoic fluid collection,

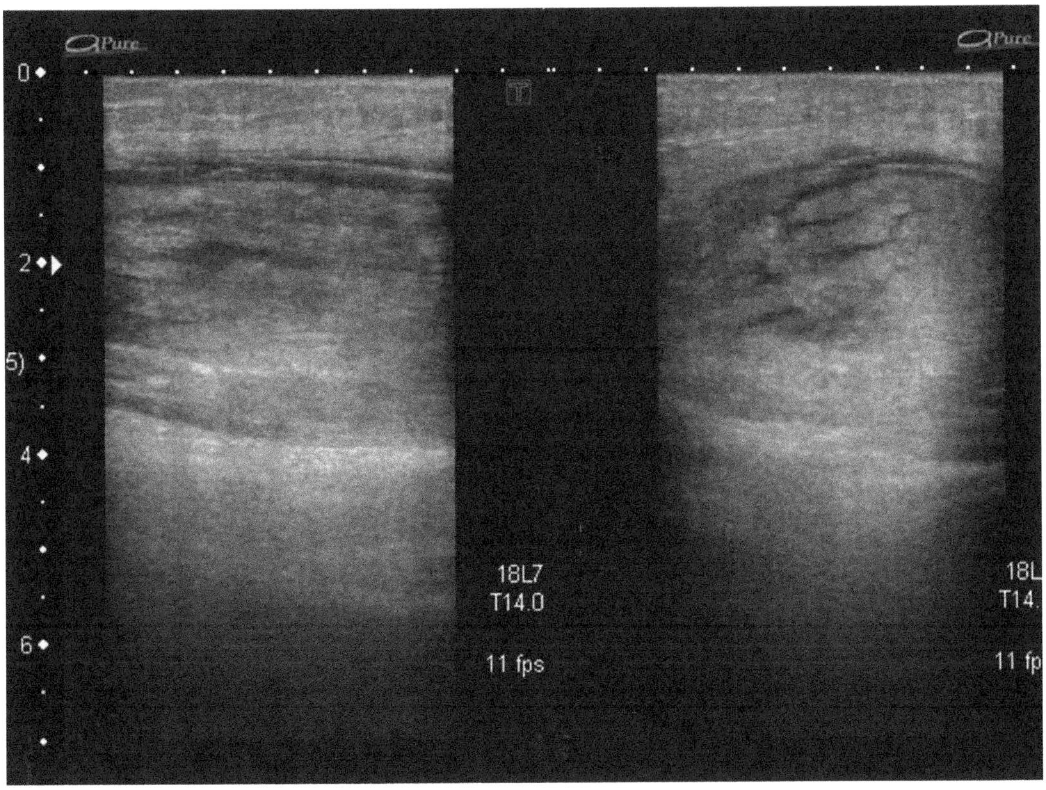

Fig. 3 Hyperechoic, oedematous appearance in the sartorius muscle belly

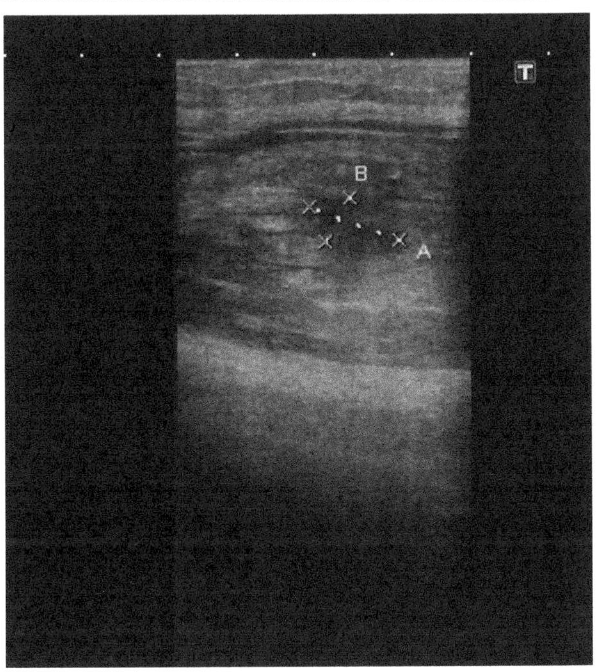

Fig. 4 **a** Hypoechoic gap in the central muscle belly, solid arrow) with haematoma. **b** Schematic drawing of tear (black confirmed on ultrasound as intramuscular tear (Grade II)

which represents loss of typical muscular striations on ultrasound (blurring of the muscle bundles with local hypoechoic blood infiltration). This confirmed an intramuscular tear (grade II). See Figs. 3, 4, 5 and Table 1.

The surrounding hyperechoic oedematous muscle fibres confirmed haemorrhagic infiltration and was confirmed with power Doppler imaging as localized inflammatory reaction. See Fig. 6. It is important during the study of vascularity in muscle injury, to have correctly set parameters. Pulse repetition frequency (PRF) should be set to a maximum of 0.8 MHz, wall filter setting should be low, and the focus should be set on the area of interest to increase sensitivity for the detection of slow blood flow [1].

The extent of the tear was evaluated with longitudinal imaging for accurate measurement.

Comparison with the contralateral leg also aids in the evaluation process due to significant swelling in the acute phase of the affected leg. See Fig. 7.

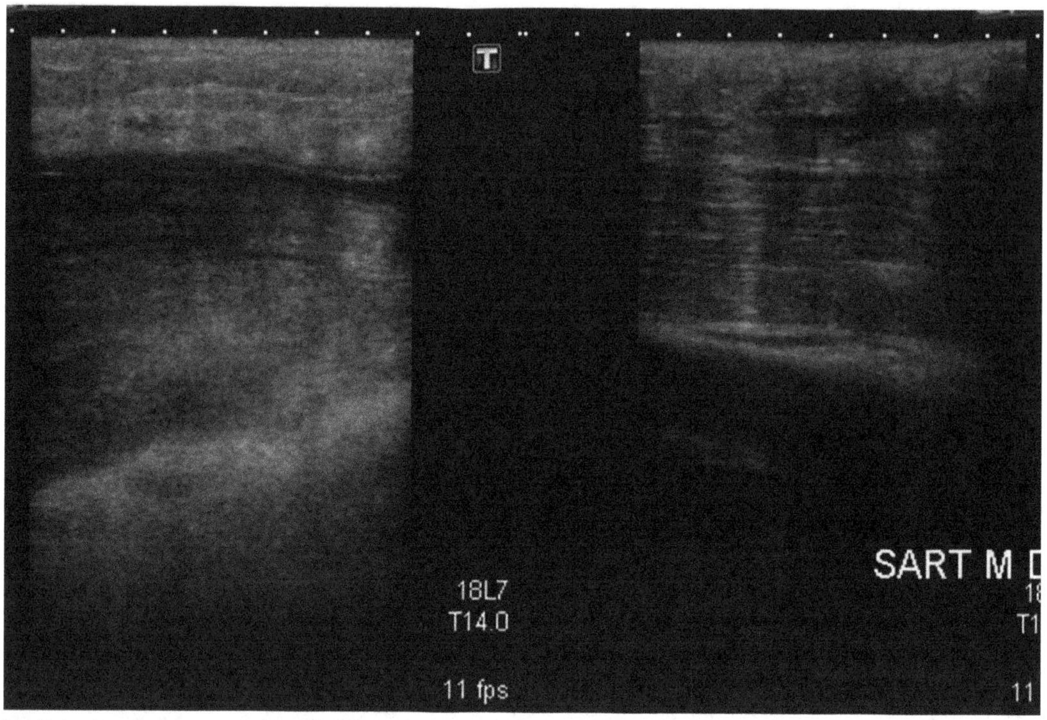

Fig. 5 Loss of typical striated appearance of muscle at site of injury (dashed arrow), more distal to the injury site, the intact sartorius muscle has a typical striated muscular appearance (double arrow)

Table 1 US grading of intrinsic muscle injuries

Grade	US findings
0	No US image suggesting muscle injury
1	Small areas of damaged muscle tissue (< 5%)
2	Partial lesion (> 5–50%), which does not involve the entire muscle
3	Complete rupture of the muscle at the myotendinous junction

Discussion and conclusion

Intramuscular tears of the sartorius muscle in the acute phase are limited in the previous research, more specifically relating to the use of ultrasound as diagnostic tool. It is an uncommon site of injury and is considered as a deficit during the differential diagnosis of acute anterior hip pain [6].

In the elderly population, the use of anticoagulant therapy should be recorded as part of the initial clinical assessment, to determine the cause of any visible bleeding and or ecchymosis on the skin surface, following intrinsic injuries of the thigh.

Ultrasound imaging is essential for correct classification of an injury, assessment of severity and to exclude associated complications. US imaging proves useful in the acute phase as well as in the chronic phase to assess the healing process of muscle injury [1, 5].

The case is considered worthy of reporting to prove the important role of ultrasound in the radiological setting for diagnosis acute intramuscular tears in lieu of MRI imaging.

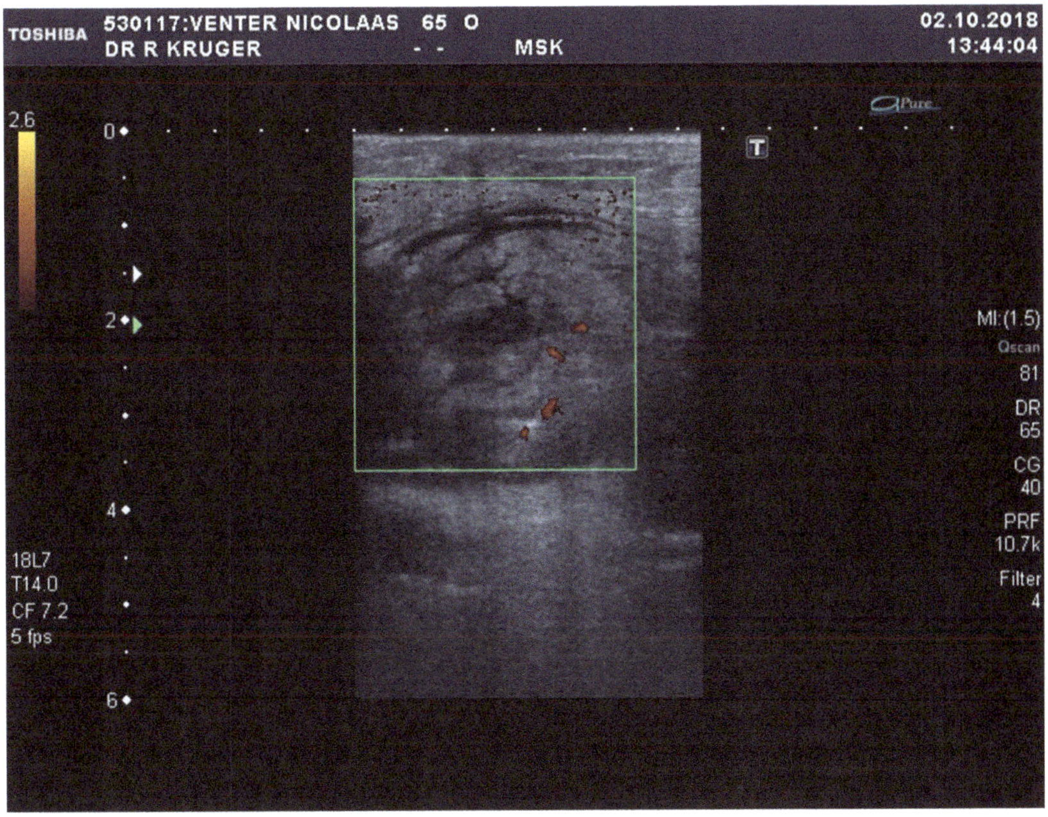

Fig. 6 Increased vascularity noted with Power Doppler imaging

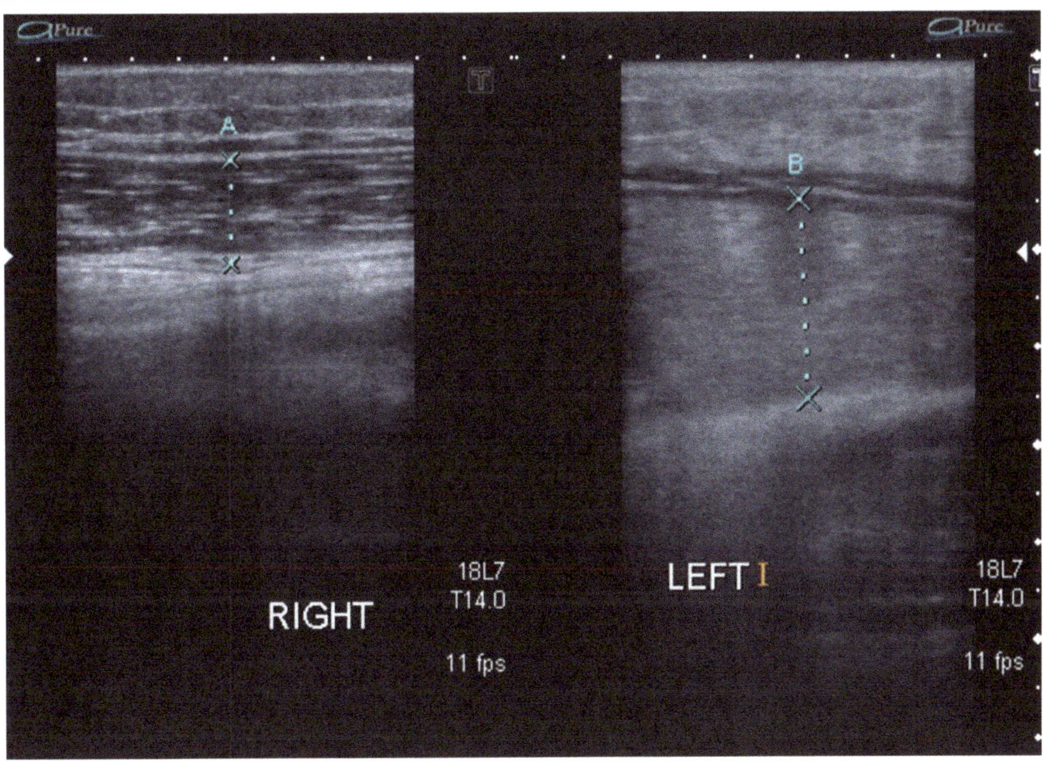

Fig. 7 Comparison to the contralateral right side proves swelling and oedema of the affected leg

Acknowledgements
Dr. E. Thomas (Ph.D. Psych- Stellenbosch University) for academic support and guidance.

Disclaimer
The views expressed in the submitted article are the author's own work and not an official position of the institution or funder.

Author's contributions
The author read and approved the final manuscript.

References

1. Lee JCHJ (2004) Sonography of lower limb muscle injury: pictorial essay. Am J Roentgenol 182:341–351
2. Roscoe M (2016) The notorius sartorius muscle—know your muscle series. SBR Sport. https://www.sbrsport.me/2016/10/13/the-notorius-sartorius-muscle
3. Wang J, Jiao J, Zhao G, Shi JXJ (2018) Case report: a rare case of focal myositis presenting as Sartorius muscle contracture. Medicine (Baltimore). 97(20):1–4
4. Valle X (2010) Clinical practice guide for muscular injuries: epidemiology, diagnosis, treatment and prevention. Br J Sports Med. https://doi.org/10.1136/bjsm.2010.0815.70.29
5. Draghi F, Zacchino M, Canepari M, Nucci PAF (2013) Muscle injuries: ultrasound evaluation in the acute phase. J Ultrasound 16:209–214
6. Kumar B, Sirisena DRM (2013) Proximal sartorius tendon rupture as a cause of traumatic anterior hip pain—a case report of a professional footballer. Br Medial J. 47:10

8

High-frequency ultrasound in clinical dermatology

Jack Levy[1], Devon L. Barrett[1], Nile Harris[1], Jiwoong Jason Jeong[2,3], Xiaofeng Yang[2,4] and Suephy C. Chen[5*]

Abstract

Background: Ultrasound was first introduced in clinical dermatology in 1979. Since that time, ultrasound technology has continued to develop along with its popularity and utility.

Main text summary: Today, high-frequency ultrasound (HFUS), or ultrasound using a frequency of at least 10 megahertz (MHz), allows for high-resolution imaging of the skin from the stratum corneum to the deep fascia. This non-invasive and easy-to-interpret tool allows physicians to assess skin findings in real-time, enabling enhanced diagnostic, management, and surgical capabilities. In this review, we discuss how HFUS fits into the landscape of skin imaging. We provide a brief history of its introduction to dermatology, explain key principles of ultrasonography, and review its use in characterizing normal skin, common neoplasms of the skin, dermatologic diseases and cosmetic dermatology.

Conclusion: As frequency advancements in ultrasonography continue, the broad applications of this imaging modality will continue to grow. HFUS is a fast, safe and readily available tool that can aid in diagnosing, monitoring and treating dermatologic conditions by providing more objective assessment measures.

Keywords: High-frequency ultrasound, Dermatology, Diagnostic imaging, Ultrasonography

Introduction

Dermatology is among the rare specialties of medicine in which the organ of interest can be readily examined and biopsied. As a consequence, histology has become the gold standard for many dermatologic diagnoses. It has also allowed for clinicopathologic correlation to guide therapeutics and advance prognostics [1]. In the last few decades, a number of imaging modalities have been introduced to augment clinical exam or obviate the need for histology [2]. Some examples include total body digital photography (TBDP), dermoscopy, reflectance confocal microscopy (RCM), optical coherence tomography (OCT), and ultrasound. In this review, we discuss how ultrasound fits into the landscape of skin imaging. We provide a brief history of its introduction to dermatology, explain key principles of ultrasonography, and review its use in characterizing normal skin, common neoplasms of the skin, dermatologic diseases and cosmetic dermatology.

History of ultrasound in medicine

Sonography dates back to the late 1700s when two Italian zoologists discovered the acoustic orientation sense of bats [3]. Nearly a century later, the Curie brothers presented the piezoelectric effect of sound waves on natural quartz [4]. It was their observation that a force applied to the crystal produced an electric discharge. Conversely, an alternating electric current applied to a crystal produces vibrations that generate high-frequency sound waves called ultrasound [4, 5]. Over a half-century later, the technique was adapted by both the American military as SONAR and by an American Neurologist, Karl Dussik, who used ultrasound to detect brain tumors in patients [5].

*Correspondence: suephy.chen@duke.edu
[5] Department of Dermatology, Duke University School of Medicine, Duke Clinic, 40 Duke Medicine Cir, Clinic 3K, Durham, NC 27710-4000, USA
Full list of author information is available at the end of the article

Ultrasound emerged in the practice of dermatology around 1980 when two independent groups used the technique to measure skin thickness in normal and diseased skin [6]. Since then, the practice has gained popularity in several European and South American countries that incorporate its use in resident training and where its application is reimbursable [7, 8]. As the technology has improved, so has its utility. In an early study of over 4300 skin lesions, Wortsman et al. demonstrated the ability of higher frequency ultrasound (7–15 MHz) to significantly improve diagnostic accuracy. Compared to clinical examination alone, ultrasound corrected the referring diagnosis in 17% of cases and detected 3 missed malignancies [9]. The application of ultrasound in dermatology is continuously evolving and increasingly studied [10, 11].

Ultrasound technology and how it works

Ultrasound allows for high-resolution imaging of the skin from the stratum corneum down to the deep fascia [12]. Newer ultrasound technologies, including high-frequency ultrasound (HFUS, between 20 and 30 MHz) and ultra high-frequency ultrasound (UHFUS, > 30 MHz), have further enhanced imaging clarity and expanded upon the myriad applications for use of ultrasound in dermatology [11, 13, 14]. With fast acquisition times, ultrasound images are produced in real-time, allowing for physical adjustments and optimal imaging. Many devices include color Doppler analysis for characterization of blood flow and vessel morphology. It is readily available and can be easily incorporated into clinical practice [10, 11, 15].

The main component of the ultrasound device is the transducer—typically a handheld device containing thousands of piezoelectric crystals. These crystals, when stimulated by an electric voltage, generate millions of acoustic waves that pass through tissue and are reflected back to the transducer. As the waves return to the transducer, they are converted back into electrical energy interpreted by a computer. The computer then generates a one-dimensional line graph in amplitude mode (A-mode) that can be used to interpret echogenicity at various distances from the probe. In brightness mode (B-mode) an image is generated with different intensities of brightness.

These varying intensities are dependent upon the ultrasound waves' ability to pass through the tissue. Bright or hyperechoic regions represent an abrupt increase in tissue density while dark or hypoechoic areas represent a decrease or no change in tissue density. A black anechoic region represents an area of tissue from which virtually no waves are reflected [5]. Although dense structures reflect a greater number of waves, resulting in a hyperechoic ultrasonographic structures, they may also generate an artifactual acoustic shadow due to attenuation of the ultrasound waves at the interface between two tissues of varying densities [13]. Another common artifact, acoustic enhancement, can appear as a result of relatively unimpeded passage of ultrasound waves through a preceding area of low acoustic impedance. This results in the appearance of a brighter structure deep to the area of low impedance [16, 17].

The resolution and penetration of an ultrasound image depends on the frequency of the acoustic waves produced. Traditional lower-frequency ultrasound devices are ideal for evaluation of internal organs like the liver and lungs due to their penetration ability. HFUS and UHFUS waves, on the other hand, are unable to travel easily through tissue, but provide higher-resolution, superficial detail. This makes HFUS and UHFUS ideal for visualizing a superficial organ like the skin [5, 10, 11, 15, 18, 19]. Given the diverse range of probe frequencies and the variation of dermal thickness in different regions of the body, specific frequencies should be considered for optimal visualization of lesions in various anatomic locations [15].

Normal skin

One of the first dermatologic applications of ultrasound measured the thickness of healthy skin [20]. While this original study used a 15-MHz transducer (and not meeting current standards for HFUS), the study was among the first to highlight the benefit of higher frequencies. Subsequent research has demonstrated that the three layers of the skin have distinct echogenicity, or corresponding levels of brightness (Fig. 1) [21]. The epidermis is mainly composed of keratin, a dense, fibrous structural protein that strongly reflects ultrasound waves; therefore, the epidermis is hyperechoic. The dermis is also hyperechoic, though to a lesser extent than the epidermis, due to its high content of collagen. Finally, the subcutis is hypoechoic due to the presence of fat lobules that allow for the unimpeded passage of ultrasound waves [2, 21].

The dermis can be further distinguished on ultrasound based on the arrangement of collagen and elastin bundles; the upper 20% of the hyperechoic dermis corresponds to the papillary dermis and contains irregularly arranged, thinner collagen and elastin bundles. The lower 80% of the dermis is made up of more regularly arranged collagen and elastin. Correspondingly, ultrasound at frequencies > 10 MHz demonstrates a reticular dermis with hyperechoic strands of thicker collagen bundles interposed with hypoechoic extracellular matrix [2, 5, 22].

An important consideration when using ultrasound to study healthy skin is persistence of a well-defined high-amplitude echo between the ultrasound gel and the corneal layer of the epidermis. This has been attributed to the impedance jump of the ultrasound waves from the

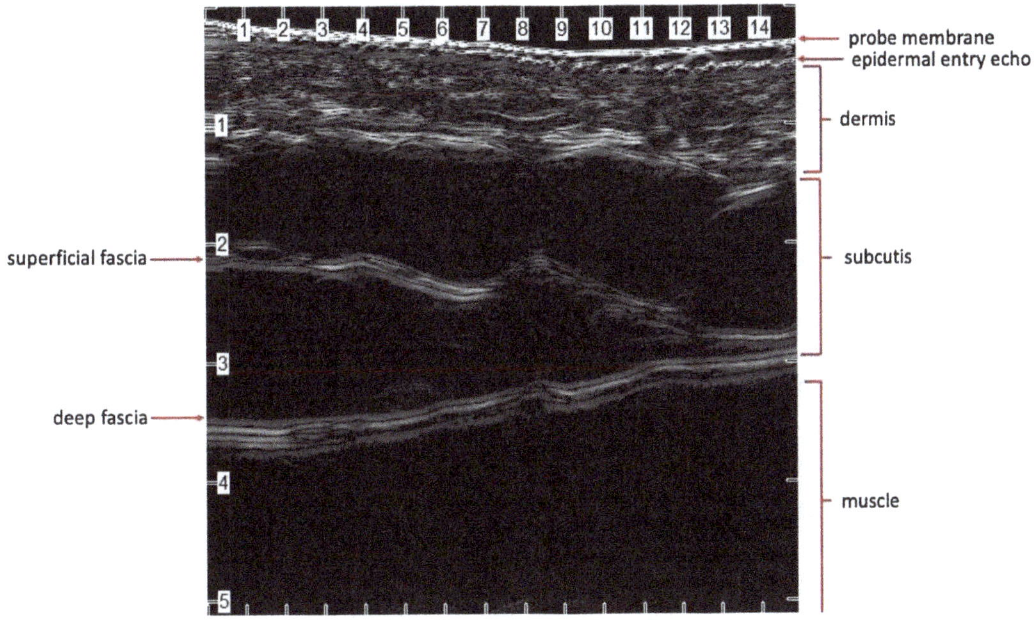

Fig. 1 Normal skin from the anterior arm using a 50-MHz HFUS probe (Longport, Inc. EPISCAN). Note the fine hyperechoic epidermal entry echo. Deep to the entry echo is the hyperechoic dermis measuring about 1 millimeter (mm) with thicker horizontal bands in the deep dermis corresponding to the organized, horizontally arrayed collagen bundles in the reticular dermis. Deep to the dermis is the subcutis composed primarily of hypoechoic fat globules. Within this layer is the hyperechoic superficial fascia. Deep to the subcutis is the hyperechoic deep fascia overlying the biceps muscle

ultrasound gel to the callused epidermal cells [2]. This reflection is thus referred to as the epidermal entry echo. Thus, the epidermal entry echo is not a direct visualization of the epidermis per se, but an artifact representing the epidermis [23].

Ultrasound studies examining healthy skin have demonstrated that while skin thickness is inversely proportional to age, echogenicity tends to increase with age corresponding to increase collagen production [24–28]. One notable exception is sun-damaged skin, as first described in 1988 by Querleux et al., where there is presence of a subepidermal low-echogenic band (SLEB). The SLEB was described as a dark band subjacent to the epidermal entry echo [29]. Though not specific to sun damage, its presence in more than 50% of adults over the age of 40 and its prominence in highly sun-exposed areas like the face and dorsal forearms have been correlated to solar elastosis, a histologic marker of cutaneous sun damage [25]. Similar findings have been recently demonstrated in patients treated with radiotherapy for head and neck cancers [30].

Glabrous skin, hair follicles, and the scalp

Compared to non-glabrous skin, glabrous epidermis appears as a bright bilaminar structure when visualized by ultrasound (Fig. 2). The bilaminar structure is thought to be caused by sound waves first entering the thick, compact stratum corneum before entering the normally hyperechoic epidermis itself [9]. This bilaminar appearance can be difficult to visualize at lower frequencies in which the stratum corneum is poorly resolved from the entry echo, but is discernable in UHFUS ranges [31]. Understanding the structure and characteristics of normal glabrous skin has allowed for differentiation between abnormalities in glabrous skin in conditions like Pachyonychia Congenita and other palmoplantar keratodermas [32–34].

At other anatomic sites, hair follicles appear as oblique hypoechoic bands on ultrasound imaging. Multiple studies have demonstrated ultrasound can be used to estimate the phase of hair follicle growth, identify inflammation of hair follicles, and assess hair density [18, 35, 36]. Hair follicle growth phase is estimated based on band termination relative to the subcutis with anagen phase hairs terminating in the deeper dermis and telogen phase hairs terminating more superficially. An inflamed hair follicle will appear thicker and darker relative to a normal hair follicle. A number of studies have suggested that the ultrasonographic findings of an inflamed hair follicle may improve diagnostics by identifying early signs of adnexal pathologies like hidradenitis suppurativa [35, 37, 38].

In addition to identifying changes in hair follicle appearance, ultrasound has also been used to characterize scalp cysts; cysts typically appear as round and dark

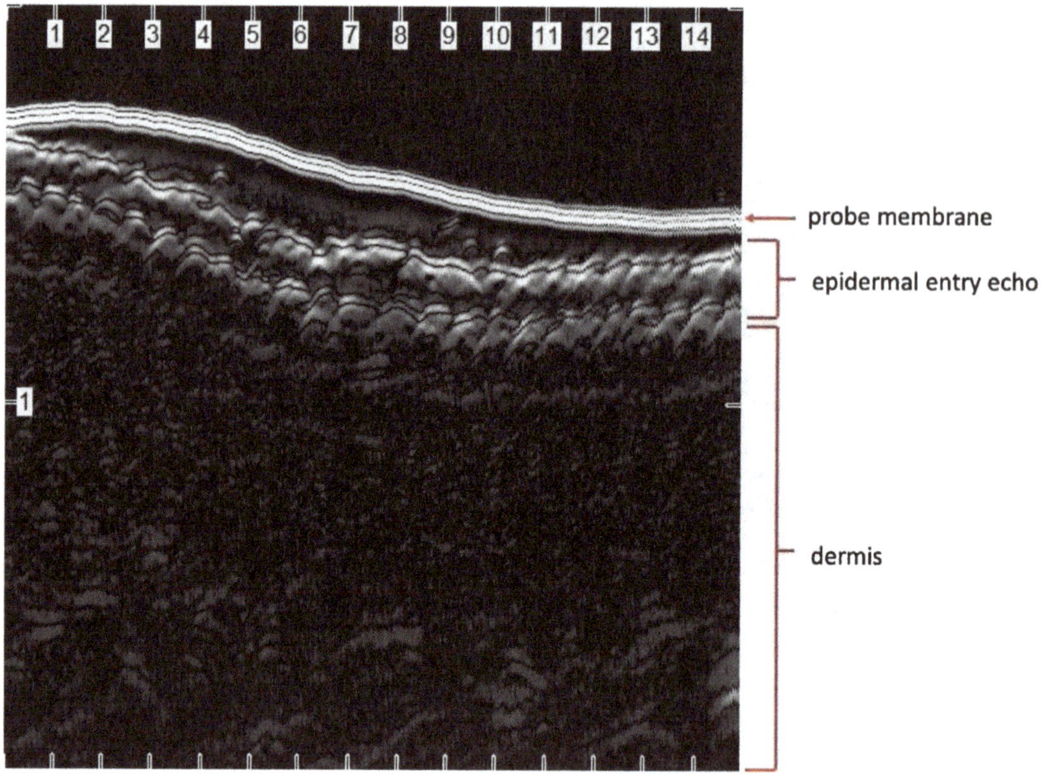

Fig. 2 Glabrous skin from the palm using a 50-MHz HFUS probe (Longport, Inc. EPISCAN). Note the bilaminar hyperechoic entry echo due to the thickened stratum corneum in this anatomic location

structures. Trichilemmal cysts characteristically contain hyperechoic areas within their round, dermal anechoic structures, corresponding to the dense keratinous and oily inner-cystic debris [35]. Pilomatricomas appear targetoid with a solid hyperechoic nodule thought to correspond to cystic calcifications or giant cells surrounded by a hypoechoic rim [35].

The nail

The dorsal and ventral plates of the nail are visible as separate entities on ultrasound, generating the second instance of a hyperechoic bilaminar linear structure (Fig. 3). The matrix of the nail is hypoechoic and ventral to the hyperechoic proximal nail fold. The nail bed is normally hypoechoic and just deep to the hyperechoic ventral nail plate. Finally, the surface of the distal phalanx appears as a hyperechoic linear structure [5, 22, 39].

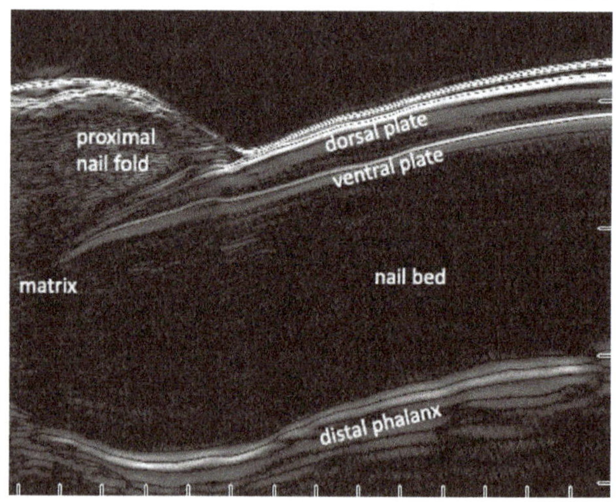

Fig. 3 Longitudinal view of a normal nail using a 50-MHz HFUS probe (Longport, Inc. EPISCAN). Note the bilaminar appearance of the nail plate consisting of the hyperechoic dorsal and ventral nail plates separated by a hypoechoic band. The top-most hyperechoic horizontal line represents the probe membrane

Ultrasonography in neoplastic disease

Nonmelanoma skin cancers

The main dermatologic use of ultrasound is in the pre-operative assessment of non-melanoma and melanoma skin cancers [40, 41] and detection of early neoplasms [42]. In general, cutaneous neoplasms appear sonographically as hypoechoic lesions in a relatively hyperechoic epidermis and/or dermis [43]. The most prevalent human malignancy, BCC, has several histologic subtypes including superficial, nodular, micronodular and morpheaform [44]. The most common BCC histologic subtype—nodular—sonographically appears as a hypoechoic lesion with well-defined borders and is usually found in the dermis, though occasionally can extend deeper into the subcutis (Fig. 4) [42, 45]. Some histologic subtypes of BCC that have demonstrated more aggressive biologic behavior have been shown to feature small hyperechoic dots seen within the hypoechoic tumor. Such spots are referred to as "flower cotton" spots [13, 46]. Though the cause of this artifactual finding is unknown, flower cotton spots are thought to correlate with clusters of apoptotic neoplastic cells within the tumor [13, 46]. Risk of aggressive BCC phenotype, such as micronodular or morpheaform, and risk of recurrence have been correlated to increasing numbers of flower cotton spots [47]. Furthermore, the presence of flower cotton spots is important in differentiating a BCC from melanoma as melanoma lacks these hyperechoic inclusions [48, 49].

The clinical relevance of ultrasound in the examination of suspected SCC is less well defined. Ultrasound has been used to identify SCCs, which also appear as hypoechoic lesions [42, 50]. However, in 2010 Wortsman et al. analyzed 75 non-melanoma skin cancers of which 18 were cutaneous SCCs. She demonstrated a modest but significant increase in diagnostic accuracy with the addition of higher frequencies of ultrasound [9]. An additional study demonstrated the accuracy of SCC measurement with HFUS by comparing SCC depth to histometry, noting a correlation to the 100th of a millimeter [51]. Despite this correlation, ultrasonographic examination of SCCs can be limited by the presence of an acoustic shadow artifact due to the reflection of ultrasound waves by thickened, hyperkeratotic stratum corneum, which may obscure lesion boundaries [48, 52]. Therefore, ultrasound has suggested use as a complementary tool to support the pre-operative evaluation of SCC but not as the sole method of diagnosis [50].

An additional form of non-melanoma skin cancer studied with HFUS is mycosis fungoides (MF) [53, 54]. MF is characterized by presence of a SLEB, which researchers have noticed can be helpful for identifying response to therapy and disease remission; in two separate studies of patients with MF, thinning or complete disappearance of the SLEB corresponded with disease severity and completion of therapy, supporting the utility of HFUS as an objective tool in routine clinical practice [53, 55].

Melanoma

In the study of melanoma, ultrasound demonstrates a homogenous hypoechoic lesion. The shape of the lesion often correlates to the histologic subtype of the melanoma. For example, nodular melanoma will typically present with a spherical hypoechoic lesion, while a superficial spreading melanoma will present with a thinner, lenticular, hypoechoic lesion subjacent to the epidermal entry echo [13]. Although no distinct ultrasonographic features of melanoma have been described, one important strength of ultrasound is its ability to predict Breslow thickness of a melanoma [48, 56]. This correlation with histologic thickness, the current gold standard on which melanoma staging and surgical planning rests, is predicted to be over 92% [57]. When compared to other techniques like OCT, ultrasound has superior correlation with histology, repeatability and inter-rater reliability [58]. Where OCT tends to underestimate Breslow

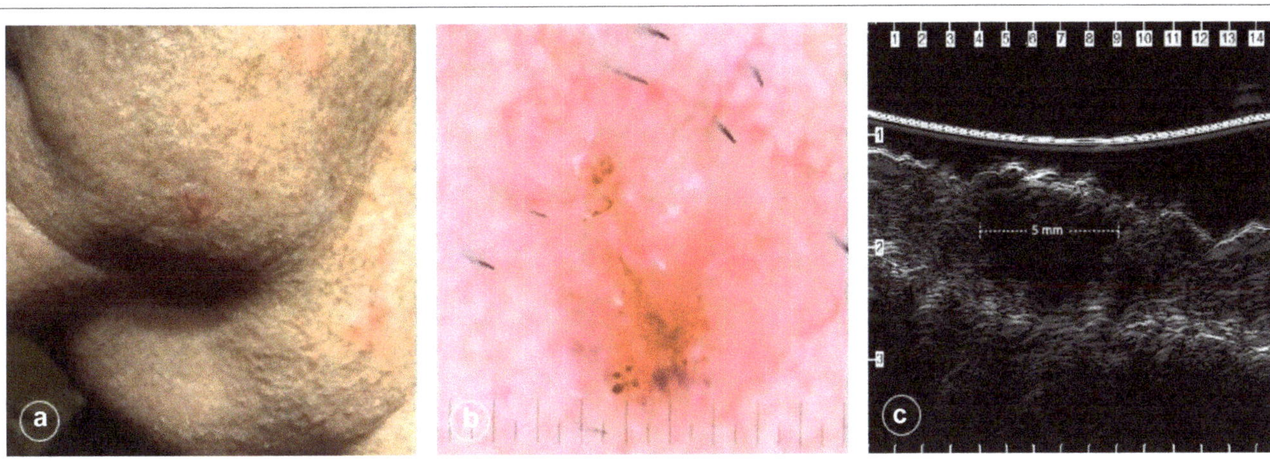

Fig. 4 Nodular basal cell carcinoma measuring 5 mm by 7 mm on the left lower cheek of a 66-year-old man. Note the pearly borders and central ulceration in the gross photograph (**a**), the polymorphous vessels and ulceration in the dermatoscopic photo (**b**), and the 5 mm hypoechoic lesion in the superficial dermis across the short axis of this biopsy-supported nodular basal cell carcinoma using a 50-MHz UHFUS probe (Longport, Inc. EPISCAN)

thickness, ultrasound has been shown to modestly overestimate tumor thickness [58]. The cause of this overestimation is thought to result from the technology's inability to distinguish an inflammatory infiltrate from melanocytic proliferation and neovascularization. Another contributing factor may be the desiccation of tissue as it is processed for histologic review. Nevertheless, its ability to resolve well beyond the dermis renders HFUS superior to other imaging modalities in predicting Breslow thickness [59].

Though melanomas have been distinguished from benign melanocytic proliferations with specificities as low as 30%, the addition of color Doppler sharply improves ultrasound as a diagnostic tool [43]. Melanomas have been shown to demonstrate more dense vascularization than benign nevi and exhibit low-flow arterioles. In another study of pigmented lesions, the direction of intralesional blood flow demonstrated a 100% specificity in distinguishing melanoma from nonmelanoma tumors [46, 60].

Single-center experience with 50-MHz ultrasound device

In a single-center experience with a 50-MHz device, the Longport, Inc. EPISCAN, the authors examined ultra-high-frequency ultrasound biomicrographs of nearly 70 cutaneous lesions as well as normal skin and adnexae. Transducer power gain and time-gain compensation (TGC) were set to the device's default settings—100% and 10%, respectively, with a TGC start of 0%. Skin position, or distance between transducer and impermeable membrane barrier, or skin, was 7.5 mm. Scanning depth ranged from 3.8 mm to 15.0 mm, with a scan length of 15 mm at a rate of 1 scan per frame per second. A standard acquisition protocol was followed. The protocol included a horizontal (cranial–caudal) scan and perpendicular scan in the center of each lesion or anatomical area with and without pressure. Then, 3D-views were simulated using two sweeps in both planes over 3–8 s for a total of three to eight 2D-slices in each plane.

Normal skin of the non-sun exposed medial upper arm of a middle-aged man demonstrated a hyperechoic epidermal entry echo and hyperechoic dermis with horizontally arrayed collagen bundles of the reticular dermis. These superficial structures are followed by the hypoechoic subcutis transected by a hyperechoic band of superficial fascia and the hypoechoic biceps muscle invested by the hyperechoic deep fascia (Fig. 1). The thickened stratum corneum over the thenar eminence demonstrated a hyperechoic bilaminar entry echo (Fig. 2). Ultrasound of a first digit nail also demonstrated a bilaminar appearance with hyperechoic dorsal and ventral plates separated by a hypoechoic band (Fig. 3). Finally, a basal cell carcinoma on the medial mandibular cheek of an elderly man demonstrated a hypoechoic lesion in the superficial dermis with subtle posterior acoustic enhancement (Fig. 4).

Inflammatory skin diseases

Sclerosing disorders

One of the earliest dermatologic applications of ultrasound was in scleroderma [61]. Due to the pathological increase in collagen deposition, ultrasound can help differentiate between the inflammatory and sclerotic phases of the disease [62]. In the inflammatory phase there is a reduction in echogenicity of the skin and dermal thickening, whereas in the sclerotic phase there is increased echogenicity and thickening [63]. Finally, ultrasonographic features of sclerodermatous skin in the atrophic phase demonstrates thinning of the dermis with an echogenicity similar to unaffected surrounding skin [64].

The modified Rodnan score is used to measure skin hardening. Skin lesions are scored on a 4-point scale from 0 to 3. This score is applied to 17 discrete areas of the body after evaluation by a clinician. A study found that 18-MHz ultrasound is more sensitive than clinical assessment in measuring skin hardening, with results of ultrasound providing the additional benefits of being quantitative, valid, and reproducible [65].

In a study of 16 patients with morphea and four with extragenital lichen sclerosis, the results of HFUS demonstrated unique features of extragenital lichen sclerosis characterized by widened, polycyclic, hyperechoic and disorganized epidermal entry echo relative to that seen in morphea [62]. Another study using UHFUS to measure response to treatment demonstrated a statistically significant decrease in dermal thickness and density after treatment with ultraviolet A1 phototherapy [66].

Psoriasis

Currently, evaluation of psoriasis in a clinical setting includes the use of the Psoriasis Epidemiology Screening Tool, a validated screening tool designed to identify patients who should be referred to a rheumatologist for possible co-existing psoriatic arthritis. Rheumatologists, on the other hand, use the Classification Criteria for Psoriatic Arthritis (CASPAR) to characterize psoriatic arthritis disease burden.

A 2015 study used ultrasound (6–18 MHz) to determine the prevalence of enthesitis, a feature in the pathogenesis of psoriatic arthritis, among psoriasis patients with and without psoriatic arthritis as defined by CASPAR criteria [67]. The study found at least one ultrasonographic sign of enthesitis in approximately half the patients with psoriatic arthritis, but also in almost half of the psoriasis patients without a diagnosis of psoriatic arthritis [67]. Furthermore, after these patients were treated for 6 months with systemic therapy, ultrasonographic features of enthesitis in both of these groups improved, suggesting subclinical joint involvement and underdiagnosis of psoriatic arthritis among psoriasis patients [67].

In a 2013 study, researchers found that 78% of patients with psoriasis had at least one nail abnormality identified by ultrasound: loss of ultrasonographic architecture, pitting, or both [68]. This study suggested that OCT was better than ultrasound at 9–14 MHz for identifying features of psoriatic nails, but both were more sensitive than clinical examination alone [68]. In a later study utilizing a UHFUS 40-MHz probe, researchers identified ventral nail plate deposits, irregular or fused nail plates, and significantly thicker nail plates in patients with psoriasis compared to controls, with Doppler-ultrasound noting increased nail blood flow and increased vascular resistance [69].

Finally, a recent study using 20-MHz HFUS to compare two treatment arms reliably demonstrated a reduction in the SLEB of psoriatic skin coinciding with clinical improvement, supporting the use of ultrasonography as a useful objective marker in patients with psoriasis [70].

Hidradenitis suppurativa

Hidradenitis suppurativa (HS) is an inflammatory disease that affects between 0.05 and 4.1% of the population [71–73]. This disease results in chronic inflammation of the hair follicle and presents with painful, erythematous nodules that often rupture, forming draining sinus tracts that eventually scar. Current HS staging tools include Hurley staging, HS severity index, HS physician global assessment and sonographic scoring of HS [74, 75]. Hurley staging is generally the most commonly used method for assessment of HS severity, but lacks the ability to effectively measure disease fluctuation and response to treatment [74].

A number of studies have demonstrated that these various staging tools underestimate the true disease severity in comparison to ultrasound-assisted staging of HS [76–79]. Ultrasound has allowed for understanding of a proposed sequence of skin changes in HS pathology with the earliest sign of follicular widening eventuating in the formation of fistulous tracts and increased vascularity over acutely inflamed lesions [78]. A meaningful association between the ultrasonographically measured diameter of an HS nodule and the patient's subjective assessment of the nodule's tenderness and the clinician's assessment of erythema have also been established [80].

Finally, ultrasound can aid in medical and surgical management of HS. One study noted a modification in the management of 82% of cases following ultrasonographic evaluation with a 24% transition from medical to surgical management [78].

Atopic dermatitis

Atopic dermatitis (AD) is a chronic inflammatory skin condition characterized by intense pruritis and abnormal skin barrier function [81]. Currently, there is a lack of standardization of core outcome measurement tools for this disease. The Harmonising Outcome Measures in Eczema initiative recommends the use of the Eczema Area and Severity Index and the Scoring Atopic Dermatitis in assessing physician-reported signs of AD, noting the utility of the latter in clinical trials [82, 83]. But these disease severity tools are subjective, cumbersome and have demonstrated poor reproducibility [84, 85].

A number of studies have attempted to better understand the severity of AD through the use of ultrasound. In particular, these studies have sought to measure the thickness of the SLEB and skin echogenicity in order to quantify disease burden. Unlike in sun damaged skin, in AD, the SLEB appears to be the result of edema and inflammatory cell infiltrate in sites of active inflammation [13]. In one 2019 study, the mean thickness of the hypoechoic band was found to be higher in lesional skin but present in both lesional and non-lesional skin of individuals with AD [81]. A separate study compared SLEB thickness in patients with AD as visualized by 20-MHz ultrasound to their EASI score and histopathological findings from 5 mm punch biopsies. The study found SLEB thickness correlated with the histologic degree of epidermal hyperkeratosis, parakeratosis, spongiosis, and intensity of inflammatory infiltrates as well as the provider-assessed EASI scores [84]. Finally, two studies using HFUS and UHFUS to examine the effect of phototherapy and tacrolimus on SLEB thickness found statistically significant reductions in mean SLEB thickness [86, 87].

Granulomatous diseases

Sarcoidosis is characterized by the formation of granulomas in a number of different organs and is associated with cutaneous induration and erythema. A pilot study in 2017 evaluated the utility of UHFUS in objectively quantifying granuloma burden in cutaneous sarcoidosis in comparison to the Cutaneous Sarcoidosis Activity and Morphology Instrument (CSAMI) and histopathological evaluation [88]. The study found a strong correlation between the mean brightness of UHFUS and the lesion CSAMI score, as well as the percent of the dermis with granulomas on histopathology; ultimately, these results highlighted the utility of ultrasound in quantifying disease burden in patients with cutaneous sarcoidosis [88].

Another granulomatous disease, idiopathic facial aseptic granuloma (IFAG), is a self-limiting pediatric disease; as such, it does not require aggressive treatment [16]. On ultrasound, IFAG can appear as a poorly defined oval shaped hypoechogenic lesion in the dermis surrounded by areas of hyperechogenicity and hypervascularization due to inflammation. Ultrasound can therefore be utilized to differentiate IFAG from its differential diagnoses that might require further management. For example, a facial abscess may exhibit a characteristic "squish sign" with ultrasound and would require incision and drainage with antimicrobial therapy [89]. Further differentiating factors include lack of calcium deposits, differentiating it from a pilomatricoma, lack of defined borders, as seen in epidermal cysts, and lack of vascularity, as seen in vascular tumors [16]. The use of ultrasound to properly diagnose, manage and monitor disease progression in IFAG is therefore important and provides a non-invasive alternative to biopsy [16].

Vascular lesions

A number of vascular lesions have been studied using ultrasound, including Port-wine stains (PWS), arteriovenous (AV) malformations and spider nevi. The first study to successfully examine PWS using ultrasound was conducted in 2018 [90]. This retrospective study utilized both 10-MHz and 22-MHz transducers with and without Doppler to assess lesional depth, echogenicity, vessel density and AV flow signals. The results of this study demonstrated a clear contrast between lesional and normal skin [90]. Furthermore, the study demonstrated ultrasound could help differentiate a PWS from other vascular anomalies due to their hypoechoic, poorly vascularized appearance with venous flow, while other capillary-arteriovenous malformations appear hyperechoic and well-vascularized with mixed arterial and venous blood flow [90].

Another type of vascular lesion known as a Spider nevus has also been characterized using ultrasound [91]. Spider nevi were historically classified as low-flow capillary malformations [92]; however, a 2017 study by Alegre-Sanchez et al. found that spider nevi demonstrated pulsatile flow on dermoscopy and ultrasound. This finding was subsequently supported by the presence of high-flow arterial-type waveform as seen on Doppler-ultrasound, suggesting that spider nevi are more similar to arteriovenous malformations, or high-flow vascular lesions [91].

Ultrasound can also be used to guide and assess response to treatment [48]. For example, researchers have used its Doppler capabilities to correctly identify venous structures and aid in guiding injectable foam sclerotherapy for the treatment of venous leg ulcers, demonstrating good healing rate and a low reflux ratio [93].

Cosmetic applications

Several cosmetic applications of ultrasound have been established. For example, botulinum toxin injections demonstrate increase subcutaneous echogenicity leading to a blurring of the normally discrete boundaries between the subcutis and underlying muscle [94]. Similarly, fillers can be visualized using ultrasound to determine locations of prior injections—an important application since a small but significant proportion of patients seeking injectable fillers fail to report prior procedures. The risk of granulomas and filler dermopathies associated with injections of multiple filler materials has been established [95–97].

The efficacy of topical vitamin C therapy in increasing collagen production, reducing ultraviolet radiation induced oxidative stress and enhancing dermal remodeling has been demonstrated in several studies [98, 99]. One notable study using HFUS evaluated the skin of patients throughout a 60-day period of topical vitamin C therapy, demonstrating increased echogenicity in both the epidermis and dermis after 40 days and to a greater extent after 60 days [98]. Ultrasound at 15-MHz and 20-MHz has also been used to evaluate the efficacy of an oral micronutrient supplement on preservation of skin quality through the measurement of skin thickness and density [99, 100].

Conclusion

While ultrasound has been used in dermatology for more than 40 years, its uses have continued to evolve with improvements in technology. Today, there are a few dermatologic lesions with pathognomonic sonographic features. One example is the "jellyfish" sign described in some cases of dermatofibrosarcoma protuberans [101]. Other examples include the "saw-tooth" pattern of cellulite [102–104]. Pathognomonic ultrasonographic features are likely to increase with integration of higher frequency ultrasound devices in clinical practice; for future work with HFUS, a core international task force group formed by 15 physicians from 11 countries called the DERMUS (dermatologic ultrasound) group recommends dermatologists use Doppler-capable ultrasound devices with a frequency of at least 15- to 22-MHz in all ultrasound examinations of the skin [18].

While there is support for use of ultrasound in future dermatological practice, there are a number of limitations associated with the use of this tool. One major limitation is the skill of the operator. Consequently, the DERMUS group suggests utilizing ultrasound at least 300 times per year to achieve minimum competency. Similarly, it is strongly advised that the dermatologist functions as the sonographer because of the years of training in dermatologic pathologies and ability to correlate histology with clinical presentation of cutaneous lesions [18].

As frequency advancements in ultrasonography continue, the broad applications of this imaging modality will continue to grow. Ultrasound is a fast, safe and readily available tool that can aid in diagnosing, monitoring and treating dermatologic conditions by providing more objective assessment measures.

Abbreviations

HFUS: High-frequency ultrasound; MHz: Megahertz; TBDP: Total body digital photography; RCM: Reflectance confocal microscopy; OCT: Optical coherence tomography; µm: Micrometers; BCC: Basal cell carcinoma; SCC: Squamous cell carcinoma; SLEB: Subepidermal low-echogenic band; MF: Mycosis fungoides; CASPAR: Classification criteria for psoriatic arthritis; HS: Hidradenitis suppurativa; AD: Atopic dermatitis; CSAMI: Cutaneous Sarcoidosis Activity and Morphology Instrument; IFAG: Idiopathic facial aseptic granuloma; PWS: Port-wine stain; AV: Arteriovenous.

Acknowledgements

Not applicable.

Authors' contributions

JL and SCC had the concept for the review article and performed the majority of the literature search, with assistance from DLB and NH. JJJ and XY contributed to the imaging and planing of the work that led to this manuscript. DLB, NH, JL and SCC drafted the article, with all authors critically revising the work. All authors read and approved the final manuscript.

Author details

[1] Department of Dermatology, Emory University School of Medicine, Atlanta, GA, USA. [2] Department of Radiation Oncology, Emory University School of Medicine, Atlanta, GA, USA. [3] Department of Biomedical Informatics, Emory University, Atlanta, GA, USA. [4] Winship Cancer Institute, Emory University, Atlanta, GA, USA. [5] Department of Dermatology, Duke University School of Medicine, Duke Clinic, 40 Duke Medicine Cir, Clinic 3K, Durham, NC 27710-4000, USA.

References

1. Bhattacharya A, Young A, Wong A, Stalling S, Wei M, Hadley D (2017) Precision diagnosis of melanoma and other skin lesions from digital images. AMIA Jt Summits Transl Sci Proc 2017:220–226
2. Schneider SL, Kohli I, Hamzavi IH, Council ML, Rossi AM, Ozog DM (2019) Emerging imaging technologies in dermatology: Part I: Basic principles. J Am Acad Dermatol 80(4):1114–1120. https://doi.org/10.1016/j.jaad.2018.11.042
3. Kane D, Grassi W, Sturrock R, Balint PV (2004) A brief history of musculoskeletal ultrasound: "From bats and ships to babies and hips." Rheumatology 43(7):931–933. https://doi.org/10.1093/rheumatology/keh004
4. Parsons SK, Chan JA, Yu WW, Obadan N, Ratichek SJ, Lee J et al. Noninvasive Diagnostic Techniques for the Detection of Skin Cancers. AHRQ Comparative Effectiveness Technical Briefs. Rockville (MD)2011.
5. Barcaui Ede O, Carvalho AC, Lopes FP, Pineiro-Maceira J, Barcaui CB (2016) High frequency ultrasound with color Doppler in dermatology. An Bras Dermatol 91(3):262–273. https://doi.org/10.1590/abd1806-4841.20164446
6. Mlosek RK, Malinowska S (2013) Ultrasound image of the skin, apparatus and imaging basics. J Ultrason 13(53):212–221. https://doi.org/10.15557/JoU.2013.0021
7. Kleinerman R, Whang TB, Bard RL, Marmur ES (2012) Ultrasound in dermatology: principles and applications. J Am Acad Dermatol 67(3):478–487. https://doi.org/10.1016/j.jaad.2011.12.016
8. Dill-Muller D, Maschke J (2007) Ultrasonography in dermatology. J Dtsch Dermatol Ges 5(8):689–707. https://doi.org/10.1111/j.1610-0387.2007.06453.x
9. Wortsman X, Wortsman J (2010) Clinical usefulness of variable-frequency ultrasound in localized lesions of the skin. J Am Acad Dermatol 62(2):247–256. https://doi.org/10.1016/j.jaad.2009.06.016
10. Bhatta AK, Keyal U, Liu Y (2018) Application of high frequency ultrasound in dermatology. Discov Med 26(145):237–242
11. Izzetti R, Oranges T, Janowska A, Gabriele M, Graziani F, Romanelli M (2020) The application of ultra-high-frequency ultrasound in dermatology and wound management. Int J Low Extrem Wounds 19(4):334–340. https://doi.org/10.1177/1534734620972815
12. Shung KK (2009) High frequency ultrasonic imaging. J Med Ultrasound 17(1):25–30. https://doi.org/10.1016/S0929-6441(09)60012-6
13. Polanska A, Danczak-Pazdrowska A, Jalowska M, Zaba R, Adamski Z (2017) Current applications of high-frequency ultrasonography in dermatology. Postepy Dermatol Alergol 34(6):535–542. https://doi.org/10.5114/ada.2017.72457
14. Izzetti R, Vitali S, Aringhieri G, Nisi M, Oranges T, Dini V et al (2020) Ultra-high frequency ultrasound, a promising diagnostic technique: review of the literature and single-center experience. Can Assoc Radiol J. https://doi.org/10.1177/0846537120940684
15. Iyengar S, Makin IR, Sadhwani D, Moon E, Yanes AF, Geisler A et al (2018) Utility of a high-resolution superficial diagnostic ultrasound system for assessing skin thickness: a cross-sectional study. Dermatol Surg 44(6):855–864. https://doi.org/10.1097/DSS.0000000000001445
16. Knopfel N, Gomez-Zubiaur A, Noguera-Morel L, Torrelo A, Hernandez-Martin A (2018) Ultrasound findings in idiopathic facial aseptic granuloma: case series and literature review. Pediatr Dermatol 35(3):397–400. https://doi.org/10.1111/pde.13324
17. Li JW, Tong YY, Zhou J, Shi ZT, Sun PX, Chang C (2020) Tumor proliferation and invasiveness derived from ultrasound appearances of invasive breast cancers: moving beyond the routine differential diagnosis. J Ultrasound Med. https://doi.org/10.1002/jum.15250
18. Wortsman X, Alfageme F, Roustan G, Arias-Santiago S, Martorell A, Catalano O et al (2016) Guidelines for performing dermatologic ultrasound examinations by the DERMUS Group. J Ultrasound Med 35(3):577–580. https://doi.org/10.7863/ultra.15.06046
19. Izzetti R, Vitali S, Oranges T, Dini V, Romanelli M, Caramella D et al (2020) Intraoral ultra-high frequency ultrasound study of oral lichen planus: a pictorial review. Skin Res Technol 26(2):200–204. https://doi.org/10.1111/srt.12777

20. Alexander H, Miller DL (1979) Determining skin thickness with pulsed ultra sound. J Invest Dermatol 72(1):17–19. https://doi.org/10.1111/1523-1747.ep12530104
21. Van Mulder TJ, de Koeijer M, Theeten H, Willems D, Van Damme P, Demolder M et al (2017) High frequency ultrasound to assess skin thickness in healthy adults. Vaccine 35(14):1810–1815. https://doi.org/10.1016/j.vaccine.2016.07.039
22. Barcaui Ede O, Carvalho AC, Pineiro-Maceira J, Barcaui CB, Moraes H (2015) Study of the skin anatomy with high-frequency (22 MHz) ultrasonography and histological correlation. Radiol Bras 48(5):324–329. https://doi.org/10.1590/0100-3984.2014.0028
23. Jemec GB, Gniadecka M, Ulrich J (2000) Ultrasound in dermatology. Part I. High frequency ultrasound. Eur J Dermatol. 10(6):492–497
24. de Rigal J, Escoffier C, Querleux B, Faivre B, Agache P, Leveque JL (1989) Assessment of aging of the human skin by in vivo ultrasonic imaging. J Invest Dermatol 93(5):621–625. https://doi.org/10.1111/1523-1747.ep12319741
25. Sandby-Moller J, Wulf HC (2004) Ultrasonographic subepidermal low-echogenic band, dependence of age and body site. Skin Res Technol 10(1):57–63. https://doi.org/10.1111/j.1600-0846.2004.00056.x
26. Seidenari S, Pagnoni A, Di Nardo A, Giannetti A (1994) Echographic evaluation with image analysis of normal skin: variations according to age and sex. Skin Pharmacol 7(4):201–209. https://doi.org/10.1159/000211295
27. Tsukahara K, Takema Y, Moriwaki S, Fujimura T, Kitahara T, Imokawa G (2000) Age-related alterations of echogenicity in Japanese skin. Dermatology 200(4):303–307. https://doi.org/10.1159/000018392
28. Gniadecka M (2001) Effects of ageing on dermal echogenicity. Skin Res Technol 7(3):204–207. https://doi.org/10.1034/j.1600-0846.2001.70310.x
29. Querleux B, Leveque JL, de Rigal J (1988) In vivo cross-sectional ultrasonic imaging of human skin. Dermatologica 177(6):332–337. https://doi.org/10.1159/000248602
30. Pazdrowski J, Danczak-Pazdrowska A, Polanska A, Kazmierska J, Barczak W, Szewczyk M et al (2019) An ultrasonographic monitoring of skin condition in patients receiving radiotherapy for head and neck cancers. Skin Res Technol 25(6):857–861. https://doi.org/10.1111/srt.12745
31. El Gammal S, El Gammal C, Kaspar K, Pieck C, Altmeyer P, Vogt M et al (1999) Sonography of the skin at 100 MHz enables in vivo visualization of stratum corneum and viable epidermis in palmar skin and psoriatic plaques. J Invest Dermatol 113(5):821–829. https://doi.org/10.1046/j.1523-1747.1999.00795.x
32. Goldberg I, Sprecher E, Schwartz ME, Gaitini D (2013) Comparative study of high-resolution multifrequency ultrasound of the plantar skin in patients with various types of hereditary palmoplantar keratoderma. Dermatology 226(4):365–370. https://doi.org/10.1159/000351321
33. Eliason MJ, Leachman SA, Feng BJ, Schwartz ME, Hansen CD (2012) A review of the clinical phenotype of 254 patients with genetically confirmed pachyonychia congenita. J Am Acad Dermatol 67(4):680–686. https://doi.org/10.1016/j.jaad.2011.12.009
34. McLean WH, Hansen CD, Eliason MJ, Smith FJ (2011) The phenotypic and molecular genetic features of pachyonychia congenita. J Invest Dermatol 131(5):1015–1017. https://doi.org/10.1038/jid.2011.59
35. Wortsman X, Wortsman J, Matsuoka L, Saavedra T, Mardones F, Saavedra D et al (2012) Sonography in pathologies of scalp and hair. Br J Radiol 85(1013):647–655. https://doi.org/10.1259/bjr/22636640
36. Wortsman X, Carreno L, Ferreira-Wortsman C, Poniachik R, Pizarro K, Morales C et al (2019) Ultrasound characteristics of the hair follicles and tracts, sebaceous glands, montgomery glands, apocrine glands, and arrector pili muscles. J Ultrasound Med 38(8):1995–2004. https://doi.org/10.1002/jum.14888
37. Wortsman X (2012) Common applications of dermatologic sonography. J Ultrasound Med 31(1):97–111. https://doi.org/10.7863/jum.2012.31.1.97
38. Wortsman X, Rodriguez C, Lobos C, Eguiguren G, Molina MT (2016) Ultrasound diagnosis and staging in pediatric Hidradenitis Suppurativa. Pediatr Dermatol 33(4):e260–e264. https://doi.org/10.1111/pde.12895
39. Wortsman X, Jemec GB (2006) Ultrasound imaging of nails. Dermatol Clin 24(3):323–328. https://doi.org/10.1016/j.det.2006.03.014
40. Schneider SL, Kohli I, Hamzavi IH, Council ML, Rossi AM, Ozog DM (2019) Emerging imaging technologies in dermatology: Part II: applications and limitations. J Am Acad Dermatol 80(4):1121–1131. https://doi.org/10.1016/j.jaad.2018.11.043
41. Pilat P, Borzecki A, Jazienicki M, Gerkowicz A, Krasowska D (2019) High-frequency ultrasound in the diagnosis of selected non-melanoma skin nodular lesions. Postepy Dermatol Alergol 36(5):572–580. https://doi.org/10.5114/ada.2019.89505
42. Bard RL (2017) High-frequency ultrasound examination in the diagnosis of skin cancer. Dermatol Clin 35(4):505–511. https://doi.org/10.1016/j.det.2017.06.011
43. Harland CC, Kale SG, Jackson P, Mortimer PS, Bamber JC (2000) Differentiation of common benign pigmented skin lesions from melanoma by high-resolution ultrasound. Br J Dermatol 143(2):281–289. https://doi.org/10.1046/j.1365-2133.2000.03652.x
44. Dinnes J, Bamber J, Chuchu N, Bayliss SE, Takwoingi Y, Davenport C et al (2018) High-frequency ultrasound for diagnosing skin cancer in adults. Cochrane Database Syst Rev. 12:CD03188. https://doi.org/10.1002/14651858.CD013188
45. Bobadilla JL, Love RB, Jankowska-Gan E, Xu Q, Haynes LD, Braun RK et al (2008) Th-17, monokines, collagen type V, and primary graft dysfunction in lung transplantation. Am J Respir Crit Care Med 177(6):660–668. https://doi.org/10.1164/rccm.200612-1901OC
46. Marmur ES, Berkowitz EZ, Fuchs BS, Singer GK, Yoo JY (2010) Use of high-frequency, high-resolution ultrasound before Mohs surgery. Dermatol Surg 36(6):841–847. https://doi.org/10.1111/j.1524-4725.2010.01558.x
47. Malvehy J, Pellacani G (2017) Dermoscopy, confocal microscopy and other non-invasive tools for the diagnosis of non-melanoma skin cancers and other skin conditions. Acta Derm Venereol. 218:22–30. https://doi.org/10.2340/00015555-2720
48. Mandava A, Ravuri PR, Konathan R (2013) High-resolution ultrasound imaging of cutaneous lesions. Indian J Radiol Imaging 23(3):269–277. https://doi.org/10.4103/0971-3026.120272
49. Uhara H, Hayashi K, Koga H, Saida T (2007) Multiple hypersonographic spots in basal cell carcinoma. Dermatol Surg 33(10):1215–1219. https://doi.org/10.1111/j.1524-4725.2007.33256.x
50. Warszawik-Hendzel O, Olszewska M, Maj M, Rakowska A, Czuwara J, Rudnicka L (2015) Non-invasive diagnostic techniques in the diagnosis of squamous cell carcinoma. J Dermatol Case Rep 9(4):89–97. https://doi.org/10.3315/jdcr.2015.1221
51. Rohrbach DJ, Muffoletto D, Huihui J, Saager R, Keymel K, Paquette A et al (2014) Preoperative mapping of nonmelanoma skin cancer using spatial frequency domain and ultrasound imaging. Acad Radiol 21(2):263–270. https://doi.org/10.1016/j.acra.2013.11.013
52. Schmid-Wendtner MH, Dill-Muller D (2008) Ultrasound technology in dermatology. Semin Cutan Med Surg 27(1):44–51. https://doi.org/10.1016/j.sder.2008.01.003
53. Polanska A, Danczak-Pazdrowska A, Olek-Hrab K, Osmola-Mankowska A, Bowszyc-Dmochowska M, Zaba R et al (2018) High-frequency ultrasonography-New non-invasive method in assessment of skin lymphomas. Skin Res Technol 24(3):517–521. https://doi.org/10.1111/srt.12450
54. Wang Y, Niu Z, Liu J, Zhu Q, Liu Z, Liu Y et al (2020) Value of high-frequency ultrasound in accurate staging of mycosis fungoides/Sezary Syndrome. J Ultrasound Med. https://doi.org/10.1002/jum.15297
55. Polanska A, Osmola-Mankowska A, Olek-Hrab K, Molinska-Glura M, Adamski Z, Zaba R et al (2017) High-frequency ultrasonography in objective evaluation of the efficacy of PUVA and UVA 1 phototherapy in mycosis fungoides. Arch Dermatol Res 309(8):645–651. https://doi.org/10.1007/s00403-017-1767-7
56. Szymanska E, Nowicki A, Mlosek K, Litniewski J, Lewandowski M, Secomski W et al (2000) Skin imaging with high frequency ultrasound - preliminary results. Eur J Ultrasound 12(1):9–16. https://doi.org/10.1016/s0929-8266(00)00097-5
57. Botar-Jid CM, Cosgarea R, Bolboaca SD, Senila SC, Lenghel LM, Rogojan L et al (2016) Assessment of cutaneous melanoma by use of very- high-frequency ultrasound and real-time elastography. AJR Am J Roentgenol 206(4):699–704. https://doi.org/10.2214/AJR.15.15182
58. Pilat P, Borzecki A, Jazienicki M, Krasowska D (2018) Skin melanoma imaging using ultrasonography: a literature review. Postepy Dermatol Alergol 35(3):238–242. https://doi.org/10.5114/ada.2018.76211

59. Kozarova A, Kozar M, Tonhajzerova I, Pappova T, Minarikova E (2018) The value of high-frequency 20 MHz ultrasonography for preoperative measurement of cutaneous melanoma thickness. Acta Dermatovenerol Croat 26(1):15–20
60. Samimi M, Perrinaud A, Naouri M, Maruani A, Perrodeau E, Vaillant L et al (2010) High-resolution ultrasonography assists the differential diagnosis of blue naevi and cutaneous metastases of melanoma. Br J Dermatol 163(3):550–556. https://doi.org/10.1111/j.1365-2133.2010.09903.x
61. Akesson A, Forsberg L, Hederstrom E, Wollheim F (1986) Ultrasound examination of skin thickness in patients with progressive systemic sclerosis (scleroderma). Acta Radiol Diagn (Stockh) 27(1):91–94. https://doi.org/10.1177/028418518602700117
62. Bialynicki-Birula R, Reszke R, Szepietowski JC (2017) High-frequency ultrasonography (HFUS) as a useful tool in differentiating between plaque morphea and extragenital lichen sclerosus lesions. Postepy Dermatol Alergol 34(5):485–489. https://doi.org/10.5114/ada.2017.71118
63. Hesselstrand R, Carlestam J, Wildt M, Sandqvist G, Andreasson K (2015) High frequency ultrasound of skin involvement in systemic sclerosis - a follow-up study. Arthritis Res Ther 17:329. https://doi.org/10.1186/s13075-015-0853-5
64. Ranosz-Janicka I, Lis-Swiety A, Skrzypek-Salamon A, Brzezinska-Wcislo L (2019) An extended high-frequency ultrasound protocol for assessing and quantifying of inflammation and fibrosis in localized scleroderma. Skin Res Technol 25(3):359–366. https://doi.org/10.1111/srt.12660
65. Li H, Furst DE, Jin H, Sun C, Wang X, Yang L et al (2018) High-frequency ultrasound of the skin in systemic sclerosis: an exploratory study to examine correlation with disease activity and to define the minimally detectable difference. Arthritis Res Ther 20(1):181. https://doi.org/10.1186/s13075-018-1686-9
66. Arisi M, Lorenzi L, Incardona P, Fusano M, Zanca A, Rossi MT et al (2019) Clinical, histological and high-frequency ultrasonographic evaluation (50 MHz) of morphoea treated with ultraviolet al phototherapy. Clin Exp Dermatol 44(3):270–276. https://doi.org/10.1111/ced.13693
67. Acquacalda E, Albert C, Montaudie H, Fontas E, Danre A, Roux CH et al (2015) Ultrasound study of entheses in psoriasis patients with or without musculoskeletal symptoms: a prospective study. Joint Bone Spine 82(4):267–271. https://doi.org/10.1016/j.jbspin.2015.01.016
68. Aydin SZ, Castillo-Gallego C, Ash ZR, Abignano G, Marzo-Ortega H, Wittmann M et al (2013) Potential use of optical coherence tomography and high-frequency ultrasound for the assessment of nail disease in psoriasis and psoriatic arthritis. Dermatology 227(1):45–51. https://doi.org/10.1159/000351702
69. Marina ME, Solomon C, Bolboaca SD, Bocsa C, Mihu CM, Tataru AD (2016) High-frequency sonography in the evaluation of nail psoriasis. Med Ultrason 18(3):312–317. https://doi.org/10.11152/mu.2013.2066.183.hgh
70. Polanska A, Gaura T, Bowszyc-Dmochowska M, Osmola-Mankowska A, Olek-Hrab K, Adamski Z et al (2019) Calcipotriol/betamethasone ointment compared to narrow-band UVB in plaque psoriasis: first clinical and ultrasonographic study. Int J Dermatol 58(1):108–113. https://doi.org/10.1111/ijd.14150
71. Jemec GB, Heidenheim M, Nielsen NH (1996) The prevalence of hidradenitis suppurativa and its potential precursor lesions. J Am Acad Dermatol 35(2 Pt 1):191–194. https://doi.org/10.1016/s0190-9622(96)90321-7
72. Revuz JE, Canoui-Poitrine F, Wolkenstein P, Viallette C, Gabison G, Pouget F et al (2008) Prevalence and factors associated with hidradenitis suppurativa: results from two case-control studies. J Am Acad Dermatol 59(4):596–601. https://doi.org/10.1016/j.jaad.2008.06.020
73. Cosmatos I, Matcho A, Weinstein R, Montgomery MO, Stang P (2013) Analysis of patient claims data to determine the prevalence of hidradenitis suppurativa in the United States. J Am Acad Dermatol 68(3):412–419. https://doi.org/10.1016/j.jaad.2012.07.027
74. Vinkel C, Thomsen SF (2018) Hidradenitis Suppurativa: causes, features, and current treatments. J Clin Aesthet Dermatol 11(10):17–23
75. Bard RL (ed) (2019) Image guided dermatologic treatments. Springer, Switzerland
76. Lacarrubba F, Dini V, Napolitano M, Venturini M, Caposiena Caro DR, Molinelli E et al (2019) Ultrasonography in the pathway to an optimal standard of care of hidradenitis suppurativa: the Italian Ultrasound Working Group experience. J Eur Acad Dermatol Venereol 33(Suppl 6):10–14. https://doi.org/10.1111/jdv.15847
77. Nazzaro G, Passoni E, Muratori S, Moltrasio C, Guanziroli E, Barbareschi M et al (2018) Comparison of clinical and sonographic scores in hidradenitis suppurativa and proposal of a novel ultrasound scoring system. G Ital Dermatol Venereol. https://doi.org/10.23736/S0392-0488.18.06196-5
78. Wortsman X, Moreno C, Soto R, Arellano J, Pezo C, Wortsman J (2013) Ultrasound in-depth characterization and staging of hidradenitis suppurativa. Dermatol Surg 39(12):1835–1842. https://doi.org/10.1111/dsu.12329
79. Loo CH, Tan WC, Tang JJ, Khor YH, Manikam MT, Low DE et al (2018) The clinical, biochemical, and ultrasonographic characteristics of patients with hidradenitis suppurativa in Northern Peninsular Malaysia: a multicenter study. Int J Dermatol 57(12):1454–1463. https://doi.org/10.1111/ijd.14210
80. Zarchi K, Yazdanyar N, Yazdanyar S, Wortsman X, Jemec GB (2015) Pain and inflammation in hidradenitis suppurativa correspond to morphological changes identified by high-frequency ultrasound. J Eur Acad Dermatol Venereol 29(3):527–532. https://doi.org/10.1111/jdv.12610
81. Sabau M, Boca AN, Ilies RF, Tataru A (2019) Potential of high-frequency ultrasonography in the management of atopic dermatitis. Exp Ther Med 17(2):1073–1077. https://doi.org/10.3892/etm.2018.6984
82. Grinich EE, Schmitt J, Kuster D, Spuls PI, Williams HC, Chalmers JR et al (2018) Standardized reporting of the Eczema Area and Severity Index (EASI) and the Patient-Oriented Eczema Measure (POEM): a recommendation by the Harmonising Outcome Measures for Eczema (HOME) Initiative. Br J Dermatol 179(2):540–541. https://doi.org/10.1111/bjd.16732
83. Schmitt J, Spuls PI, Thomas KS, Simpson E, Furue M, Deckert S et al (2014) The Harmonising Outcome Measures for Eczema (HOME) statement to assess clinical signs of atopic eczema in trials. J Allergy Clin Immunol 134(4):800–807. https://doi.org/10.1016/j.jaci.2014.07.043
84. Polanska A, Danczak-Pazdrowska A, Silny W, Wozniak A, Maksin K, Jenerowicz D et al (2013) Comparison between high-frequency ultrasonography (Dermascan C, version 3) and histopathology in atopic dermatitis. Skin Res Technol 19(4):432–437. https://doi.org/10.1111/srt.12064
85. Charman CR, Venn AJ, Williams HC (1999) Measurement of body surface area involvement in atopic eczema: an impossible task? Br J Dermatol 140(1):109–111. https://doi.org/10.1046/j.1365-2133.1999.02617.x
86. Polanska A, Silny W, Jenerowicz D, Kniola K, Molinska-Glura M, Danczak-Pazdrowska A (2015) Monitoring of therapy in atopic dermatitis–observations with the use of high-frequency ultrasonography. Skin Res Technol 21(1):35–40. https://doi.org/10.1111/srt.12153
87. Osmola-Mankowska A, Polanska A, Silny W, Zaba R, Adamski Z, Danczak-Pazdrowska A (2014) Topical tacrolimus vs medium-dose ultraviolet al phototherapy in the treatment of atopic dermatitis-a preliminary study in relation to parameters of the epidermal barrier function and high-frequency ultrasonography. Eur Rev Med Pharmacol Sci 18(24):3927–3934
88. Noe MH, Rodriguez O, Taylor L, Sultan L, Sehgal C, Schultz S et al (2017) High frequency ultrasound: a novel instrument to quantify granuloma burden in cutaneous sarcoidosis. Sarcoidosis Vasc Diffuse Lung Dis 34(2):136–141
89. Chen KC, Lin AC, Chong CF, Wang TL (2016) An overview of point-of-care ultrasound for soft tissue and musculoskeletal applications in the emergency department. J Intensive Care 4:55. https://doi.org/10.1186/s40560-016-0173-0
90. Gong X, Yu W, Li J, Ding A, Xiong P, Lin X (2019) High-Frequency Ultrasound investigation of port-wine stains: hemodynamic features revealed by 10- and 22-MHz transducers. J Ultrasound Med 38(3):641–648. https://doi.org/10.1002/jum.14732
91. Alegre-Sanchez A, Bernardez C, Fonda-Pascual P, Moreno-Arrones OM, Lopez-Gutierrez JC, Jaen-Olasolo P et al (2018) Videodermoscopy and doppler-ultrasound in spider naevi: towards a new classification? J Eur Acad Dermatol Venereol 32(1):156–159. https://doi.org/10.1111/jdv.14602
92. Wassef M, Blei F, Adams D, Alomari A, Baselga E, Berenstein A et al (2015) Vascular anomalies classification: recommendations from the

International Society for the Study of Vascular Anomalies. Pediatrics 136(1):e203–e214. https://doi.org/10.1542/peds.2014-3673
93. Lloret P, Redondo P, Cabrera J, Sierra A (2015) Treatment of venous leg ulcers with ultrasound-guided foam sclerotherapy: healing, long-term recurrence and quality of life evaluation. Wound Repair Regen 23(3):369–378. https://doi.org/10.1111/wrr.12288
94. Wortsman X, Wortsman J (2011) Sonographic outcomes of cosmetic procedures. AJR Am J Roentgenol 197(5):W910–W918. https://doi.org/10.2214/AJR.11.6719
95. Giovagnorio F, Drudi FM, Valentini C, Paonessa A (2004) Ultrasonography in follow-up of soft tissue augmentation of the face with synthetic materials: a pilot study. Acta Radiol 45(7):746–750. https://doi.org/10.1080/02841850410008207
96. Schelke LW, Van Den Elzen HJ, Erkamp PP, Neumann HA (2010) Use of ultrasound to provide overall information on facial fillers and surrounding tissue. Dermatol Surg 36(Suppl 3):1843–1851. https://doi.org/10.1111/j.1524-4725.2010.01740.x
97. Wortsman X, Wortsman J, Orlandi C, Cardenas G, Sazunic I, Jemec GB (2012) Ultrasound detection and identification of cosmetic fillers in the skin. J Eur Acad Dermatol Venereol 26(3):292–301. https://doi.org/10.1111/j.1468-3083.2011.04047.x
98. Crisan D, Roman I, Crisan M, Scharffetter-Kochanek K, Badea R (2015) The role of vitamin C in pushing back the boundaries of skin aging: an ultrasonographic approach. Clin Cosmet Investig Dermatol 8:463–470. https://doi.org/10.2147/CCID.S84903
99. Addor FAS, Cotta Vieira J, Abreu Melo CS (2018) Improvement of dermal parameters in aged skin after oral use of a nutrient supplement. Clin Cosmet Investig Dermatol 11:195–201. https://doi.org/10.2147/CCID.S150269
100. Fanian F, Mac-Mary S, Jeudy A, Lihoreau T, Messikh R, Ortonne JP et al (2013) Efficacy of micronutrient supplementation on skin aging and seasonal variation: a randomized, placebo-controlled, double-blind study. Clin Interv Aging 8:1527–1537. https://doi.org/10.2147/CIA.S43976
101. Rodriguez Bandera AI, Moreno Bonilla G, Feito Rodriguez M, Beato Merino MJ, de Lucas LR (2019) Jellyfish-like sonographic pattern can help recognition of dermatofibrosarcoma protuberans. Report of 3 new cases and review of the literature. Australas J Dermatol. 60(2):e148–e150. https://doi.org/10.1111/ajd.12922
102. Bousquet-Rouaud R, Bazan M, Chaintreuil J, Echague A (2009) High-frequency ultrasound evaluation of cellulite treated with the 1064 nm Nd:YAG laser. J Cosmet Laser Ther 11(1):34–44. https://doi.org/10.1080/14764170802612968
103. Lucassen GW, van der Sluys WL, van Herk JJ, Nuijs AM, Wierenga PE, Barel AO et al (1997) The effectiveness of massage treatment on cellulite as monitored by ultrasound imaging. Skin Res Technol 3(3):154–160. https://doi.org/10.1111/j.1600-0846.1997.tb00180.x
104. Rosenbaum M, Prieto V, Hellmer J, Boschmann M, Krueger J, Leibel RL et al (1998) An exploratory investigation of the morphology and biochemistry of cellulite. Plast Reconstr Surg 101(7):1934–1939. https://doi.org/10.1097/00006534-199806000-00025

9

The role of ultrasound imaging in vascular compression syndromes

Renato Farina*, Pietro Valerio Foti, Andrea Conti, Francesco Aldo Iannace, Isabella Pennisi, Luigi Fanzone, Corrado Inì, Federica Libra, Francesco Vacirca, Giovanni Failla, Davide Baldanza, Stefano Palmucci, Serafino Santonocito and Antonio Basile

Abstract

Vascular compression syndromes are rare alterations that have in common the compression of an arterial and/or venous vessel by contiguous structures and can be congenital or acquired. The best known are the Thoracic Outlet Syndrome, Nutcracker Syndrome, May–Thurner Syndrome, and Dunbar Syndrome. The incidence of these pathologies is certainly underestimated due to the non-specific clinical signs and their frequent asymptomaticity. Being a first-level method, Ultrasound plays a very important role in identifying these alterations, almost always allowing a complete diagnostic classification. If in expert hands, this method can significantly contribute to the reduction of false negatives, especially in the asymptomatic population, where the finding of the aforementioned pathologies often happens randomly following routine checks. In this review, we briefly discuss the best known vascular changes, the corresponding ultrasound anatomy, and typical ultrasound patterns.

Keywords: May–Thurner syndrome, Dunbar syndrome, Nutcracker syndrome, Color Doppler ultrasound, Duplex Doppler ultrasound, Abdominal ultrasound

Thoracic Outlet Syndrome (TOS)

Introduction

Thoracic Outlet Syndrome (TOS) [1, 2] is a rare pathology of neuro-vascular compression caused by the bilateral (Fig. 1a) or unilateral cervical rib (Fig. 1b) [3] or by hypertrophy of the scalene muscles [4]. The cervical rib is a congenital alteration, often asymptomatic, while hypertrophy of the scalene muscles is generally acquired, frequent in some sports that involve the shoulder muscles. TOS can therefore be bilateral, due to the presence of two cervical ribs and/or to bilateral hypertrophy of the scalene muscles. In most cases, TOS is unilateral. Very rare is the combination of bilateral compression of the artery and subclavian vein, due to the coexistence of two cervical ribs and bilateral hypertrophy of the scalene muscles [5]. The incidence of the disease is higher in females aged between 20 and 50. In TOS, for anatomical reasons, compression of the subclavian vein always takes place at the "cost-clavicular space" [6](Fig. 2a), while compression of the subclavian artery at the level of the "inter-scalene triangle" [7](Fig. 2b). The subclavian artery is almost always compressed by the cervical rib, while the subclavian vein by hypertrophy of the anterior scalene muscle.

Clinical implications

The cervical rib can compress both the brachial plexus (neurological form) with tingling and/or paresthesia, and the subclavian artery (vascular form) with consequent hypo-perfusion and cyanosis of the upper limb. If compression is caused by hypertrophy of the scalene muscles, it always involves the subclavian vein and causes venous stasis with hypertension, cyanosis, swelling (often in the morning), and pain in the upper limbs. The diagnosis of TOS can be clinical: Adson test [8], Allen test [9], Wright test [10], Halstead maneuver [11], and/or instrumental.

*Correspondence: radfaro@hotmail.com
Radiodiagnostic and Radiotherapy Unit, Department of Medical and Surgical Sciences and Advanced Technologies "GF Ingrassia", Via Santa Sofia 78, 95123 Catani, Italy

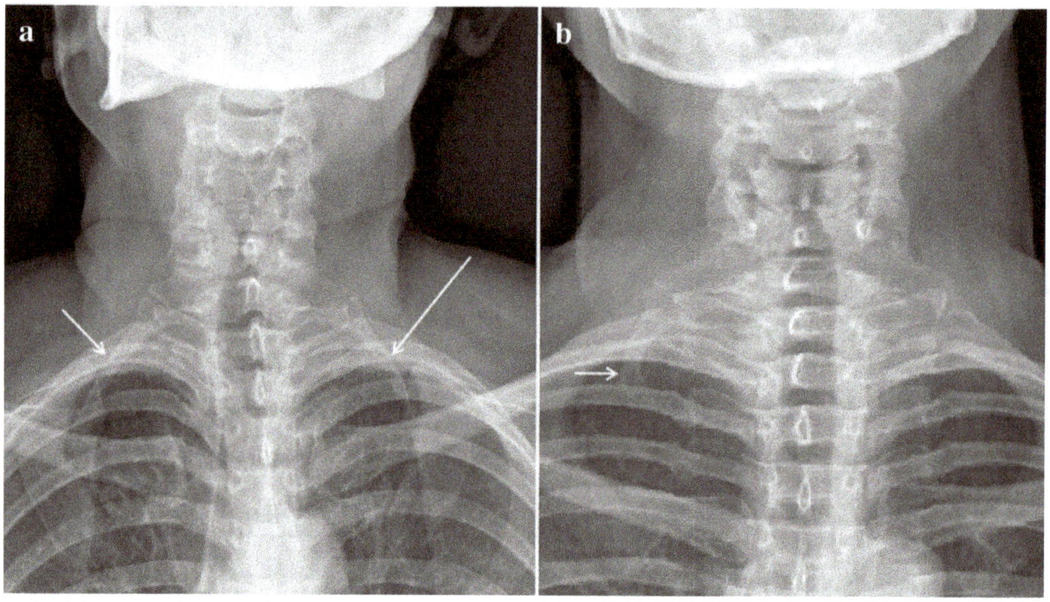

Fig. 1 TOS. Standard chest X-ray. Patient with bilateral cervical ribs: **a** right (short arrow) and left (long arrow) cervical rib. Patient with unilateral cervical rib: **b** right cervical rib (arrow)

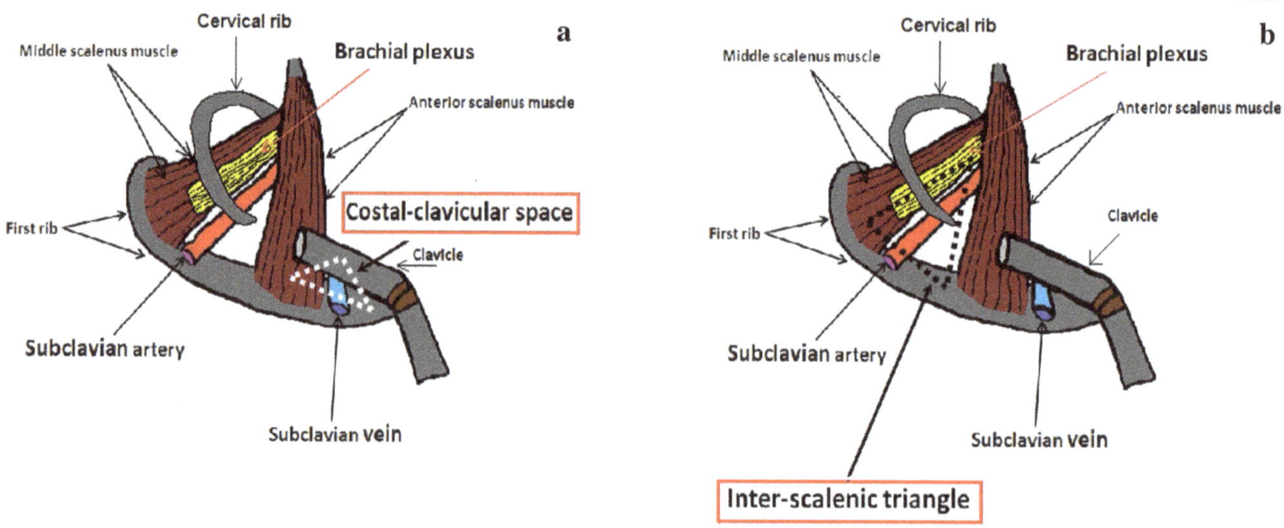

Fig. 2 Scheme summarizing the anatomical relationships between the shoulder structures in TOS. **a** Cost-clavicular space delimited inferiorly by first rib, superiorly by clavicle, and anteriorly by anterior scalene muscle. **b** Inter-scalene triangle delimited inferiorly by clavicle, medially by anterior scalene muscle, and laterally by middle scalene muscle

Instrumental diagnosis

The imaging is entrusted to Standard Radiography to ascertain the presence of the cervical ribs and to ultrasound for the study of vascular alterations [12]. The Ultrasound is the first-level examination and must be performed with arms raised to 90° and arms lowered (Adson test), to measure the changes in the caliber and flow of the artery and subclavian vein. Generally, by raising the arms to 90°, the arterial and/or venous compression appears or accentuates and with them the symptomatology. The Ultrasound examination must be performed using both B-Mode Ultrasound (US) for the scalene muscles and cervical ribs morphological study (Fig. 3); Color Doppler US and Duplex Doppler US for the flowmeter study [13].

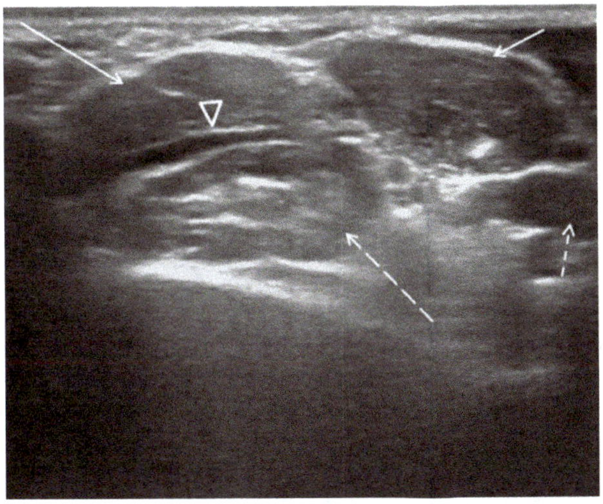

Fig. 3 B-Mode US: transverse scan of the cost-clavicular space which highlights the anterior scalene muscle (short arrow), the middle scalene muscle (long arrow), and the posterior scalene muscle (long-dashed arrow). Subclavian artery (head of arrow). Subclavian vein (dashed short arrow)

Color Doppler US of the subclavian vein must be performed at the level of the "costal-clavicular space", where compression occurs, which is delimited below by first rib, above by clavicle and anteriorly by anterior scalene muscle. The subclavian artery study must instead be carried out at the level of the "inter-scalene triangle" which is delimited inferiorly by clavicle, medially by anterior scalene muscle and laterally by middle scalene muscle. During the Adson test, the caliber and the flow of the vessels must be measured.

In subclavian vein compression upstream of the stenosis, a slowing of the peak flow with consequent venous hypertension is observed (Fig. 4a–e). When the compression involves the subclavian artery, it is possible to observe a progressive reduction in the caliber of the vessel passing from the position with lowered arms to that with raised arms and an increase in the peak speed proportional to the degree of stenosis; if the stenosis is severe, very high speeds and aliasing artifacts are observed with Color Doppler US and Duplex

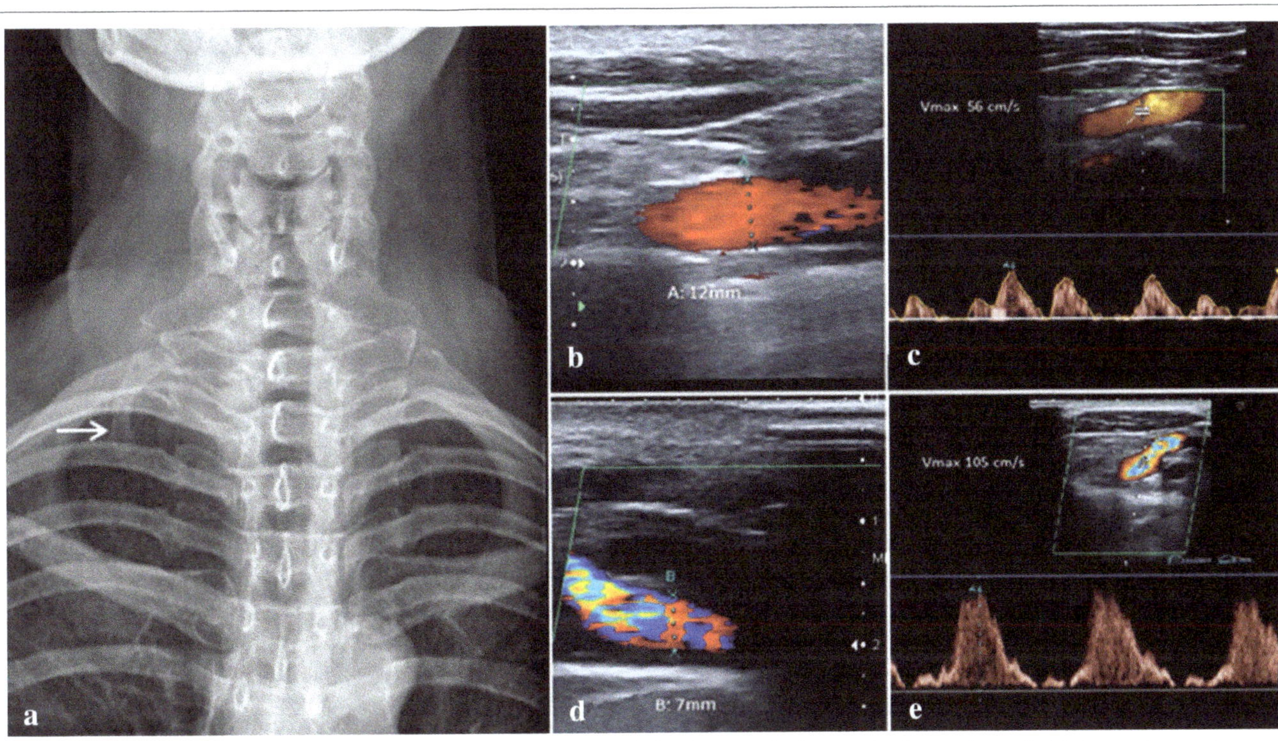

Fig. 4 **a** Standard radiography showing a cervical rib on the right (arrow). **b** Color Doppler US examination, performed with lowered arms, shows a regular diameter (12 mm) and a regular flow-C of the right subclavian artery. **d** Color Doppler US examination with raised arms shows artifacts due to turbulent flux. E: Duplex Doppler US shows increase in peak speed (105 cm/s)

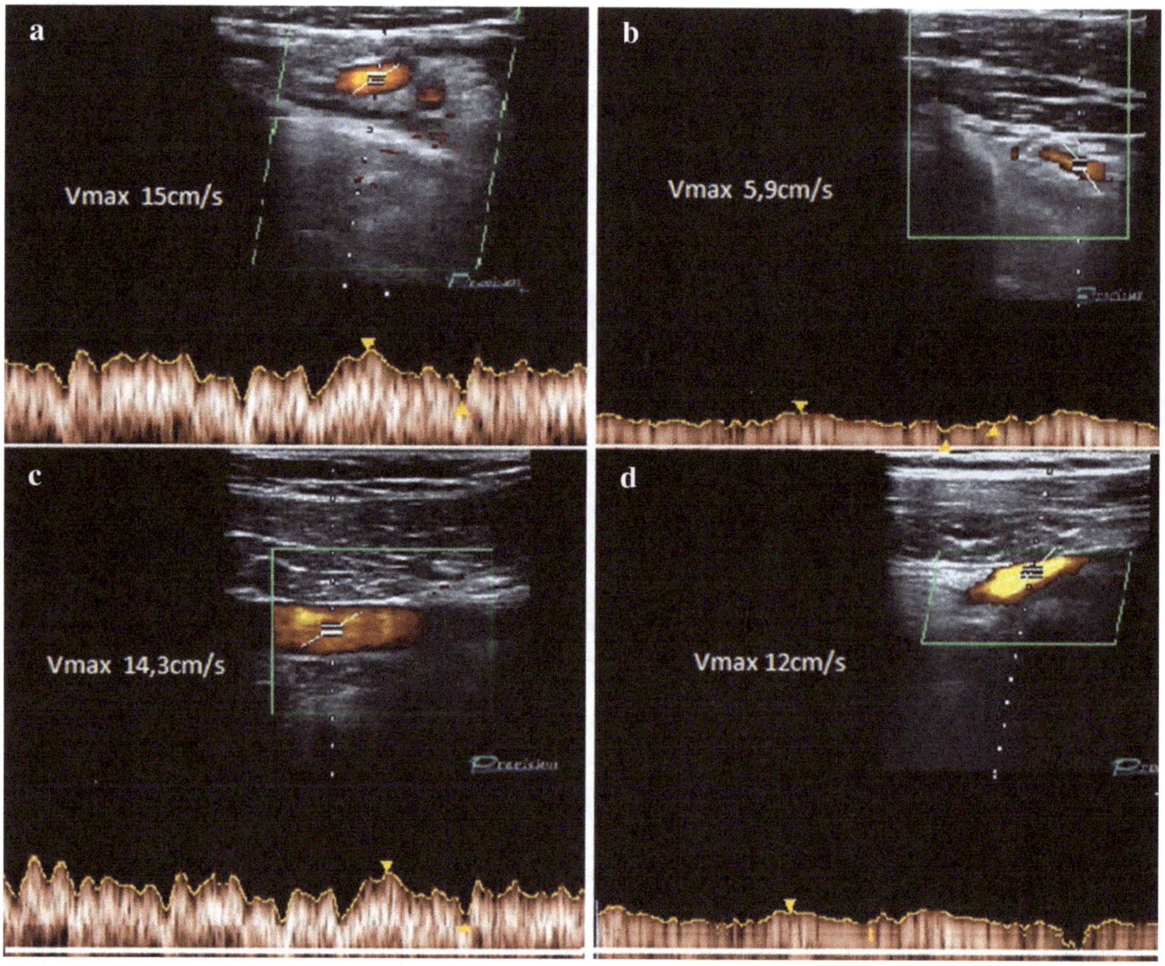

Fig. 5 Hypertrophy of the right anterior scalene muscle. **a** Duplex Doppler US examination of the right subclavian veins, with lowered arms, shows a regular diameter and flow. **b** With arms raised to 90° Duplex Doppler US shows a peak speed reduction due to compression by the anterior scalene muscle. **c** Duplex Doppler US of left subclavian vein, with lowered arms, shows a regular caliber and flow. **d** Which remain regular even with arms raised to 90°

Doppler US, due to the turbulent flow in the stenotic tract (Fig. 5a–d) Magnetic Resonance Imaging (MRI) can highlight the main signs of TOS, but is mainly used in children to avoid the radiological risk related to the ionizing radiation [14]. Multidetector Computed Tomography (MDCT) is used in the diagnosis of TOS for its overview and high accuracy for vascular structures [15]; moreover, even if burdened by radiological risk, recent technological developments have made it possible to lower radiation doses, without compromising image quality [16].

Treatment

Patient treatment can be surgical with cervical rib resection [17] and scalenectomy [18], or conservative with physiotherapy, orthotics, and taping [19]. The above treatments are all aimed at reducing arterial and/or venous vascular compression.

Nutcracker Syndrome (NCS)

Introduction

NCS, also known as left renal vein entrapment syndrome, is a rare vascular alteration due to compression of the left renal vein in the transition between the abdominal aorta and the superior mesenteric artery [20]. It was first described by Wilkie [21]. This disease is caused by the reduction in the angle between the abdominal aorta and the superior mesenteric artery that originates at an angle of less than 22 degrees, maintaining a distance to the aorta of less than 8 mm. The reduced angle involves

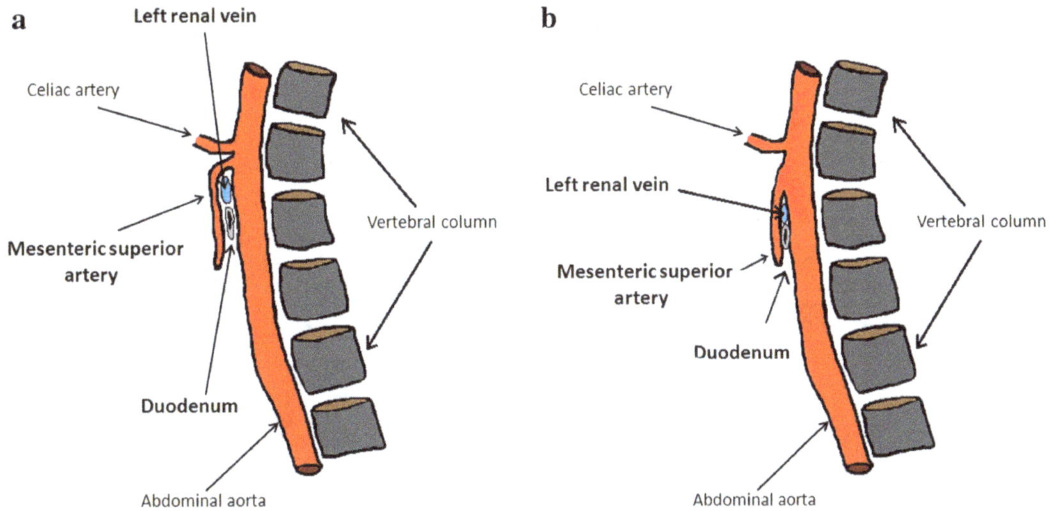

Fig. 6 NCS. Scheme summarizing that describes the relationships between the aorto-mesenteric angle, left renal vein, and duodenum. **a** Healthy patient with regular aorto-mesenteric angle. **b** Aorto-mesenteric angle lower than 22° which causes compression of the left renal vein

the structures that pass through this anatomical space, namely the duodenum and the left renal vein which undergo compression proportionate to the reduction of the aorto-mesenteric angle (Fig. 6a, b). Isolated stenosis of the left renal vein is commonly called "NCS ", while isolated compression of the duodenum "Wilkie Syndrome" (WS). The two alterations can combine or occur in isolation. In most cases, the compression of the renal vein arises anteriorly to the aorta, while in much rarer cases, it occurs posteriorly and happens when the renal vein is retro-aortic; in this case, compression occurs between the spine and the abdominal aorta [22]. The incidence of the disease is probably underestimated considering that compression is often asymptomatic and that there are cases of unknown proteinuria and hematuria that could be caused by NCS. NCS can affect all age groups, but it prevails in very thin young people [23]. The Syndrome can be congenital or acquired. In the acquired form, the greatest prevalence is in anorexic patients and is due to the reduction of the peri-vascular adipose tissue which results in a narrowing of the aorto-mesenteric angle; in these patients, vomiting, which is initially self-induced, following the onset of duodenal compression (WS), becomes organic and contributes to the progressive worsening of clinical conditions [24].

Clinical implications

In NCS not combined with WS, clinically patients may have different clinical manifestations, ranging from asymptomatic hematuria to proteinuria, nephrovascular hypertension, left flank pain, and secondary varicocele [25]. The most commonly reported symptom is hematuria due to rupture of thin-walled varices due to venous hypertension [26]. If compression involves the duodenum, vomiting, sub-occlusive crisis, and weight loss may occur and the most constant symptom is post-prandial vomiting. The combination of the two syndromes can manifest with all the above symptoms.

Instrumental diagnosis

Ultrasound is the first-level examination for the diagnosis of NCS, it allows you to accurately measure the aorto-mesenteric angle and the aorto-mesenteric distance (Fig. 7a) (Clip 1. NCS. B-Mode US of the AO) [27]; it can also measure the flow (Fig. 7b) and the caliber of pre-stenotic tract of the left renal vein (Fig. 7c). Pelvic Ultrasound examination can highlight varicosities of the pampiniform and/or gonadal plexus (Fig. 7d) due to stasis and hypertension of the left renal vein. Ultrasound therefore allows a complete diagnostic framework of the NCS but not of the WS, for the diagnosis of which integration with other imaging methods such as MR-Enterography [28], Fluoroscopy [29], and Ecoendoscopy [30] is necessary. MDCT can demonstrate compression and pre-stenotic dilation of the left renal vein, as well as the presence of varicocele. An advantage of MDCT is the possibility of highlighting also the stenosis of the duodenum and the intestinal dilation upstream of the stenosis. A pathognomonic sign of NCS in MDCT is the "Beak sign" that is the origin of the superior mesenteric artery from the

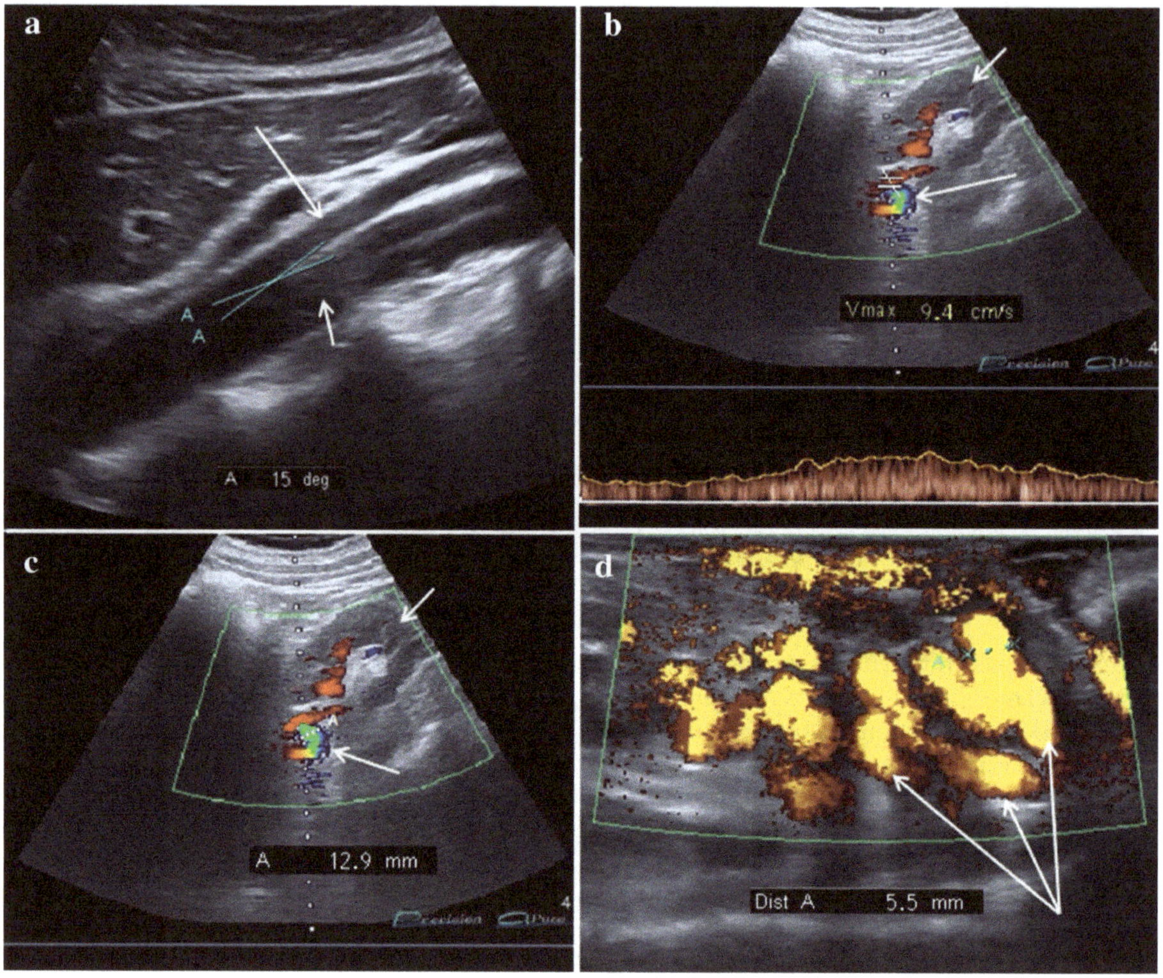

Fig. 7 B-Mode US: longitudinal sub-xiphoid scan of the abdominal aorta performed in supine decubitus. **a** Measurement of the aorto-mesenteric angle "A" in patient with NCS. Abdominal aorta (short arrow). Superior mesenteric artery (long arrow). **b** Duplex Doppler US shows a peak speed reduction in left renal vein. **c** Measurement of the left renal vein diameter. **d** Power Doppler US shows varicosity of the gonadal plexus (vein diameter 5.5 mm)

aorta with an acute angle also known as "hooked appearance" evident in the sagittal reconstructions (Fig. 8a–d) [31]. MRI can highlight all pathognomonic signs of NCS (Fig. 9a–d); compared to MDCT, it is not burdened by radiological risk, but is less sensitive for the evaluation of duodenal stenosis [32, 33].

Treatment

The choice of treatment should be based on the clinical presentation, physical condition, and severity of left renal vein stenosis. Conservative treatment, of choice, when possible, consists in restoring the normal layer of perivascular fat tissue with a high calorie diet [34]. The other two therapeutic approaches are surgical treatment [35, 36] and endovascular stenting treatment [37]. The surgical treatment consists in overcoming the stenosis with the resection of the first jejunal loop and the retrovascular duodenum followed by the anastomosis between the duodenum and the second jejunal loop which are anteriorized. In recent years, however, the use of interventional procedures with stenting of the left renal vein [38] has led to a significant reduction in surgical treatments, much more invasive and with greater complications. The positioning of the endovascular stent in the left renal vein causes the restoration of the normal aorto-mesenteric angle with resolution of the venous compression and all

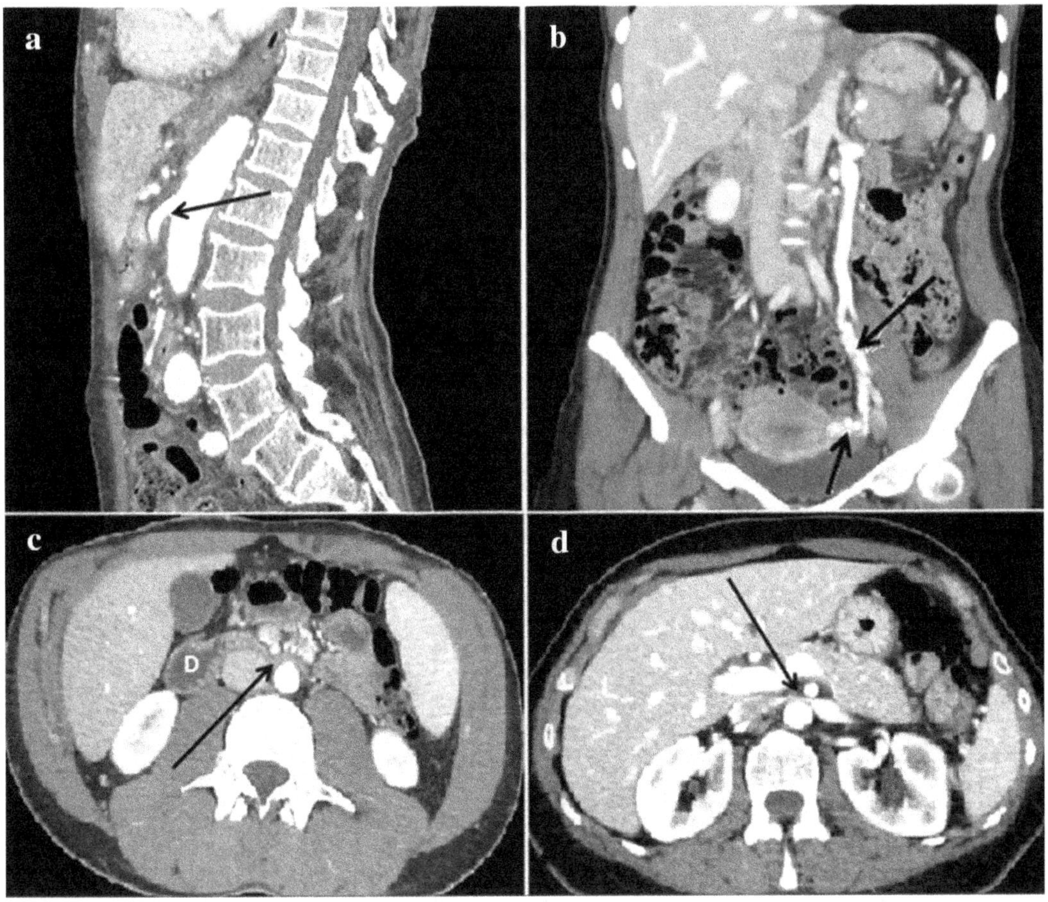

Fig. 8 Abdomen MDCT examination. **a** The reconstruction according to a sagittal plane shows the characteristic pattern with aorta and superior mesenteric artery "beak-like" appearance (black arrow). **b** The coronal plane reconstruction shows dilation of the gonadal vein and gonadal plexus (arrow). **c** The axial plane reconstruction shows a stenosis of duodenum (arrow). "D": Duodenum. **d** The axial plane reconstruction shows a stenosis of the left renal vein (arrow)

the alterations related to it (Fig. 10a–d). Power Doppler US (Clip 2. NCS. After stenting, power Doppler US that shows flow inside the stent), Duplex Doppler US (Clip 3. NCS. After stenting, duplex Doppler US that shows flow inside the stent), and selective Angiography (Clip 4. NCS. Selective Angiography demonstrates stent patency) can be used to check the patency of the endovascular stent. The absence of treatment can predispose to left renal venous thrombosis with consequent renal damage up to the loss of the organ.

May–Thurner Syndrome (MTS)

Introduction

MTS [39] also known as Cockett Syndrome [40] is caused by chronic compression of the left common iliac vein against the lumbar spine by the right common iliac artery (Fig. 11a, b). Compression of the left common iliac vein can generate various degrees of venous hypertension and can predispose the left lower limb to thrombosis. The exact incidence of the disease is unknown both, because it can be asymptomatic

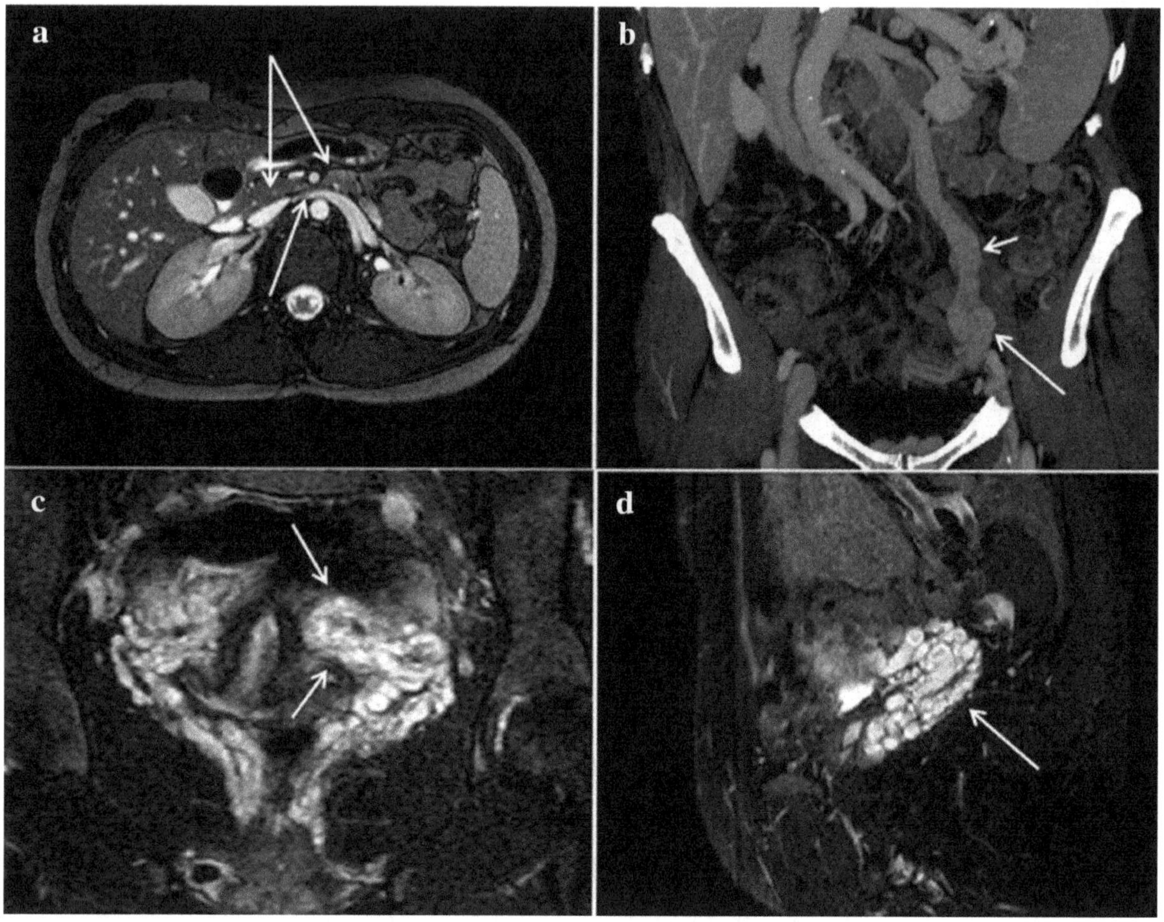

Fig. 9 Abdomen MRI examination. **a** The axial plane reconstruction shows a stenosis of the left renal vein and duodenum (arrows) in the aorto-mesenteric angle (arrow). **b** The coronal plane reconstruction shows gonadal vein (short arrow) and gonadal plexus (long arrow) dilatation. **c** The coronal plane reconstruction shows the varicosities of the gonadal plexus (arrow), also evident in the reconstruction according to a sagittal plane (arrow)—D

[41] and due to the specificity of the symptoms. In 1851, Virchow noted a five times higher incidence of deep vein thrombosis on the left side than deep vein thrombosis on the right side. The anatomical variant responsible for this discovery was described in 1908 by McMurrich; however, it was May and Thurner in 1957 to better frame the mechanisms of the Syndrome, describing the formation of "spurs" in the left common iliac vein as a consequence of chronic compression at work of the right common iliac artery against the spine. The combination of arterial pulsations and mechanical compression by the right common iliac artery would cause hypertrophy of the intimate, with consequent accumulation of elastin and collagen that form the so-called "spurs" responsible for the narrowing of the vascular lumen. In most cases (84%), the right common iliac artery compresses the left common iliac vein, but compression of the right common iliac vein by the ipsilateral common iliac artery has also been described [42]. Compression generally occurs against the fifth lumbar vertebra, but also against the fourth lumbar vertebra has been described [43]. Other causes of compression of the left common iliac vein caused by the bladder [44], endometriosis [45], a

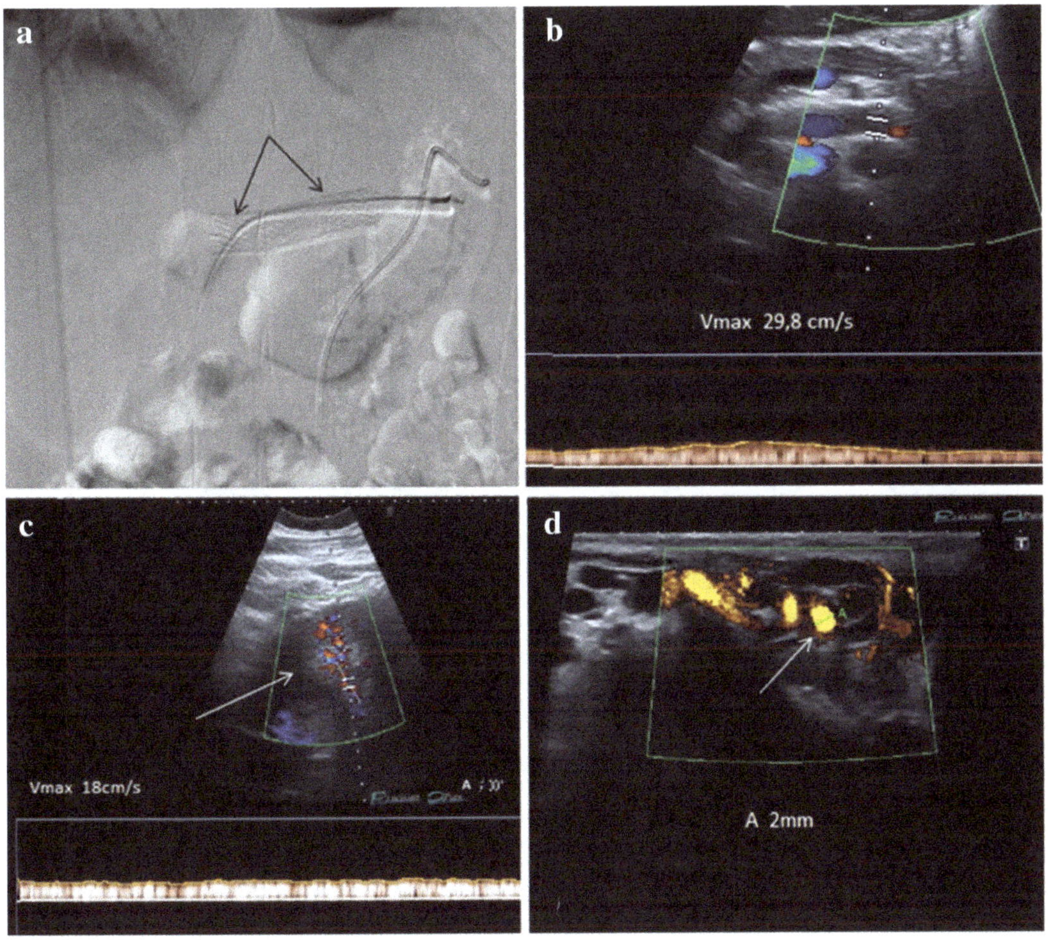

Fig. 10 **a** This angiographic image shows the endovascular stent after positioning into the left renal vein (arrows). **b** Duplex Doppler US highlights the patency of the vascular stent showing a flow with a peak velocity of about 29.8 cm/s. **c** After stenting, Color Doppler US show a increased flow of the left renal vein (18 cm/s). **d** Power Doppler US shows a regular caliber of the pampiniform plexus vein (diameters of 2 mm)

penile prosthesis reservoir [46], and aneurysm of the common iliac artery [47, 48] have been described in the literature.

Clinical implications

Symptomatology in MTS is related to the degree of stenosis of the left common iliac vein and the presence or absence of deep vein thrombosis. In the milder degrees of compression, it can be asymptomatic, while in the most severe degrees, patients can experience: swelling of the left lower limb, pain, venous claudication, deep vein thrombosis, and up to the most serious complication which is pulmonary embolism.

Instrumental diagnosis

Ultrasound represents the first-level imaging method thanks to the high sensitivity, low costs, equipment availability, and absence of risks. Color Doppler US, Power Doppler US, and Duplex Doppler US can highlight deep venous thrombosis and measure their extension. Unlike other imaging methods, Ultrasound allows you to measure the left common iliac vein flow by providing an estimate of stenosis severity and

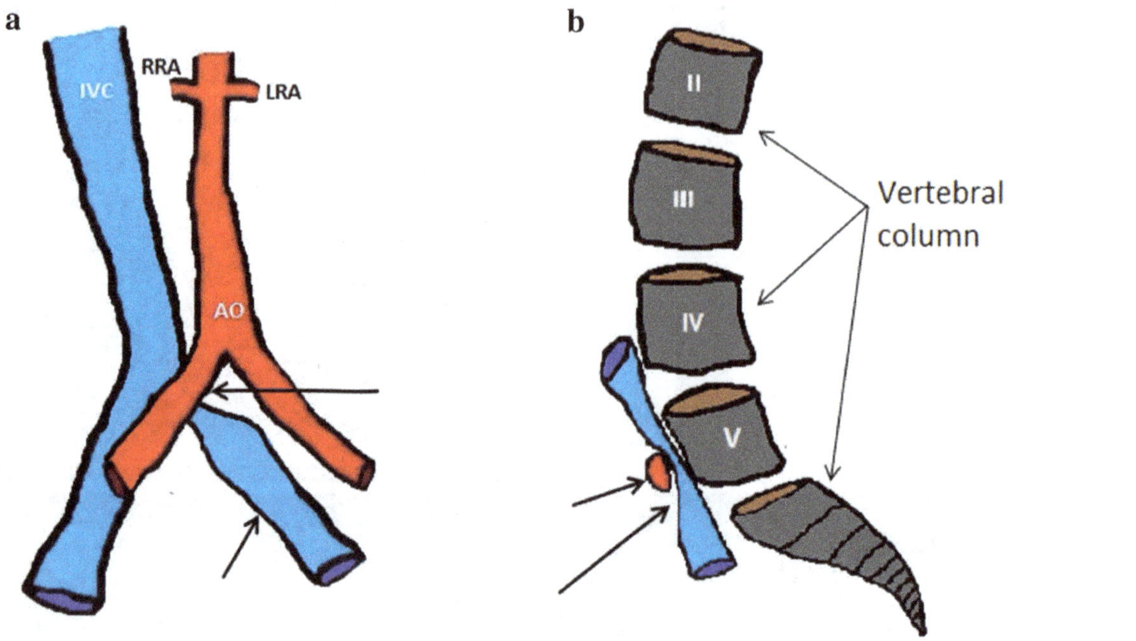

Fig. 11 MTS. Scheme summarizing describing the main anatomical structures involved in the syndrome. **a** Left common iliac vein compression (short arrow) by the right common iliac artery (long arrow). *AO* Abdominal aorta. IV **c** Inferior cava vein. RR **a** Right renal artery. *LRA* Left renal artery. **b** This illustration shows the right common short iliac artery which compresses the left common iliac vein (long arrow) against the spinal column

venous hypertension degree: the ratio between downstream flow and upstream flow of the stenosis can in fact give an indirect measure of the stenosis degree [49] (Fig. 12a–d). Lower limb MDCT can demonstrate compression of the left common iliac vein by the right common iliac artery (Fig. 13a, b) (Clip 5. MTS. Power Doppler US showing stenosis of the left common iliac vein) and allows to exclude other causes of compression, and it can also highlight the presence of venous thrombosis (Fig. 14a, b).

Intravenous ultrasound venography is the most accurate way to define the extension and type of morphological lesions of the iliac vein [50]. MRI, like MDCT, can demonstrate compression of the left common iliac vein by the right common iliac artery and rule out other causes of compression.

Treatment

Endovascular stenting [51–53] has progressively replaced surgical thrombectomy, because it is less invasive and also represents the best therapeutic approach when pharmacological thrombolysis has contraindications. Short-term or long-term thrombolytic, anticoagulant prophylaxis, and vascular stenting currently seem to represent the treatment of choice for symptomatic MTS and hemodynamically significant stenosis of the left common iliac vein. According to the authors, in patients with thrombosis and edema of the lower limb, endovascular treatment is successful in 91% of patients. In patients with acute thrombosis, however, direct trans-catheter thrombolysis is still performed [54]. Other types of intervention have recently been reported, such as "radiofrequency thermocoagulation" [55] not yet supported, however, by sufficient case studies.

Dunbar Syndrome (DS)

Introduction

DS [56], also known as median arcuate ligament syndrome (MALS) [57], is a vascular alteration caused by compression of the celiac artery (CA) and/or surrounding neural ganglion by the median arcuate ligament (MAL) of the diaphragm. In healthy patients, the MAL

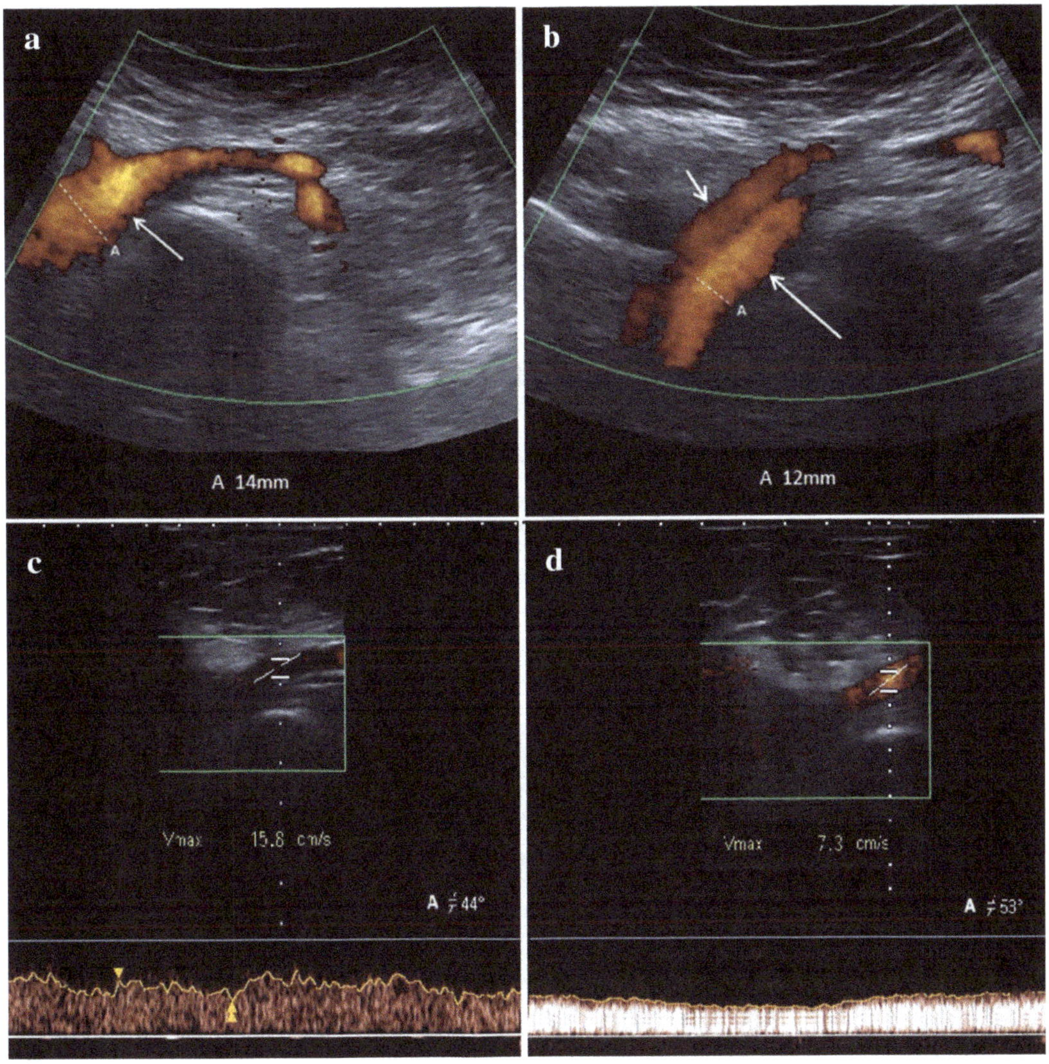

Fig. 12 Power Doppler US and Duplex Doppler US of common iliac veins. **a** Left common iliac vein (arrow) dilatation in the pre-stenotic tract (14 mm). **b** Right common iliac vein (long arrow) with regular diameter (12 mm). Right common iliac artery (short arrow). **c** Duplex Doppler US shows a regular peak speed in the post-stenotic tract of the left common iliac vein (15.8 cm/s) and peak speed reduction in the pre-stenotic tract (7.3 cm/s) -D

runs cranially to the ostium of the CA; in some patients, however, it runs more caudally, always above the origin of the CA, causing stenosis (Fig. 15). The cause of this alteration is still unknown. There are congenital factors in the literature [58], but cases in which it occurred following surgery [59] are also reported. The syndrome prevails in women between the ages of 30 and 50 [60]. The incidence is estimated at around 2 for every 100,000 patients.

Clinical implications

This vascular alteration is very difficult to diagnose, since the clinical manifestations depend on the degree

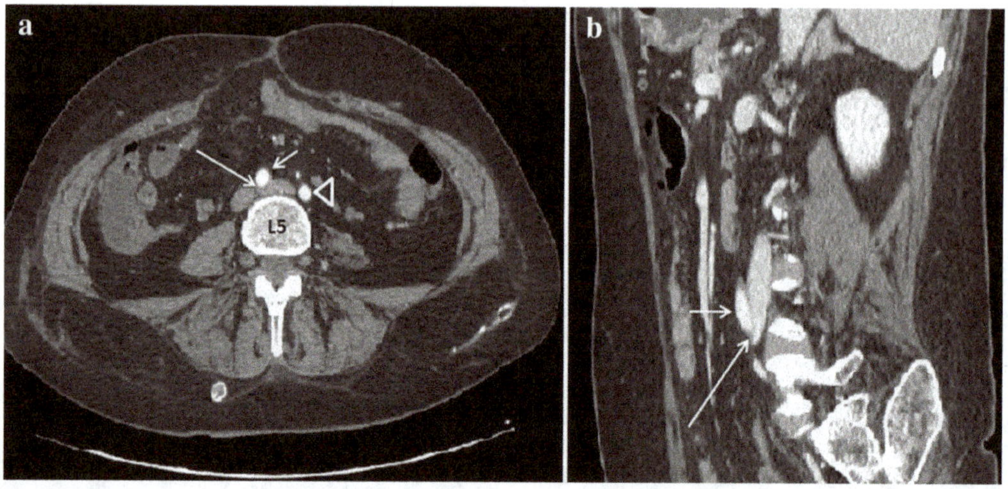

Fig. 13 Abdomen MDCT examination. **a** The axial plane reconstruction shows a stenosis of the left common iliac vein (long arrow) by the right common iliac artery (short arrow) against the vertebral column. Fifth lumbar vertebra (L5). Left common iliac artery (head arrow). **b** The sagittal plane reconstruction shows the point where the right common iliac artery (short arrow) compresses the left common iliac vein (long arrow) against the vertebral column

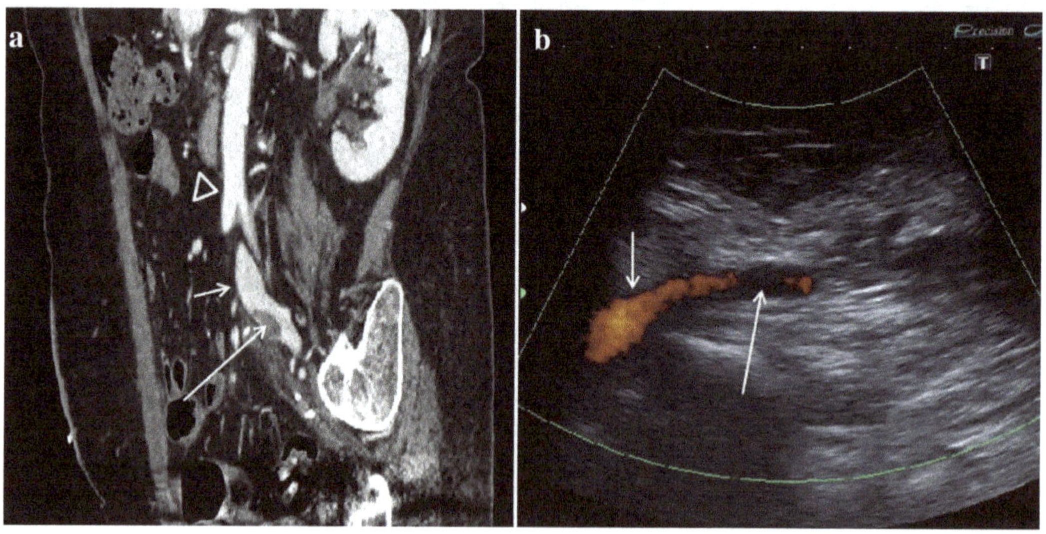

Fig. 14 Abdominal MDCT examination. **a** The sagittal plane reconstruction shows an enhancement defect (long arrow) in the left common iliac vein (short arrow) due to a thrombus. Abdominal aorta (head arrow). **b** Power Doppler US shows a thrombus (long arrow) in the left common iliac vein (short arrow)

of stenosis and are often non-specific; moreover, this disease is not well known by operators. Compression of the CA, if mild, can be asymptomatic and can go unnoticed in simple routine checks. When stenosis is significant, the resulting chronic ischemia becomes symptomatic and can change with the respiratory acts; in fact, it generally increases with forced exhalation which causes a relaxation in the diaphragm and a

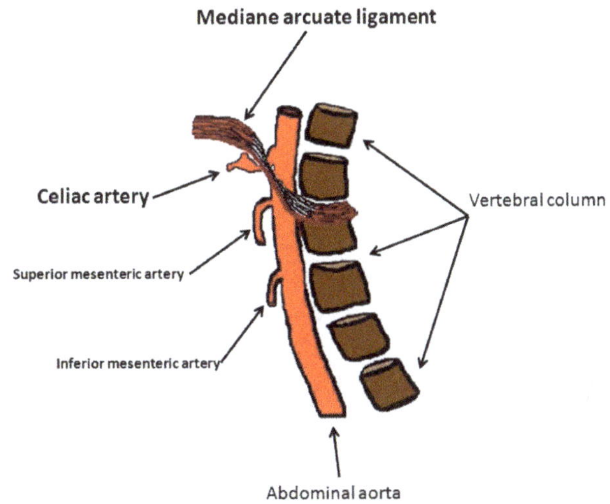

Fig. 15 DS. Scheme summarizing of the anatomical structures involved in DS. More caudal course of the MAL that compresses the CA in the expiratory apnea phase

lowering of the MAL. In more severe cases, ischemia no longer changes with respiratory acts. Symptomatology can include non-specific symptoms such as diarrhea, back-sternal pain, vomiting, swelling, and nausea, but there is a typical clinical presentation represented by a triad: weight loss, post-prandial abdominal pain (94.4%), and epigastric murmur [61, 62]. The first two symptoms are more frequent and linked to each other, because the transient functional ischemia that occurs during digestion causes pain and induces patients to limit meals causing weight loss.

Instrumental diagnosis

The diagnosis must be based on imaging and clinic, and must exclude pathologies that have a similar clinical presentation, such as cholecystitis, pancreatitis, neoplasms of the digestive tract, peptic ulcer, gastritis, appendicitis, hepatitis, intestinal ischemia, etc. To be considered DS, it must be symptomatic; therefore, in asymptomatic patients, there is no mention of DS but only of a vascular alteration well compensated by collateral circulation. Color Doppler US and Duplex Doppler US are considered to be first-level tests for diagnosis [63]. Second-level exams are represented by MDCT [64], MRI [65], and selective Angiography [66].

Color Doppler US can highlight the CA stenosis and Duplex Doppler US the consequent fluximetric variations such as the increase in the peak speed in the stenotic tract that can reach and exceed values of 200 cm/s (Fig. 16a–d) [Clip 6. DS. Duplex Doppler US which demonstrates the high-speed peaks (> 150 cm/s) due to stenosis of the CA]. MDCT can highlight the stenosis of the CA and the characteristic "Hooked appearance" that the CA assumes when it is compressed by the MAL (Fig. 17a, b). MRI can demonstrate both stenosis of the CA and the lower implant of the MAL (Fig. 18a, b).

Treatment

Therapy consists of surgical treatment with open ligament release and celiac ganglionectomy [67, 68]. Surgery allows for rapid regression of symptoms in 85% of patients. In cases of recurrence (7%), treatment with endovascular stenting may be indicated [69].

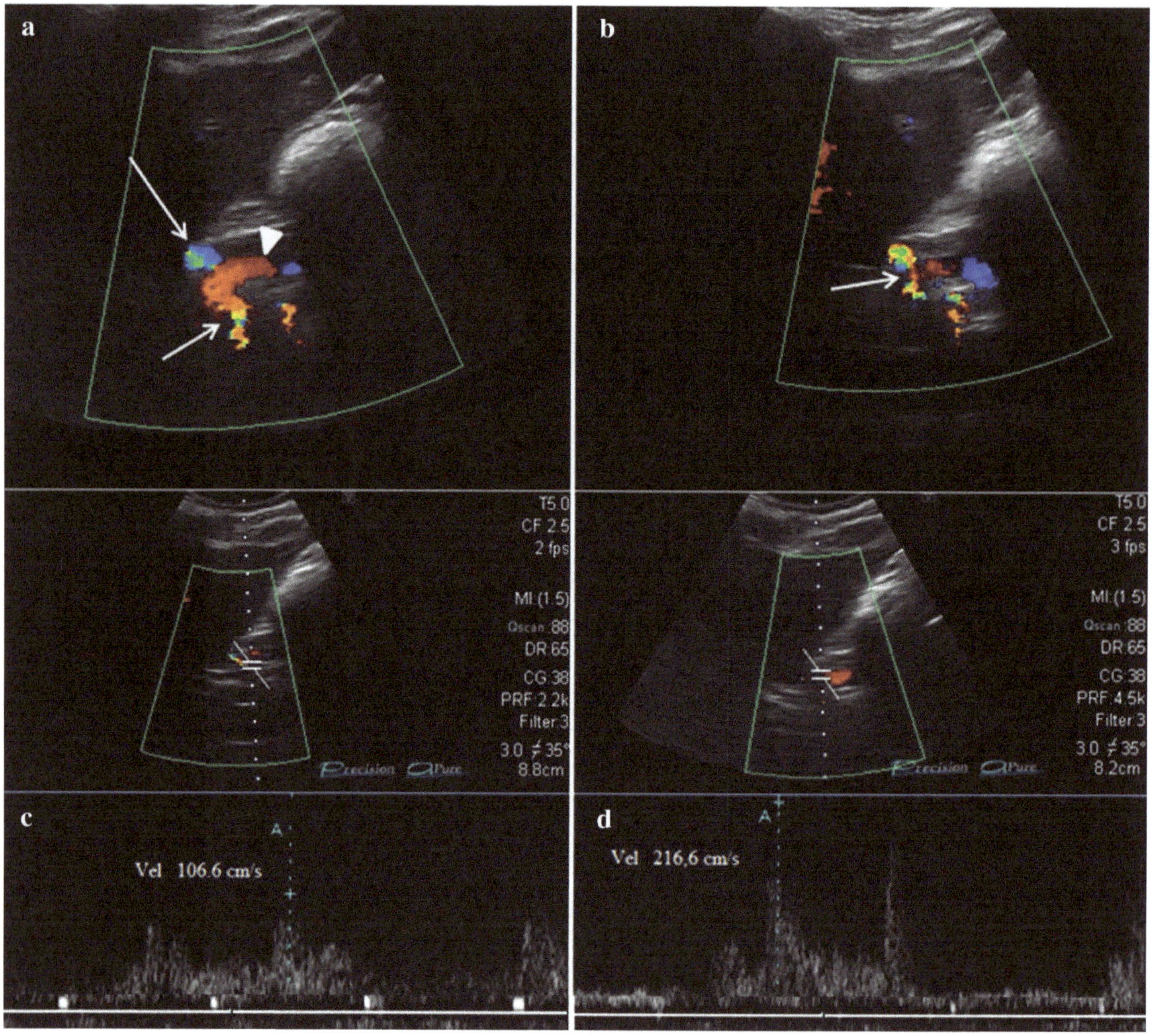

Fig. 16 Abdominal MDCT examination. **a** The axial plane reconstruction shows a stenosis of CA (arrow), origin off the abdominal aorta. **b** The sagittal plane reconstruction shows stenosis of CA with the "Hooked appearance" (long arrow). AO: Abdominal aorta. Superior mesenteric artery (short arrow)

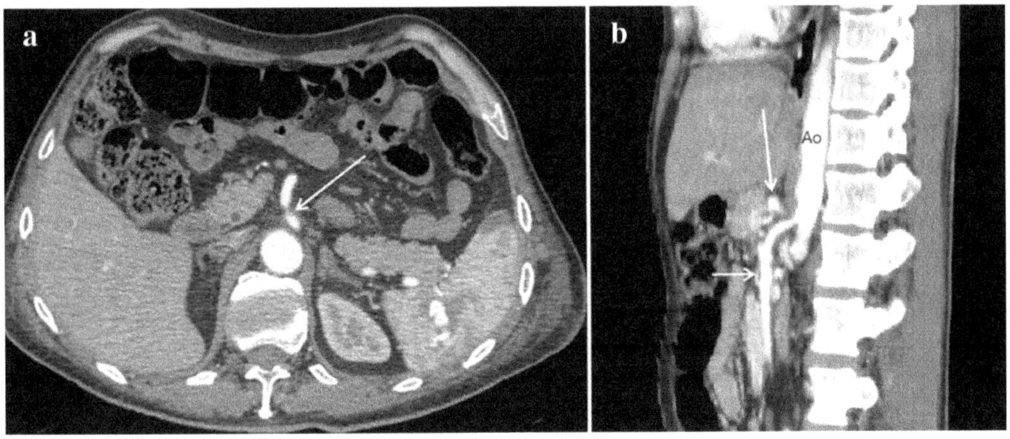

Fig. 17 Abdomen MRI examination. **a** The axial plane reconstruction shows a stenosis of CA (long arrow); origin off the abdominal aorta (short arrow). **b** The axial plane reconstruction, cranially to the CA origin, shows the MAL (arrows). Abdominal aorta (short arrow)

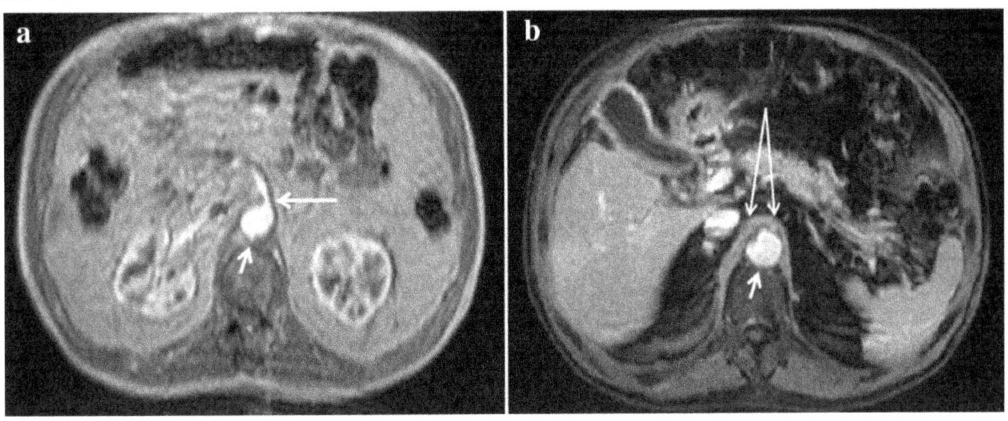

Fig. 18 Transverse sub-xiphoid Ultrasonographic scan. **a** Color Doppler US performed in inspiratory apnea that shows a regular diameter of the CA (short arrow). Epatic artery (long arrow). Splenic artery (head of arrow). **b** Color Doppler US performed in expiratory apnea that shows severe stenosis at the origin of the CA with aliasing due to turbulent flow and high-speed peak. **c** Duplex Doppler US of the CA performed in inspiratory apnea that shows a slight increase in peak speed. **d** Duplex Doppler of the CA performed in expiratory apnea that shows very high peak speeds (> 200 cm/s) due to severe stenosis

Conclusions

Ultrasound imaging plays an important role in the diagnosis of vascular compression syndromes. It allows you to significantly reduce false negatives and, in doubtful cases, provides indications for any further diagnostic analysis with second level methods. Failure to diagnose and treat, in these patients, could have serious consequences for their health.

Abbreviations

TOS: Thoracic Outlet syndrome; US: Ultrasound; MRI: Magnetic Resonance Imaging; MDCT: Multidetector Computed Tomography; NCS: Nutckracker Syndrome; WS: Wilkie Syndrome; DS: Dunbar Syndrome; MALS: Mediane Arcuate Ligament Syndrome; CA: Celiac Artery; MAL: Mediane Arcuate Ligament; AO: Abdominal Aorta.; IVC: Inferior Cava Vein.; RRA: Right Renal Artery.; LRA: Left Renal Artery.

Acknowledgements

The authors thank Lucia Zuccarello (Radiodiagnostic and Radiotherapy Unit, Department of Medical and Surgical Sciences and Advanced Technologies "GF Ingrassia" Catania Italy) for her technical assistance.

Authors' contributions

RF study design/planning collected data, preparation of manuscript, data analysis/statistics, data interpretation, and involved in project development, literature analysis/search. PVF, AC, FAI, IP, CI, FL, and SS collected data, wrote the manuscript, literature analysis/search. LF, FV, GF, DB, SP, and AB: collected data and wrote the manuscript. All authors read and approved the final manuscript.

References

1. Jones MR, Prabhakar A, Viswanath O et al (2019) Thoracic outlet syndrome: a comprehensive review of pathophysiology, diagnosis, and treatment. Pain Ther 8(1):5–18
2. Pesser N, Teijink JAW, Vervaart K et al. (2020) Value of Ultrasound in the Diagnosis of Neurogenic Thoracic Outlet Syndrome. Eur J Vasc Endovasc Surg.
3. Schut PC, Eggink AJ, Cohen-Overbeek TE et al (2020) Miscarriage is associated with cervical ribs in thoracic outlet syndrome patients. Early Hum Dev 144:105027
4. Benzon HT, Rodes ME, Chekka K et al (2012) Scalene muscle injections for neurogenic thoracic outlet syndrome: case series. Pain Pract 12(1):66–70
5. Farina R, Foti PV, Iannace FA et al. (2019) Thoracic outlet syndrome: a rare case with bilateral cervical ribs and bilateral anterior scalene hypertrophy. J Ultrasound.
6. Kaplan T, Comert A, Esmer AF et al (2018) The importance of costoclavicular space on possible compression of the subclavian artery in the thoracic outlet region: a radio-anatomical study. Interact Cardiovasc Thorac Surg 27(4):561–565
7. Sharma P, Rasheed I, Ansari MA et al (2010) Cervical rib causing thrombosis of subclavian artery. JNMA J Nepal Med Assoc 49(178):161–163
8. Fried SM, Nazarian LN (2013) Dynamic neuromusculoskeletal ultrasound documentation of brachial plexus/thoracic outlet compression during elevated arm stress testing. Hand (N Y) 8(3):358–365
9. Bigler MR, Buffle E, Siontis GCM et al (2019) Invasive assessment of the human arterial palmar arch and forearm collateral function during transradial access. Circ Cardiovasc Interv 12(7):e007744
10. Fuhrman TM, Pippin WD, Talmage LA et al (1992) Evaluation of collateral circulation of the hand. J Clin Monit 8(1):28–32
11. Hixson KM, Horris HB, McLeod TCV et al (2017) The diagnostic accuracy of clinical diagnostic tests for thoracic outlet syndrome. J Sport Rehabil 26(5):459–465
12. Wilson MP, Low G, Katlariwala P et al (2020) Ultrasound for eurogenic thoracic outlet obstruction remains theoretical. Diagnostics (Basel) 10:4
13. Wadhwani R, Chaubal JN, Sukthankar R et al (2001) Color Doppler and duplex sonography in 5 patients with thoracic outlet syndrome. Ultrasound Med. 20(7):795–801
14. Chavhan GB, Batmanabane V, Muthusami P et al (2017) MRI of thoracic outlet syndrome in children. Pediatr Radiol 47(10):1222–1234
15. Ghouri MA, Gupta N, Bhat AP et al (2019) CT and MR imaging of the upper extremity vasculature: pearls, pitfalls, and challenges. Cardiovasc Diagn Ther 9(Suppl 1):S152–S173
16. Svensson A, Brismar TB, Brehmer K (2020) Computed tomography venography of the upper extremities - Using low dose bilateral contrast media injection in a patient with suspected venous thoracic outlet syndrome. Radiol Case Rep 15(3):302–305
17. Chang KZ, Likes K, Davis K et al (2013) The significance of cervical ribs in thoracic outlet syndrome. J Vasc Surg 57(3):771–775
18. Rochlin DH, Orlando MS, Likes KC et al (2014) Bilateral first rib resection and scalenectomy is effective for treatment of thoracic outlet syndrome. J Vasc Surg 60(1):185–190
19. Vanti C, Natalini L, Romeo A et al (2007) Conservative treatment of thoracic outlet syndrome. A review of the literature. Eura Medicophys. 43(1):55–70
20. Oh MJ (2017) Superior mesenteric artery syndrome combined with renal nutcracker syndrome in a young male: a case report. Korean J Gastroenterol 70(5):253–260
21. Wilkie DPD (1927) Chronic duodenal ileus. Am J Med Sci 173:643
22. De Macedo GL, Dos Santos MA, Sarris AB et al (2018) Diagnosis and treatment of the Nutcracker syndrome: a review of the last 10 years. J Vasc Bras 17(3):220–228
23. Gebhart T (2015) Superior mesenteric artery syndrome. Gastroenterol Nurs 38:189–193
24. Farina R, Pennisi F, Politi G et al (1999) Color Doppler-echo in Wilkie's syndrome. A case report. Radiol Med 98(3):206–207
25. Gulleroglu K, Gulleroglu B, Baskin E (2014) Nutcracker syndrome. World. J Nephrol 4:277–281
26. Genov PP, Kirilov IV, Hristova IA et al (2019) Management and diagnosis of Nutcracker syndrome-a case report. Urol Case Rep 29:101103
27. Mauceri B, Misseri M, Tsami A et al (2010) Ultrasound in diagnosis of superior mesenteric artery syndrome. Clin Ter 161(1):35–37
28. Cicero G, D'Angelo T, Bottari A et al (2018) Superior mesenteric artery syndrome in patients with crohn's disease: a description of 2 cases studied with a novel magnetic resonance enterography (MRE) procedure. Am J Case Rep 19:431–437
29. Warncke ES, Gursahaney DL, Mascolo M et al (2019) Superior mesenteric artery syndrome: a radiographic review. Abdom Radiol (NY) 44(9):3188–3194
30. Di Matteo F, Picconi F, Sansoni I et al (2010) Superior mesenteric artery syndrome diagnosed with linear endoscopic ultrasound. Endoscopy. 42(Suppl 2):E67–E68
31. Agrawal GA, Johnson PT, Fisherman EK (2007) Multidetector row CT of superior mesenteric artery syndrome. J Cin Gastroenterol 41(1):62–65
32. Er A, Uzunlulu N, Guzelbey T, Yavuz S et al (2019) The nutcracker syndrome: The usefulness of different MRI sequences for diagnosis and follow-up. Clin Imaging 55:144–147
33. Wong HI, Chen MC, Wu CS et al (2010) The usefulness of fast-spin-echo T2-weighted MR imaging in Nutcracker syndrome: a case report. Korean J Radiol 11(3):373–377
34. Farina R, Foti PV, Cocuzza G et al (2017) Wilkie's syndrome. J Ultrasound 20(4):339–342
35. Shin JI, Baek SY, Lee JS et al (2007) Follow-up and treatment of nutcracker syndrome. Ann Vasc Surg 21:402
36. Jain N, Chopde A, Soni B et al. (2020) SMA syndrome: management perspective with laparoscopic duodenojejunostomy and long-term results. Surg Endosc.
37. Agle CG, Amorim DS, De Almeida LC et al (2019) Endovascular treatment of Nutcracker syndrome: case report. J Vasc Bras 18:e20180135
38. Wang He, Guo Y-T, Jiao Y et al (2019) A minimally invasive alternative for the treatment of nutcracker syndrome using individualized three-dimensional printed extravascular titanium stents. Chin Med J (Engl) 132(12):1454–1460
39. May R, Thurner J (1957) The cause of the predominantly sinistral occurrence of thrombosis of the pelvic veins. Angiology 8(5):419–427
40. Du Pont B, Verbist J, Van den Eynde W et al (2016) Right-sided Cockett's syndrome. Acta Chir Belg 116(2):114–118
41. Cheng L, Zhao H, Zhang FX (2017) Iliac vein compression syndrome in an asymptomatic patient population: a prospective study. Chin Med J (Engl) 130(11):1269–1275
42. Molloy S, Jacob S, Buckenham T et al (2002) Arterial compression of the right common iliac vein; an unusual anatomical variant. Cardiovasc Surg 10:291–292
43. Farina R, Foti PV, Iannace FA et al. (2020) May Thurner syndrome: description of a case with unusual clinical onset. J Ultrasound.
44. Palma L, Peterson MD, Ingebretsen R (1995) Iliac vein compression syndrome from urinary bladder distension due to prostatism. South Med J 88:959–960
45. Rosengarten AM, Wong J, Gibbons S (2002) Endometriosis causing cyclic compression of the right external iliac vein with cyclic edema of the right leg and thigh. J Obstet Gynaecol Can 24:33–35
46. Justa DG, Bianco FJ Jr, Ogle A et al (2003) Deep venous thrombosis due to compression of external iliac vein by the penile prosthesis reservoir. Urology 61:462
47. Janczak D, Rucinski A, Skora J et al (2000) Iliac-femoral vein thrombosis as a first symptom of the isolated common and internal illiac artery aneurysm. Wiad Lek 53(458–61):18
48. Rosenthal D, Matsuura JH, Jerius H et al (1998) Iliofemoral venous thrombosis caused by compression of an internal iliac artery aneurysm: a minimally invasive treatment. J Endovasc Surg 5:142–145
49. Liyanage AM, Shafiq T, Wadekar VR et al (2018) An Unusual Presentation of Deep Vein Thrombosis. Eur J Case Rep Intern Med 5(8):000899
50. Qian AM, Cai ZX, Zhang S et al (2019) Endovascular treatment for non-thrombotic right iliac vein compression syndrome with intravascular ultrasound. Zhonghua Yi Xue Za Zhi 99(46):3633–3637
51. Bondarev S, Keller EJ, Han T et al (2019) Predictors of Disease Recurrence after Venoplasty and Stent Placement for May-Thurner Syndrome. J Vasc Interv Radiol 30(10):1549–1554
52. Gavrilov SG, Vasilyev AV, Krasavin GV et al. (2020) Endovascular interventions in the treatment of pelvic congestion syndrome caused by May-Thurner syndrome. J Vasc Surg Venous Lymphat Disord.

53. Barge TF, Wilton E, Wigham A (2020) Endovascular treatment of an extensive iliocaval and renal vein thrombosis secondary to inferior vena cava stenosis and May-Thurner type iliac vein compression: a case report. Vasc Endovascular Surg 54(3):297–300
54. Lopez R, DeMartino R, Fleming M et al (2019) Aspiration thrombectomy for acute iliofemoral or central deep venous thrombosis. J Vasc Surg Venous Lymphat Disord 7(2):162–168
55. Xu F, Tian Z, Huang X et al (2019) A case report of May-Thurner syndrome induced by anterior lumbar disc herniation: Novel treatment with radiofrequency thermocoagulation. Medicine (Baltimore) 98(44):e17706
56. Santos GM, Viarengo LMA, Oliveira MDP (2019) Celiac artery compression: Dunbar syndrome. J Vasc Bras 18:e20180094
57. Camacho N, Alves G, Bastos Gonçalves F et al (2017) Median arcuate ligament syndrome - literature review and case report. Rev Port Cir Cardiotorac Vasc 24(3–4):111
58. Bech F, Loesberg A, Rosenblum J et al (1994) Median arcuate ligament compression syndrome in monozygotic twins. J Vasc Surg 19(5):934–938
59. Ali M, Patel J (2016) Dunbar syndrome following liver transplantation. BMJ Case Rep. 2016:bcr2015214168
60. Köhler M, Schardey HM, Bettels R et al (2018) Median arcuate ligament syndrome - imaging presentation and interdisciplinary management. Rofo 190(10):907–914
61. Sunkara T, Caughey M, Cai ZK et al (2017) Dunbar syndrome- a rare cause of foregut ischemia. J Clin Diagn Res. 11(7):OD13–OD14
62. Saleem T, Baril DT (2020) Celiac artery compression syndrome. StatPearls. StatPearls Publishing, Treasure Island (FL)
63. Acampora C, Di Serafino M, Iacobellis F et al. (2020) Insight into Dunbar syndrome: color-Doppler ultrasound findings and literature review. J Ultrasound. 2020.
64. Patel MV, Dalag L, Weiner A et al (2019) Inability of conventional imaging findings to predict response to laparoscopic release of the median arcuate ligament in patients with celiac artery compression. J Vasc Surg 69(2):462–469
65. Klimas A, Lemmer A, Bergert H et al (2015) Laparoscopic treatment of celiac artery compression syndrome in children and adolescents. Vasa 44(4):305–312
66. Berek P, Kopolovets I, Dzsinich, et al (2018) Celiac axis compression syndrome - diagnostic and surgical treatment. Rozhl Chir Summer 97(9):423–426
67. Grus T, Klika T, Grusová G et al (2018) Dunbar syndrome - single-center experience with surgical treatment. Rozhl Chir Winter 97(11):514–517
68. Torres OJM, Gama-Filho OP, Torres CCS et al (2017) Laparoscopic treatment of Dunbar syndrome: a case report. Int J Surg Case Rep 37:230–232
69. Hongsakul K, Rookkapan S, Sungsiri J et al (2012) A severe case of median arcuate ligament syndrome with successful angioplasty and stenting. Case Rep Vasc Med 1:129870

10

Routine lung ultrasound to detect postoperative pulmonary complications following major abdominal surgery: a prospective observational feasibility study

H. R. Touw[1,4*], A. E. Schuitemaker[1], F. Daams[3], D. L. van der Peet[3], E. M. Bronkhorst[5], P. Schober[1], C. Boer[1] and P. R. Tuinman[2]

Abstract

Background: Postoperative pulmonary complications after major abdominal surgery are associated with adverse outcome. The diagnostic accuracy of chest X-rays (CXR) to detect pulmonary disorders is limited. Alternatively, lung ultrasound (LUS) is an established evidence-based point-of-care diagnostic modality which outperforms CXR in critical care. However, its feasibility and diagnostic ability for postoperative pulmonary complications following abdominal surgery are unknown. In this prospective observational feasibility study, we included consecutive patients undergoing major abdominal surgery with an intermediate or high risk developing postoperative pulmonary complications according to the Assess Respiratory risk In Surgical patients in CATalonia (ARISCAT) score. LUS was routinely performed on postoperative days 0–3 by a researcher blinded for CXR or other clinical findings. Then, reports were drawn up for LUS concerning feasibility and detection rates of postoperative pulmonary complications. CXRs were performed on demand according to daily clinical practice. Subsequently, we compared LUS and CXR findings.

Results: A total of 98 consecutive patients with an ARISCAT score of 41 (34–49) were included in the study. LUS was feasible in all patients. In 94 (95%) patients, LUS detected one or more postoperative pulmonary complications during the first four postoperative days. On day 0, LUS detected 31 out of 43 patients (72.1%) with one or more postoperative pulmonary complications, compared to 13 out of 36 patients (36.1%) with 1 or more postoperative pulmonary complications detected with CXR RR 2.0 (95 CI [1.24–3.20]) ($p = 0.004$). The number of discordant observations between both modalities was high for atelectasis 23 (43%) and pleural effusion 29 (54%), but not for pneumothorax, respiratory infection and pulmonary edema 8 (15%), 3 (5%), and 5 (9%), respectively.

Conclusions: This study shows that LUS is highly feasible and frequently detects postoperative pulmonary complications after major abdominal surgery. Discordant observations in atelectasis and pleural effusions for LUS and CXR can be explained by a superior diagnostic ability of LUS in detecting these conditions. The effects of LUS as primary imaging modality on patient outcome should be evaluated in future studies.

Keywords: Surgical procedures, Abdominal surgery, Postoperative complications, Chest X-ray and lung ultrasound

*Correspondence: h.touw@amsterdamumc.nl; hugo.touw@radboudumc.nl
[1] Department of Anaesthesiology, Amsterdam UMC, Vrije Universiteit Amsterdam, Amsterdam Cardiovascular Sciences, De Boelelaan 1117, 1081 HV Amsterdam, The Netherlands
Full list of author information is available at the end of the article

Introduction

There is increasing interest in early detection of postoperative pulmonary complications (PPCs) to reduce patient morbidity and mortality [1]. Furthermore, in patients unexpectedly admitted to the intensive care unit (ICU), insufficient diagnostic imaging was often performed on the general ward and inadequate treatments were initiated [2]. Early PPC detection would enable physicians to start treatment in time and, therefore, prevent its negative impact on patient outcome.

Respiratory failure following anaesthesia and surgery typically starts with atelectasis, due to diaphragmatic dysfunction, inability to clear secretions and immobility. Chest auscultation and chest X-ray (CXR) are frequently used as diagnostic modalities to detect PPCs, but have limited diagnostic accuracy [3–6]. Moreover, ideally, radiography requires an upright position of the patient, and multiple concomitant lung abnormalities further complicate the two-dimensional interpretation [7–9]. Computed tomography (CT) is the gold standard for pulmonary pathology but requires significant ionizing radiation and the need for transfers within the hospital, which is not without risk [3].

Alternatively, lung ultrasound (LUS) is a quick, point-of-care and radiation free technique. It has an excellent diagnostic accuracy for atelectasis, pulmonary effusions, pulmonary edema, and/or pneumonia in critically ill patients compared to the gold standard CT [3, 4, 6]. Therefore, LUS is well established in these pathologies, and practical approaches to perform LUS have been described extensively elsewhere [10, 11]. We previously showed that, in cardiothoracic surgery patients, LUS detected more (clinically relevant) PPCs compared to CXR and at an earlier time point [12]. Following major abdominal surgery, the feasibility could be limited by dressings, chest drains, or subcutaneous emphysema.

Daily routine CXR has been largely abandoned in ICU and cardiothoracic patients due to its limitations, costs, and radiation burden. On demand, CXR performance has led to a significant decrease in the number of CXRs without any increase in adverse events in ICU patients [13]. Studies comparing on-demand strategies with routine strategies are lacking in patients after major abdominal surgery. However, performing CXR on demand does not facilitate early detection of postoperative pulmonary complications. Potentially, routine LUS can detect PPCs early and with higher accuracy to improve perioperative management in major abdominal surgery patients [4, 10, 14].

The primary objective of this pilot study was to test the feasibility of routine LUS following major abdominal surgery and to report the detected PPCs with LUS in these postoperative patients. Subsequently, PPC detection rates for LUS and CXR were compared.

Methods

We conducted this prospective, observational feasibility study in the Amsterdam UMC—VU University Medical Center Amsterdam (VUmc Amsterdam, The Netherlands), a tertiary hospital. The local Human Subjects Committee of the VUmc approved the study (METc 16/128), and written informed consent was obtained from all participants. Patient inclusion started June 2016 and ended March 2017. Patients were included on the general ward. The study included consecutive adult patients (age ≥ 18 years) scheduled for elective major abdominal (e.g., gastrointestinal, vascular, or renal) surgery with an intermediate or high risk for the development of postoperative pulmonary complications according to the Assess Respiratory risk In Surgical patients in CATalonia (ARISCAT) risk score ≥ 26 (https://www.mdcalc.com/ariscat-score-postoperative-pulmonary-complications) [15, 16]. Exclusion criteria were trauma or emergency surgery.

Patient characteristics

Patient characteristics were retrieved from the patient data management system and included age, gender, weight, length and body mass index (BMI), American Society of Anesthesiology (ASA) classification, the ARISCAT score, co morbidities, alcohol use, and smoker status. Perioperative parameters were also retrieved and included type of surgery, ICU referral, and total in-hospital length of stay. Patient and laboratory data included the following: arterial oxygen saturation, mode of ventilation, O_2 supplementation, sputum cultures, temperature, and leukocyte count.

Chest X-ray

CXR was performed according to standard clinical practice (e.g., after placement of chest tube or central venous line placement) and when demanded by the treating physician for clinical reasons. Anteroposterior bedside CXRs were obtained using a DRX-Revolution mobile X-ray unit (Carestream Health, Inc. © Toronto, Canada). CXR findings, assessed by a radiologist blinded to the LUS findings, were retrospectively retrieved from the patient data management system (PDMS). The Nomenclature Committee of the Fleischner Society recommended terminology was used to describe pathological entities according to the diagnostic criteria for bedside CXR [17, 18].

Lung ultrasound

LUS was routinely performed by a trained member of the research team ($n = 3$), which consisted of two dedicated investigators and one ICU fellow. LUS was performed upon admission after surgery on postoperative day (POD) 0, and on all consecutive PODs 1–3. Daily LUS was intended, but ultimately could not be performed in a large proportion of the time because of limited researcher availability, e.g., admission after working hours and follow-up days in the weekends. All ultrasonographers were trained according to The Netherlands Society of Intensive Care Programme for Intensive Care Ultrasound (NVIC ICARUS) training course (https://www.nvic.nl). The ultrasonographer was blinded to clinical details and CXR findings, and did not contribute to the diagnostic and treatment strategy of the patient. We used a CX50 ultrasound machine (Koninklijke Philips NV®, Eindhoven, The Netherlands) with both the cardiac phased array (1-5 MHz) and the linear vascular probe (> 10 MHz). The ultrasonographer could choose a particular probe for a particular view in a particular patient, according to individual preference. Lung sliding was determined using the vascular probe. LUS views were obtained according to the BLUE protocol [13, 19].

LUS was performed according the BLUE protocol and adjusted for the postoperative setting [12]. BLUE profile for each BLUE point (Fig. 1) and BLUE profile per hemithorax (BLUE 1 and 2) was determined as follows: A; B; A′; B′; or C profile. A profile means predominantly A lines (Fig. 2). B profile means predominantly multiple (> 2) anterior diffuse B lines indicating interstitial syndrome (Fig. 3). A′ or B′ means the corresponding BLUE profile with absence of, or abolished lung sliding. C profile means anterior alveolar consolidation (Fig. 4). Furthermore, we determined the postero-lateral alveolar and/or pleural syndrome (PLAPS) (Figs. 1, 5) at the lateral sub-posterior sides of the chest and scored them as positive or negative. When positive, consolidation and/or pleural effusion were scored separately and the diagnosis of atelectasis was added to the flowchart. The final conclusion was made according to the bedside LUS protocol in cardiothoracic patients, as published in the previous research [12]. For differentiation between pneumonia and atelectasis, the ultrasonographer was also allowed to look for fever, leukocyte count, and C-reactive protein (CRP) in the PDMS (data also available to the radiologist).

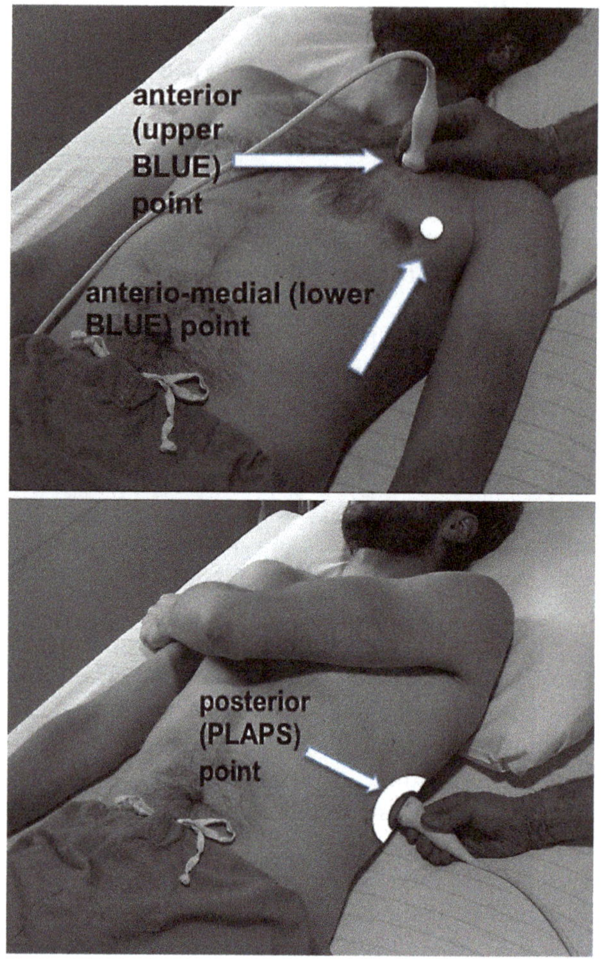

Fig. 1 BLUE and PLAPS points. Anterior (upper BLUE) point. Anteromedial (lower BLUE) point. Posterior (PLAPS) point

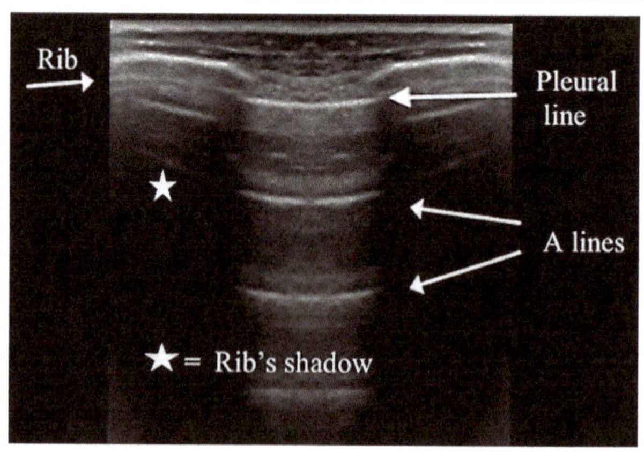

Fig. 2 A profile according to the BLUE protocol showing multiple A lines

Postoperative pulmonary complications

The incidence of PPCs detected with CXR was retrieved by a research team member using the PDMS. PPCs were scored according to reported radiology findings of on-demand CXR studies ordered by the treating physician at the ward. PPCs were scored as previously defined by Canet et al.: respiratory infection defined as treatment with antibiotics for a suspected respiratory infection and at least one of the following criteria: new or changed sputum, new or changed lung opacities, fever, leukocyte count > 12,000/mm^3; pleural effusion defined by blunting of the costophrenic angle, loss of the sharp silhouette of the ipsilateral hemidiaphragm in upright

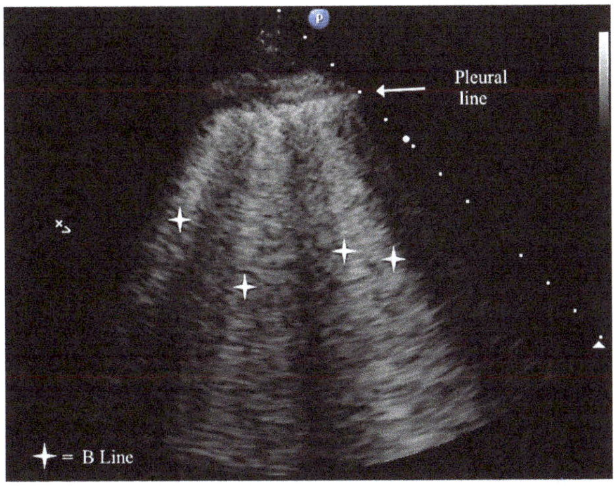

Fig. 3 B profile according to the BLUE protocol showing multiple B lines

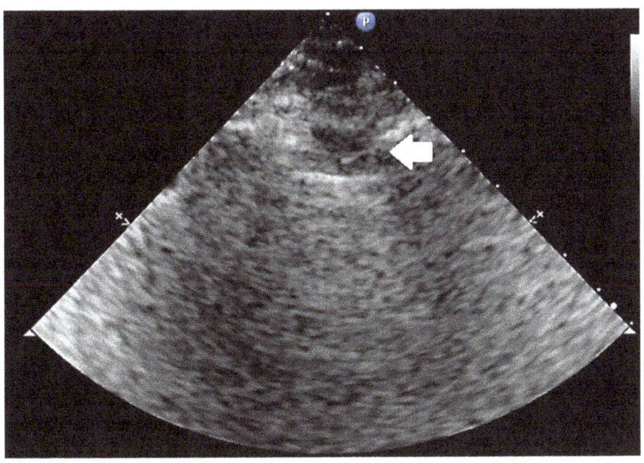

Fig. 4 C profile according to the BLUE protocol showing a C line. Arrow indicates a hypoechoic subpleural focal image generated by consolidated lung tissue

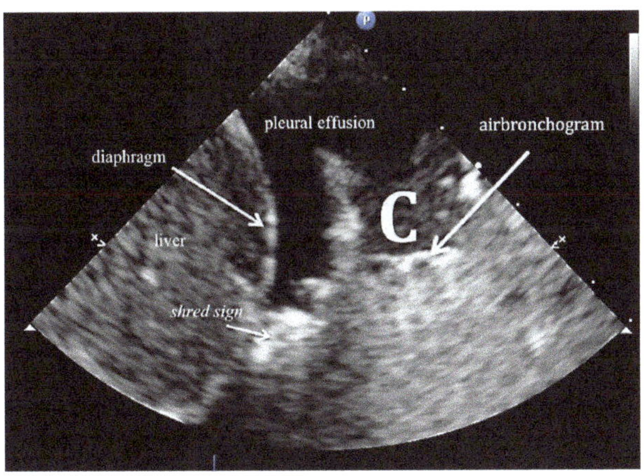

Fig. 5 Posterolateral alveolar and/or pleural syndrome

position, evidence of displacement of adjacent anatomical structures, or (in supine position) a hazy opacity in one hemithorax with preserved vascular shadows; atelectasis defined by lung opacification with shift of the mediastinum, hilum, or hemidiaphragm towards the affected area and compensatory over-inflation in the adjacent non-atelectatic lung; and pneumothorax defined by the air in the pleural space with no vascular bed surrounding the visceral pleura, all demonstrated by the CXR [15, 16].

Clinically relevant postoperative pulmonary complications

Clinically relevant PPCs, defined as a PPC that required treatment, as judged by the treating physician, were also reported [12]. We considered the following initiated treatments for scoring clinically relevant PPCs: re-intubation; ICU admission; bronchoscopy; extra bronchodilator therapy; thoracic drain placement; and the use of diuretics and/or antibiotics. Scores of clinically relevant PPCs were retrospectively retrieved from the PDMS according to initiated treatment by the treating physicians for PPCs at the ward. For example: a found pneumothorax which did not require drainage was counted as a PPC but not as a crPPC. The physician who diagnosed clinically relevant PPCs took the following into account: physical examination, conventional monitoring, laboratory results, CXR, and/or CT scan results when available. This reflected daily clinical practice. The treating physicians were blinded to LUS findings.

Statistical analysis

We included as many consecutive patients as possible in the study period. We planned to include more than 90 patients to detect around 30 PPCs based on incidence rates of PPCs after surgery [16]. Results of this study will be used to plan a larger study on the effects of LUS on patient outcome after major abdominal surgery. We performed statistical data analyses using SPSS statistical software package version 22.0 (IBM, New York, NY, USA). Feasibility was reported as percentage of patients in which LUS was possible. Detection rates of PPCs during the study period were reported as frequencies. A PPC could only develop once. For example, if a pleural effusion was detected on POD1, it could not be scored again on POD2. However, a patient could develop more than one PPC during the study period and during 1 day. In addition, detection rates were compared according to both imaging modalities. Furthermore, an aggregated analysis was performed to compare the detection of PPCs in patients who had both; CXR and LUS were performed the same day during the study period. Relative risk was calculated comparing PPC detection with LUS and CXR. Discordant observations were compared for PPCs detected with LUS and CXR.

Table 1 Perioperative patient characteristics

Patient characteristics	Values
N	98
Males/females (*n*)	59/39
Age (years)	64 ± 11.7
Body mass index (kg/m^2)	26.1 ± 4.6
Hypertension	39 (39.8)
COPD	11 (11.2)
Oncology	79 (81.4)
Median ASA physical status	2 [2, 3]
Median ARISCAT score	41 [34-49]
Types of surgery, *n* (%)	
Esophageal	14 (14.3)
Gastric	9 (9.2)
Hepatic	19 (19.4)
Pancreatic	12 (12.2)
Vascular	6 (6.1)
Renal	16 (16.3)
Other gastrointestinal	22 (22.4)

Data represent mean ± standard deviation, median with [interquartile range] or number of cases (percentage)

ASA American Society of Anesthesiologists, *ARISCAT* Assess Respiratory risk In Surgical patients in CATalonia

Results

115 patients were considered eligible for inclusion. 110 patients signed informed consent, 12 were excluded because of postoperative correction of initial ARISCAT score ($n = 7$) or cancelling informed consent ($n = 5$). Overall, 98 consecutive patients were included in the study. Table 1 shows the patient characteristics of included patients. One patient died within the 30 day follow-up period.

Routine lung ultrasound: feasibility and incidence of PPCs

In 100% of patients, LUS was feasible. In total, routine LUS detected in 94 out of 98 patients (96%) one or more PPCs in the study period. Table 2 shows the incidence rates of newly detected PPCs with LUS.

Lung ultrasound compared with chest X-ray

CXR examinations performed and incidence rates of PPCs detected are shown in Table 3. 36 out of 98 patients (37%) with one or more PPCs were detected with on-demand CXR in the study period. On POD 0, LUS detected 31 out of 43 patients (72.1%) with one or more PPCs, compared to 13 out of 36 patients (36.1%) with one or more PPCs detected with CXR ($p = 0.004$) RR 2.0 (95% CI [1.24–3.20]). LUS and CXR mainly identified atelectasis and pleural effusion, as shown in Tables 2 and 3. However, the number of discordant observations between CXR and LUS for atelectasis and pleural effusion was much higher: 23 and 29 (43% and 54%), respectively. (Table 4) For pneumothorax, respiratory infection and

Table 2 Incidence rates per day of newly detected postoperative pulmonary complications with point-of-care lung ultrasound after major abdominal surgery

Day	Number of patients in which LUS is performed (*N*)	Patients with ≥ 1 PPC [*N* (%)]	Respiratory infection	Pneumothorax	Pulmonary edema	Atelectasis	Pleural effusion
POD 0	43	31 (72%)	2	2	0	29	10
POD 1	92	64 (70%)	0	4	2	55	31
POD 2	87	21 (24%)	4	0	1	9	9
POD 3	56	8 (14%)	1	0	2	1	5

Patients can develop multiple PPCs. Total amount of PPCs can be higher than the number of patients

LUS lung ultrasound, *PPC* postoperative pulmonary complication, *POD* postoperative day

Table 3 Incidence rates of newly detected postoperative pulmonary complications with 'on-demand' chest X-ray after major abdominal surgery according to daily clinical practice

Day	Number of patients in which CXR is performed (on demand)	Patients with *N* ≥ 1 PPC [*N* (%)]	Respiratory infection	Pneumothorax	Pulmonary edema	Atelectasis	Pleural effusion
POD 0	36	13 (36%)	0	2	3	9	4
POD 1	19	13 (72%)	0	4	3	9	6
POD 2	13	7 (54%)	0	2	0	3	5
POD 3	9	3 (33%)	0	1	1	1	3

Patients can develop multiple PPCs. Total amount of PPCs can be higher than the number of patients

CXR chest X-ray, *PPC* postoperative pulmonary complication, *POD* postoperative day

Table 4 Discordant pairs of newly detected atelectasis and pleural effusion for lung ultrasound and chest X-ray when concomitantly performed ($n = 54$) between days 0 and 4 in 98 patients after abdominal surgery

Atelectasis	LUS			Pleural Effusion	LUS		
	No	Yes	Total		No	Yes	Total
CRX				CRX			
No	10	17	27	No	15	15	30
Yes	6	11	17	Yes	14	10	24
Total	16	28	54	Total	29	25	54

Table 5 Incidence of newly detected clinically relevant postoperative pulmonary complications on days 0, 1, 2, 3, and 4–30 in 98 patients after abdominal surgery

Clinically relevant PPCs	Day 0	Day 1	Day 2	Day 3	Day 4-30
Pneumonia	0	0	0	3	5
Pneumothorax	0	0	0	1	0
Pulmonary edema	0	1	3	3	0
Atelectasis	0	0	2	1	0
Pleural effusion	0	2	1	2	2

Data represent number of cases (percentage)

PPCs postoperative pulmonary complications

pulmonary edema the number of discordant pairs were 8, 3, and 5 (15%, 5%, and 9%), respectively.

The incidence of clinically relevant postoperative pulmonary complications

In total, 13 patients (13%) developed a clinically relevant PPC. Six patients were readmitted to the ICU and 1 was re-intubated for respiratory failure. The incidence of new clinically relevant PPCs during the study period POD 0–4 is shown in Table 5. The incidence of new clinically relevant PPCs increased over the first 4 days, with a maximum of 10 PPCs on POD 3. For 8 patients, the incidence of respiratory infection could be followed up to 30 days postoperatively. LUS detected consolidations in 7 out of 8 patients treated for respiratory infection and CXR detected consolidations in 5 out of 8 patients during the study period.

Discussion

This pilot study demonstrates that routine LUS is highly feasible and frequently detects PPCs in patients following major abdominal surgery. In addition, LUS detected more PPCs when compared to CXR when both modalities were performed on POD 0. Importantly, the discordant observations for LUS and CXR were highest for atelectasis and pleural effusion.

We confirm that LUS is highly feasible in postoperative patients [12, 20, 21]. Goudy et al. found that LUS was feasible in 97% of the hemi thoraxes in 252 ultrasound examinations after cardiothoracic surgery, despite the presence of chest drainage tubes or applied dressings [21]. To the best of our knowledge, we are the first to report high feasibility following major abdominal surgery. Following major abdominal surgery, dressings, chest drains, or subcutaneous emphysema or limited patient mobility could have prohibited the feasibility in this setting.

We cannot compare our results with the previous research, because this is the first study to report PPC rates detected by LUS following major abdominal surgery. The rates found with LUS are high in comparison with PPC rates previously reported with other diagnostic modalities [15]. However, in the cardiothoracic surgery population, it was previously reported that the rate of PPCs detected with LUS was up to 100% [12, 22]. Detection of PPCs with CXR in our study (37%) is in line with preoperative risk scores [16]. In addition, Mazo et al. recently showed incidence rates of PPCs ranging from 38 to 50% in a large validation study in Western Europe in a comparable study population [16].

We found that LUS and CXR, when performed at the same time, identified pleural effusion and atelectasis in different patients (discordant pairs) following major abdominal surgery. These discordant pairs were detected in up to 50% of the patients who had both imaging modalities performed on the same day. This difference can be explained by a higher sensitivity and specificity of LUS in detecting pleural effusion and atelectasis compared to CXR [3, 6, 20]. In a recent systematic review and meta-analysis, LUS had an overall sensitivity of 95% (92–96%) and specificity of 94% (90–97%) compared to CT in adult critically ill patients with respiratory symptoms [6]. CXR had an overall sensitivity of 49% (40-58%) and specificity of 92% (86–95%) in the same systematic review and meta-analysis. Therefore, LUS is being considered by others as the bedside gold standard for pulmonary pathology in critically ill patients with respiratory symptoms [4, 14].

In a recent pilot study performed in cardiothoracic surgery evaluating effectiveness of LUS as the primary diagnostic imaging technique, LUS was exhaustive in up to 80% of the patients. Subsequent CXR was not required in the postoperative management of these patients to assist decision making in this study and LUS was considered effective in perioperative patient management. Furthermore, LUS allowed further discrimination of lung abnormalities mainly between atelectasis and pleural effusions. [22, 23].

Other advantages of LUS are that the time to perform LUS was significantly shorter than for CXR in the postoperative setting [12] and LUS had excellent interobserver agreement [4, 12]. Furthermore, LUS can be used to guide central venous catheter placement and position [24], thoracentesis, and the management of fluid administration in acute circulatory failure [11]. However, if routine LUS findings are inconclusive in patients with respiratory symptoms, additional imaging is warranted; we do suggest using additional CT imaging to make a final diagnosis.

Our study has important limitations. LUS examinations could not be performed on all postoperative days. On POD 0, patients were frequently admitted after working hours, and, on POD 3, was frequently during weekends. Consequently, researchers were not always available to perform LUS. Therefore, the predictive value of detected complications to become clinically relevant PPCs could not be analysed. Another important limitation is the absence of the gold standard (computed tomography) for lung pathology to relate our LUS findings. We chose to use and adjust the most practical, succinct, but well validated and accurate LUS protocol (BLUE protocol) [14, 19]. However, detection rates could even be increased more by further quantifying B lines and to scan 8 or even 28 separate intercostal spaces instead of 4 [25]. The clinical importance of using LUS is unknown with regard to detecting PPCs that do not require therapy according to the treating physician. This should be studied in further studies. We strongly believe that not all atelectasis or pleural effusion need treatment. However, LUS findings, similar to other clinical findings, should always be seen in light of patient's symptoms and health status. Our findings indicate to further study LUS as a primary screening tool for detecting PPCs in major abdominal surgery patients. Future studies should focus on patient outcome and cost effectiveness.

Strength of this study is that we have demonstrated that LUS is indeed feasible and frequently detects PPCs in patients following major abdominal surgery. The protocol we propose is easy to use, also for physicians newly trained in LUS. The protocol is based on limited, standardized signs, a major advantage of LUS, because the risk of wrong interpretations is thereby decreased.

Developing competence in LUS is considered straightforward. Surgeons and anaesthesiologists active in the postoperative period should consider training in LUS as part of their point-of-care ultrasound skills. Furthermore, adding this useful tool into resident training would parallel its broader use in other medicine specialties. Teaching the basics of LUS to perioperative physicians and residents would be fairly easy. For example, in nephrology, a 4-h course that includes pre-course cognitive preparation, a didactic lecture and training in image acquisition/interpretation is sufficient to provide the learner a strong foundation in LUS. However, the course alone is not sufficient to provide competence [26]. Competence in LUS requires additional bedside scanning of patients under the supervision of capable faculty as outlined before [10].

Conclusions

This pilot study shows that LUS is highly feasible and detects PPCs frequently in patients after major abdominal surgery. LUS findings should be evaluated in combination with all available clinical data when considering initiating treatment. Closely monitoring patients and detecting PPCs with LUS could create a window of opportunity to limit the impact of PPCs on patient outcome. This needs to be studied in future trials.

Abbreviations

ARISCAT score: Assess Respiratory risk In Surgical patients in CATalonia score; ASA: American Society of Anesthesiology; BMI: body mass index; BLUE protocol: bedside lung ultrasound in emergency protocol; CT: computed tomography; CRP: C-reactive protein; CPAP: continuous positive airway pressure; CXR: chest X-ray; ICU: intensive care unit; LUS: lung ultrasound; PDMS: patient data management system; PEEP: positive end-expiratory pressure; PLAPS: postero-lateral alveolar and/or pleural syndrome; POD: postoperative day; PPCs: postoperative pulmonary complications.

Acknowledgements

We would like to thank Chantal Stockem for her help with the data collection.

Authors' contributions

Conception and design: HRT, FD, DLP, PS, CB, and PRT. Collection of data: HRT, AS, CS, FD, DLP, PS, and PRT. Statistical analysis: HRT, AS, EB, CB, and PRT. Drafting: HRT, AS, and PRT. All authors read and approved the final manuscript.

Author details

[1] Department of Anaesthesiology, Amsterdam UMC, Vrije Universiteit Amsterdam, Amsterdam Cardiovascular Sciences, De Boelelaan 1117, 1081 HV Amsterdam, The Netherlands. [2] Department of Intensive Care Medicine, Amsterdam UMC, Vrije Universiteit Amsterdam, Amsterdam Cardiovascular Sciences, De Boelelaan 1117, 1081 HV Amsterdam, The Netherlands. [3] Department of Surgery, Amsterdam UMC, Vrije Universiteit Amsterdam, Amsterdam Cardiovascular Sciences, De Boelelaan 1117, 1081 HV Amsterdam, The Netherlands. [4] Department of Intensive Care Medicine, Radboud University Medical Center, Geert Grooteplein Zuid 10, 6525 GA Nijmegen, The Netherlands. [5] Department of Health Evidence, Radboud University Medical Center, Geert Grooteplein Zuid 10, 6525 GA Nijmegen, The Netherlands.

References

1. Ricciardi R, Roberts PL, Read TE, Hall JF, Marcello PW, Schoetz DJ (2013) Which adverse events are associated with mortality and prolonged length of stay following colorectal surgery? J Gastrointest Surg. 17:1485–1493
2. Van Galen LS, Struik PW, Driesen BE et al (2016) Delayed recognition of deterioration of patients in general wards is mostly caused by human related monitoring failures: a root cause analysis of unplanned ICU admissions. PLoS ONE 11:e0161393
3. Lichtenstein D, Goldstein I, Mourgeon E, Cluzel P, Grenier P, Rouby JJ (2004) Comparative diagnostic performances of auscultation, chest radiography, and lung ultrasonography in acute respiratory distress syndrome. Anesthesiology 100:9–15
4. Lichtenstein DA (2014) Lung ultrasound in the critically ill. Clinical Intensive Care. 4:1–12
5. Hammon M, Dankerl P, Voit-Hohne HL, Sandmair M, Kammerer FJ, Uder M et al (2014) Improving diagnostic accuracy in assessing pulmonary edema on bedside chest radiographs using a standardized scoring approach. BMC Anesthesiol 14:94
6. Winkler MH, Touw HR, van de Ven PM, Twisk J, Tuinman PR (2018) Diagnostic accuracy of chest radiograph, and when concomitantly studied lung ultrasound, in critically ill patients with respiratory symptoms: a systematic review and meta-analysis. Crit Care Med 46:e707–e714
7. Self WH, Courtney DM, McNaughton CD, Wunderink RG, Kline JA (2013) High discordance of chest X-ray and computed tomography for detection of pulmonary opacities in ED patients: implications for diagnosing pneumonia. J Emerg Med 31:401–405
8. Halperin BD, Feeley TW, Mihm FG, Chiles C, Guthaner DF, Blank NE (1985) Evaluation of the portable chest roentgenogram for quantitating extravascular lung water in critically ill adults. Chest 88:649–652
9. Tasci O, Hatipoglu ON, Cagli B, Ermis V (2016) Sonography of the chest using linear-array versus sector transducers: correlation with auscultation, chest radiography, and computed tomography. J Clin Ultrasound 44:383–389
10. Touw HR, Tuinman PR, Gelissen HP, Lust E, Elbers PW (2015) Lung ultrasound: routine practice for the next generation of internists. Neth J Med 73:100–107
11. Miller A (2016) Practical approach to lung ultrasound. BJA Educ 16(2):39–45
12. Touw HR, Parlevliet KL, Beerepoot M, Schober P, Vonk A, Twisk JW, Elbers PW, Boer C, Tuinman PR (2018) Lung ultrasound compared with chest X-ray in diagnosing postoperative pulmonary complications following cardiothoracic surgery: a prospective observational study. Anaesthesia 73:946–954
13. Hejblum G, Chalumeau-Lemoine L, Ioos V, Boëlle PY, Salomon L, Simon T, Vibert JF, Guidet B (2009) Comparison of routine and on-demand prescription of chest radiographs in mechanically ventilated adults: a multicentre, cluster-randomised, two-period crossover study. Lancet 374:1687–1693
14. Lichtenstein DA (2015) BLUE-protocol and FALLS-protocol: two applications of lung ultrasound in the critically ill. Chest 147:1659–1670
15. Canet J, Gallart L, Gomar C et al (2010) ARISCAT Group. Prediction of postoperative pulmonary complications in a population-based surgical cohort. Anesthesiology 113:1338–1350
16. Mazo V, Sabaté S, Canet J, Gallart L, Gama de Abreu M, Belda J, Langeron O, Hoeft A, Pelosi P (2014) Prospective external validation of a predictive score for postoperative pulmonary complications. Anesthesiology 121:219–231
17. Tuddenham WJ (1984) Glossary of terms for thoracic radiology: recommendations of the Nomenclature Committee of the Fleischner Society. AJR Am J Roentgenol 143:509–517
18. Rubinowitz AN, Siegel MD, Tocino I (2007) Thoracic imaging in the ICU. Crit Care Clin 23:539–573
19. Lichtenstein DA, Mezière GA (2008) Relevance of lung ultrasound in the diagnosis of acute respiratory failure: the BLUE protocol. Chest 134:117–125
20. Vezzani A, Manca T, Brusasco C, Santori G, Valentino M, Nicolini F et al (2014) Diagnostic value of chest ultrasound after cardiac surgery: a comparison with chest X-ray and auscultation. J Cardiothorac Vasc Anesth 28:1527–1532
21. Goudie E, Bah I, Khereba M, Ferraro P, Duranceau A, Martin J, Thiffault V, Liberman M (2012) Prospectivetrialevaluatingsonographyafterthoracicsurgeryinpostoperativecareanddecisionmaking. Eur J Cardiothorac Surg 41:1025–1030
22. Chiappetta M, Meacci E, Cesario A, Smargiassi A, Inchingolo R, Petracca Ciavarella L, Lopatriello S, Contegiacomo A, Congedo MT, Margaritora S (2018) Postoperative chest ultrasound findings and effectiveness after thoracic surgery: a pilot study. Ultrasound Med Biol 44:1960–1967
23. Nooitgedacht J, Haaksma M, Touw HRW, Tuinman PR (2018) Perioperative care with an ultrasound device is as Michael Jordan with Scotty Pippen: at its best! J Thorac Dis 10:6436–6441
24. Smit JM, Raadsen R, Blans MJ, Petjak M, Van de Ven PM, Tuinman PR (2018) Bedside ultrasound to detect central venous catheter misplacement and associated iatrogenic complications: a systematic review and meta-analysis. Crit Care 22:65
25. Volpicelli G, Elbarbary M, Blaivas M, Lichtenstein DA, Mathis G, Kirkpatrick AW, Melniker L, Gargani L, Noble VE, Via G, Dean A, Tsung JW, Soldati G, Copetti R, Bouhemad B, Reissig A, Agricola E, Rouby JJ, Arbelot C, Liteplo A, Sargsyan A, Silva F, Hoppmann R, Breitkreutz R, Seibel A, Neri L, Storti E, Petrovic T, International Liaison Committee on Lung Ultrasound (ILC-LUS) for International Consensus Conference on Lung Ultrasound (ICC-LUS) (2012) International evidence-based recommendations for point-of-care lung ultrasound. Intensive Care Med 38:577–591
26. Ross DW, Abbasi MM, Jhaveri KD, Sachdeva M, Miller I, Barnett R, Narasimhan M, Mayo P, Merzkani M, Mathew AT (2018) Lung ultrasonography in end-stage renal disease: moving from evidence to practice—a narrative review. Clin Kidney J 11:172–178

11

Applications of intraoperative Duplex ultrasound in vascular surgery

Pasha Normahani[1,3*], Bilal Khan[2], Viknesh Sounderajah[1], Sepideh Poushpas[1], Muzaffar Anwar[1] and Usman Jaffer[1]

Abstract

Objective: This review aims to summarise the contemporary uses of intraoperative completion Duplex ultrasound (IODUS) for the assessment of lower extremity bypass surgery (LEB) and carotid artery endarterectomy (CEA).

Methods: We performed a systematic literature search using the databases of MEDLINE. Eligible studies evaluated the use of IODUS during LEB or CEA.

Results: We found 22 eligible studies; 16 considered the use of IODUS in CEA and 6 in LEB. There was considerable heterogeneity between studies in terms of intervention, outcome measures and follow-up. In the assessment of CEA, there is conflicting evidence regarding the benefits of completion imaging. However, analysis from the largest study suggests a modest reduction in adjusted risk of stroke/mortality when using IODUS selectively (RR 0.74, CI 0.63–0.88, $p=0.001$). Evidence also suggests that uncorrected residual flow abnormalities detected on IODUS are associated with higher rates of restenosis (range 2.1% to 20%). In the assessment of LEB, we found a paucity of evidence when considering the benefit of IODUS on patency rates or when considering its utility as compared to other imaging modalities. However, the available evidence suggests higher rates of thrombosis or secondary intervention in grafts with uncorrected residual flow abnormalities (up to 36% at 3 months).

Conclusions: IODUS can be used to detect defects in both CEA and LEB procedures. However, there is a need for more robust prospective studies to determine the best scanning strategy, criteria for intervention and the impact on clinical outcomes.

Keywords: Duplex ultrasound, Carotid artery endarterectomy, Lower limb revascularisation, Completion imaging

Introduction

Despite recent advances in the provision of enhanced risk factor modification strategies and personalised post-operative patient care, open arterial surgery remains a risky endeavour. In addition to its technical complexity, it is a practice that harbours, in relative terms, a high degree of morbidity and mortality.

*Correspondence: p.normahani@imperial.ac.uk
[1] Imperial Vascular Unit, Imperial College Healthcare NHS Trust, London, UK
Full list of author information is available at the end of the article

In elective infra-inguinal arterial, lower extremity bypass surgery (LEB), early post-operative graft failure, can occur in up to 5% of cases [1], requiring further surgical intervention, and increased length of hospital stay. For carotid artery endarterectomy (CEA), there has been reported, 7% peri-operative risk of stroke/mortality in patients with symptomatic carotid artery disease [2].

Although the aetiology of such early complications is often multifactorial, it is estimated that up to 25% are caused by technical errors and are thus preventable [3–5]. To minimise preventable technical errors, intraoperative assessments of technical adequacy may be useful. Intra-operative assessments aim to identify technical problems that may need to be immediately revised. Visual inspection, palpation and continuous-wave Doppler assessment are limited by subjectivity. In contrast, completion angiography objectively evaluates technical adequacy and arterial run-off. However, complications of arterial puncture, the use of nephrotoxic contrast agents, time taken to perform and radiation exposure limit its use.

Duplex ultrasonography (DUS) incorporates both B-mode ultrasound and pulsed-wave Doppler to allow for non-invasive anatomical imaging as well as assessment of flow through colour Doppler, and qualitative assessment of graphically displayed waveforms. Although possibly less anatomically precise compared to angiography, it can identify defects in arterial anastomoses and can also identify low velocity flow which may be undetected by angiography.

This review aims to summarise the effectiveness of intraoperative completion DUS (IODUS) for the assessment of CEA and LEB.

Methods

Search strategy

Following Preferred Reporting Items for Systematic Reviews and Meta-Analyses (PRISMA) recommendations, an electronic database search was conducted using MEDLINE to include articles from January 1950 through to February 2020 written in English. Reference lists were examined from the retrieved full-text articles. ClinicalTrials.gov was searched for in-progress trials.

In our search strategy, we used the following key terms: "ultrasonography", "Doppler", "duplex", "completion imaging", "vascular surgical procedures", "bypass grafting", "lower limb arterial bypass", "carotid artery endarterectomy" and "intra-operative". Titles and abstracts were reviewed for relevance by two investigators (PN and BK) independently. Conference abstracts and protocol papers were not included. Full-text articles were then reviewed, and data collected on technique used, participants, interventions performed, outcomes and findings. Disagreements were resolved by consensus discussion with the senior author (UJ).

Eligibility criteria

We sought studies that evaluated the use of IODUS during LEB or CEA. Restrictions were not placed on study type. However, studies only considering the natural progression of lesions (i.e., results not used to inform management decisions peri-operatively) were excluded.

Outcomes measured

For the use of IODUS for CEA, outcomes of interest included (1) stroke/mortality at 30 days and (2) flow abnormalities on follow-up imaging. For LEB, the outcome of interest was primary graft patency at 30 days. For both CEA and LEB, we also consider the natural history of cases with normal and abnormal completion imaging.

Results

Through our initial search strategy, we identified 96 papers (Fig. 1). Of these, 36 papers were shortlisted for full-text review based on their title and abstract. A full-text screening resulted in a final selection of 22 studies. Of these studies, 16 considered the use of IODUS in CEA (Table 1) and 6 in LEB (Table 2).

Quality of studies

There were no randomised controlled trials comparing IODUS with no completion imaging or other completion imaging techniques. Sixteen studies investigated the role of IODUS in CEA: 3 were based on prospectively maintained registries; 9 were prospective single-centre studies; and 4 retrospective studies. Six studies investigated the role of IODUS for LEB: 4 were prospective (in one study data was Registry analysis); 2 were retrospective studies. There was considerable heterogeneity in terms of intervention, outcome measures and follow-up.

Carotid artery endarterectomy

Study characteristics and designs

IODUS was performed routinely in 9 of 16 studies and selectively in 7 of 16. Criteria for selective use of IODUS was left to surgeons' discretion and was not specified in any of these studies.

Revision rates were available for 14 out of 16 studies and ranged between 0 and 23%. In 9 studies, the IODUS criteria for revision of the carotid reconstruction were unspecified and left to the discretion of the operating surgeon. In the remaining 7 studies, criteria for revision were variable depending upon the vessels scanned and were based-upon (1) spectral waveform criteria for flow disturbance and (2) B-mode criteria for determining significance of defects. In the majority of studies, all the three carotid vessels [6–10] were scanned. However, one paper only considered flow abnormalities in the presence of internal carotid artery (ICA) kinking [11] and another did not consider abnormalities of the external carotid artery (ECA) [12].

1. Spectral waveform criteria

   Criteria for defining severe flow abnormality were based on velocity readings (thresholds ranged from 120 to 150 cm/s) and qualitative arterial waveform features such as spectral broadening, colour mosaic and infilling of the spectral window. In three studies,

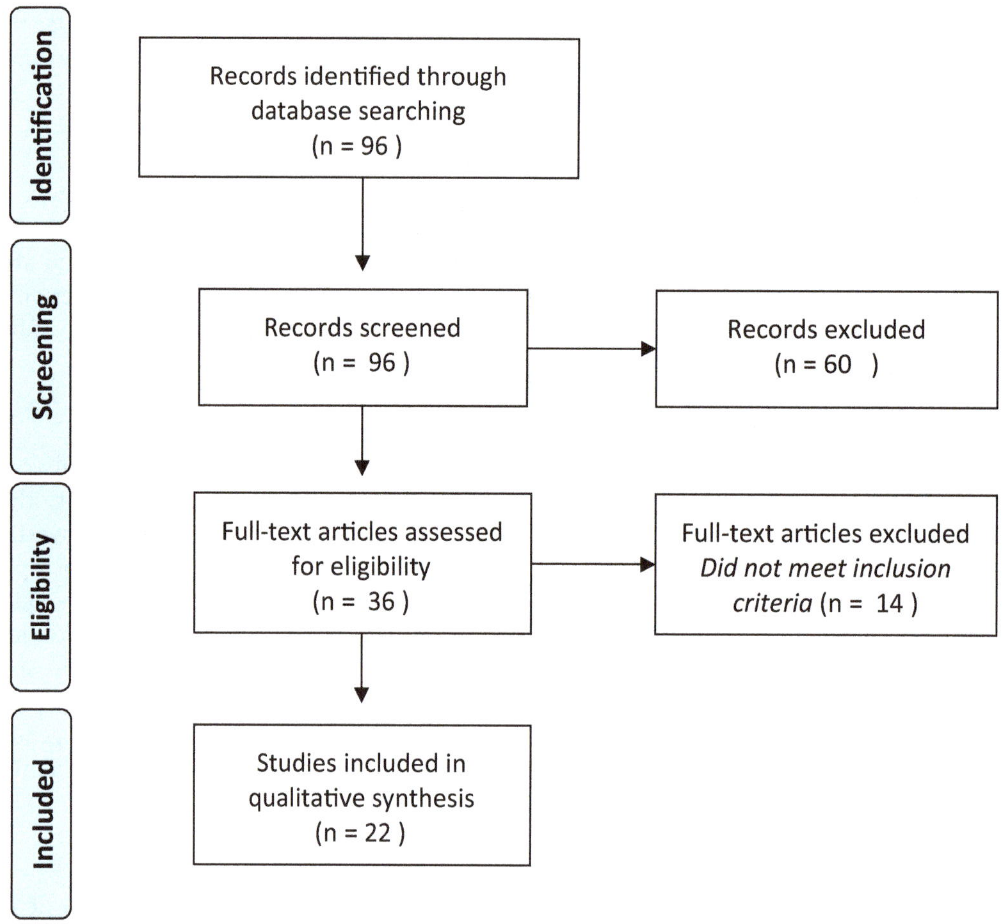

Fig. 1 PRISMA systematic review flow diagram

vessels with flow abnormalities in the absence of an identifiable cause on B-mode ultrasound were surgically revised [7, 9, 10]. In two other studies, flow abnormalities with no identifiable cause on B-mode ultrasound were first assessed with an intraoperative angiogram prior to any revision [6, 12]. In one of these studies, an elevated peak systolic velocity (PSV) was measured in 27 cases (between 151 and 421 cm/s) with no evident technical defect or residual disease. In such cases, repeated measurements 15 to 20 min later were often improved (between 62 and 199 cm/s). If values were persistently abnormal, an intraoperative angiogram was then obtained.

2. B-mode criteria

   B-mode thresholds for revision were also variable and included the presence of ICA kinking, occlusion, thrombus, marked residual plaque, dissection or flap. Thresholds for determining the significance of flaps were also variable. Mays et al. [6] immediately revised all distal ICA flaps, and common carotid artery (CCA) or bulb defects > 2 mm in the presence of flow abnormalities. Panneton et al. [8] revised cases with intimal flaps or dissections > 3 mm in the presence of significant flow abnormalities. Ascher and colleagues [12] revised all cases with mobile flaps > 2 mm in ICA or > 3 mm in the CCA.

Comparing outcomes from completion imaging vs no completion imaging

The largest studies comparing utilisation of completion imaging vs no completion imaging are the retrospective analysis of large data sets from Knappich [13], Wallaert [14] and Rockman [15].

In the largest of these data sets, Knappich [13] demonstrated an association between completion imaging with lower rates of stroke/mortality (relative risk (RR) 0.86 (CI 0.80–0.93)). Rockman and colleagues, on the other hand, demonstrate no statistically significant difference in the rates of stroke [2.8% with imaging, 2.4% without imaging, $p=$ not significant (NS)] or combined stroke/mortality rates (3.6% with imaging, 3.3% without imaging, $p=$ NS) between cases in which intraoperative imaging was used

Table 1 Summary of results from studies evaluating IODUS in CEA

Carotid endarterectomy

First author	Year	Study design	No of procedures	Imaging criteria (selective or routine)/ revision criteria	Revision rate	Stroke (30 days)	Mortality (30 days)	Follow-up imaging; residual or recurrent stenosis
Studies comparing (a) completion imaging vs no imaging or (b) different completion imaging modalities								
Knappich C	2017	Retrospective analysis of registry data; *German statutory nationwide quality assurance database*	142,074	Selective; Imaging in 66.9% (95 044/142 074) of cases. Mix of DUS/angiogram/ flowmetry or other unspecified modalities. Differential count for imaging modalities not presented in data Criteria for revision: Surgeons discretion	*Not known*	Combined stroke/mortality rate Scan: 1.7% (1654/95,044), RR 0.86 (CI 0.80–0.93) No scan: 2% (957/47,030) Adjusted risk of any stroke or mortality Intraoperative completion study Angiogram: RR 0.8 (CI 0.71–0.9) $p<0.001$ DUS: RR 0.74 (CI 0.63–0.88) $p=0.001$ Flowmetry: RR 0.87 (CI 0.74–1.04) $p=0.121$ Other: RR 0.97 (CI 0.80–1.17) $p=0.756$		*Not known*
Wallaert JB	2011	Retrospective analysis of registry data; *Vascular Study Group of New England (VSGNE) Registry*	6115	Selective; Completion imaging only performed in 2033 cases. DUS in 94% (1919/2033) of cases Amongst 73 surgeons; completion imaging used rarely (51%), selectively (22%) or routinely (27%) Criteria for revision: Surgeon's discretion Practice pattern defined as routine (imaging used in ≥ 90% of cases), selective (5% to 90%) and rare (< 5%)	Routine: 7.6% Selective: 0.8%, Rare: 0.9%	Combined stroke/mortality rates Routine: 2.4% (42/1763) Selective: 1.2% (12/1018) Rare: 1.7% (55/3334) *Routine v selective v rare; $p=0.048$* *Risk adjusted; Selective (OR, 0.75; 95% CI 0.40–1.41; $p=.366$), routine OR, 1.42; 95% CI .93–2.17; $p=.106$* Revised cases: 3.9% (7/178) Not revised cases: 1.7% (102/5937) *Revised v not revised; $p=0.028$* *Risk adjusted; OR 2.1; 95% CI, 0.9–5.0; $p=.076$* Completion imaging: 2.6% No completion imaging: 1.3% *Completion imaging v no completion imaging; $p<0.001$* *Risk adjusted; OR, 1.9; 95% CI, 1.2–2.7; $P=.002$*		Restenosis (> 70%) at 1 year Routine: 1.1% Selective: 1.1% Rare: 2.8% Routine v selective v rare; $p=0.09$
Rockman CB et al	2007	Retrospective analysis of data from the *New York Carotid Artery Surgery (NYCAS) study*	9278	Selective; Imaging in 35.8% (3318/9278) Angiogram 5.4% (178/3318), continuous wave Doppler 70.3% (2331/3318), DUS 17.6% (585/3318), combination of angio ± Doppler or DUS 5.9% (196/3318) Criteria for revision: Surgeons discretion	*Not known*	Combined stroke/mortality rate No scan: 3.8% Any scan: 4.3% Angiogram: 5.2% Doppler: 4.3% DUS: 4.3% *No statistical significance when comparing 'no scan' with 'any scan' or when comparing individual modalities with 'no scan'*		*Not known*

Table 1 (continued)

Carotid endarterectomy								
First author	**Year**	**Study design**	**No of procedures**	**Imaging criteria (selective or routine)/ revision criteria**	**Revision rate**	**Stroke (30 days)**	**Mortality (30 days)**	**Follow-up imaging; residual or recurrent stenosis**
Kinney EV	1993	Prospective single center study	461	Selective; DUS in 410 cases Criteria for revision: Severe flow disturbance (PSV > 150 cm/s and spectral broadening) or occlusion in the CCA/ICA/ECA	6.3% (26/410)	Stroke rate Combined: 2.2% (10/461) No scan: 0% (0/51) *Normal scan: 2.1% (7/337) *Abnormal scan: 4.1% (3/73) Revisions: 3.8% (1/26) *(*at completion)*	Mortality rate Combined: 2.6% (12/461) No scan: 0% (0/51) *Normal scan: 3.3% (11/337) * Abnormal scan: 1.4% (1/73)	Flow abnormality at 3 months (> 50% category): Combined: 2.4% (11/461) No scan: 9.8% (5/51) *No flow abnormality: 0.3% (1/337) *Residual flow disturbance: 6.8% (5/73)
Lingenfelter KA	1995	Prospective single center study	53	Routine; combination of hand-held Doppler, DUS and angiogram in all cases Criteria for revision: Surgeon's discretion	11.3% (6/53)	Stroke rate Combined: 1.8% (1/53) DUS detected all 6 defects requiring revision. Audible Doppler assessment detected only 1 and DSA 4	Mortality rate Combined: 0% (0/53)	*Not known*
Lipski DA	1996	Retrospective study	86	Selective (at surgeons discretion); DUS in 39 procedures Criteria for revision: Surgeon's discretion	23.1% (9/39)	Stroke rate Combined: 3.5% (3/86) Scan: 2.6% (1/39) No scan: 4.3% (2/47)	Mortality rate Combined: 0% (0/86)	Residual stenosis (> 50%): Combined: 8.1% (7/86) Scan: 0% (0/39) No scan: 14.9% (7/47) Restenosis (< 50%) at mean follow up of 20 months Combined: 4.7% (4/86) Scan: 5.1% (2/39) No scan: 4.3% (2/47) *Note: significant variation in patch vs primary closure*
Lane RJ	1987	Prospective single center study	380	Selective; DUS in 175 cases Criteria for revision: Unspecified criteria for 30% stenosis	6.9% (12/175)	Stroke rate Combined: 2.1% (8/380) No scan: 2.4% (5/205) Normal scan: 2.2% (3/136) Abnormal scan: 0% (0/39)	Mortality rate Combined: 0.5% (2/380) No scan: 0.4% (1/205) Normal scan: 0.7% (1/136) Abnormal scan: 0% (0/39)	Restenosis at mean follow up of 22 months Combined: not available No scan: not available Abnormal scan: 6.3% (1/16) Restenosis at mean follow up of 16 months Normal scan: 9.2% (8/87) **Only 103 patients followed up*

Table 1 (continued)

Carotid endarterectomy

First author	Year	Study design	No of procedures	Imaging criteria (selective or routine)/ revision criteria	Revision rate	Stroke (30 days)	Mortality (30 days)	Follow-up imaging; residual or recurrent stenosis
Descriptive studies								
Dorffner R	1997	Prospective single center study	50	Routine; DUS in all cases Criteria for revision: Surgeons' discretion	18% (9/50)	Stroke rate Combined: 4% (2/50) *Normal scan: 0% (0/32) Abnormal scan but not revised: 20% (2/10) Revised: 0% (0/9) **Normal at completion*	Mortality rate Combined: 0% (0/50)	Restenosis at mean follow up of 10 months Normal scan: 6.3% (2/32) Abnormal scan but not revised: 20% (2/10) Revised: 0% (0/9)
Mays BW	2000	Prospective single center study	100	Routine; DUS in all cases Criteria for revision: PSV > 150 cm/s and spectral broadening indicating severe flow disturbance in CCA, ICA or ECA. If no obvious cause for flow disturbance was identified then angiogram was performed prior to revision. In addition, flaps in distal ICA and defects > 2 mm in the CCA or bulb were revised in the presence of a PSV > 125 cm/s colour mosaic or loss of spectral window	21% (21/100)	Stroke rate Combined: 1% (1/100)	Mortality rate Combined: 1% (1/100)	At 6 weeks: Revisions: 1/21 showed an occluded ICA and 2/21 showed residual stenosis No abnormality on completion: 10/79 showed recurrent stenosis (16% to 49% category)
Yuan	2014	Prospective single surgeon series	285	Routine; DUS in all cases Criteria for revision: Visible ICA kinking with PSV ≥ 120 cm/s	3.9% (11/285)	Stroke rate Combined: 1.1% (3/285) Repaired ICA kinking: 0% (0/11) Unrepaired ICA kinking: 0% (0/16)	Mortality rate Combined: *0% (0/285)* Repaired ICA kinking: 0% (0/11) Unrepaired ICA kinking: 0% (0/16)	By 9–24 months: Combined: *1.8% (5/284)* Repaired ICA kinking: 9.1% (1/11) restenosis (60–79%), 9.1% (1/11) occlusion Unrepaired ICA kinking: 0% (3/15*) mild 0–40% stenosis *(*one patient lost to f/u)*

Table 1 (continued)

Carotid endarterectomy								
First author	**Year**	**Study design**	**No of procedures**	**Imaging criteria (selective or routine)/ revision criteria**	**Revision rate**	**Stroke (30 days)**	**Mortality (30 days)**	**Follow-up imaging; residual or recurrent stenosis**
Baker	1994	Retrospective single center study	316	Selective; DUS in 283 cases Criteria for revision: Surgeon's discretion	2.8% (9/316)	Stroke rate Combined: 1.6% (5/316) Normal scan: 1.6% (4/254) Unrepaired minor defects: 1.9% (1/53) Revised defects: 0% (0/9)	Mortality rate Combined: 0.3% (1/283) *(Single death was in the normal scan group)* **316 cases in 283 patients*	Stenosis (> 75%) at mean follow up of 21.6 months: Combined: 5.7% (18/316) Normal scan: 3.2% (8/251*) Unrepaired minor defects: 17.3% (9/52*). One of these arteries later occluded Revised defects: 11.1% (1/9) *Note: restenosis was correlated with primary and patch closure (p = 0.025)* **No of patent vessels in surviving patients*
Panneton JM	2001	Retrospective single center study	155	Routine; DUS in all cases Criteria for revision: PSV > 125 cm/s and marked plaque/thrombus or large intimal flap/dissection in the CCA, IC or ECA	9% (14/155)	Stroke rate Combined: 1.9% (3/155) Normal scan: 1.1% (1/91) Minor defects: 0% (0/47) Revised major defects: 0% (0/14) Unrevised major defects: 66.7% (2/3)	Mortality rate Combined: 0.7% (1/149*) (1 death in patient with unrevised major defect) **155 cases in 149 patients*	Restenosis at 6 months*: Normal scan: 1.1% (1/91) restenosis Minor defects: 2.1% (1/47) Revised major defects: 0% (0/14) **(Asymptomatic > 50%)*
Steinmetz OK	1998	Retrospective single surgeon series	100	Routine; DUS in all cases Criteria for revision: Intraluminal thrombosis or focal elevation of PSV > 120 cm/s and marked spectral broadening in either CCA, ICA or ECA	2% (2/100)	Stroke rate Combined: 2% (2/100)	Mortality rate Combined: 1% (1/100)	Abnormality at mean follow up of 9.2 months Combined: 13.6% (12/88) *(< 50% stenosis in 6, > 50% stenosis in 5, asymptomatic occlusion in 1)* **Follow up scans available in 88 patients*

Table 1 (continued)

Carotid endarterectomy								
First author	**Year**	**Study design**	**No of procedures**	**Imaging criteria (selective or routine)/ revision criteria**	**Revision rate**	**Stroke (30 days)**	**Mortality (30 days)**	**Follow-up imaging; residual or recurrent stenosis**
Ascher E	2004	Prospective single center study	650	Routine; DUS in all cases Criteria for revision: Mobile flap > 2 mm in ICA, flap > 3 mm in the CCA and technical defects causing > 30% luminal ICA stenosis	2.3% (15/650)	Stroke rate Combined: 0.3% (2/650) Revised: 0% (0/15)	Mortality rate Combined: 0.3% (2/590) **650 cases in 590 patients*	Flow abnormality at 2 weeks: Combined: 3% (2/625*)—ICA occlusion in both cases *Revised*: 0% (0/15) Flow abnormality at 3 months: Revised: 0% (0/15) **625 f/u scan available for 650 patients*
Mullenix PS	2003	Prospective single center study	100	Routine; DUS in all cases Criteria for revision: Surgeon's discretion	7% (7/100)	Stroke rate Combined: 2% (2/100) *Both stroked occurred in cases with an abnormal completion scan that was left unrepaired. However, one stroke was contralateral and likely unrelated*	Mortality rate Combined: 0% (0/100)	Re-stenosis* at follow up (range 6–45 months) Combined: 10/100 3 of these regressed and 1 was high grade (> 80%) *Defined as > 50%
Bandyk DF	1994	Prospective single center study	368 in total, of which 210 were CEA's	Routine; DUS in all cases Criteria for revision: Defect on B mode with a PSV > 150 cm/s in CCA, ICA or ECA	8.1% (17/210)	Combined: 0% (0/210)	*Not specified*	*Not specified*

Table 2 Summary of results from studies evaluating IODUS in LEB

First author	Year	Study design	No procedures	Imaging criteria (selective or routine)/revision criteria	Revision rate	Graft thrombosis/revision
Lower limb revascularisations						
Studies comparing a) completion imaging vs no imaging or b) different completion imaging modalities						
Taze-Woei T	2014	Retrospective analysis of registry data; *Vascular Study Group of New England (VSGNE) Registry*	2032	Selective: completion imaging performed in 67% of cases (1368/2032). Angiography performed in in 89% and DUS in 11% of cases Criteria for revision: Surgeons discretion		No breakdown results for completion imaging strategy (i.e., DUS and angiography) ***Selective vs routine completion imaging*** The surgeon's strategy of performing routine *vs* selective CIM was not associated with primary graft patency at discharge (RR, 0.8; 95% CI 0.6–1.1; $p = .31$) and at 1-year follow-up (RR, 1.1; 95% CI 0.9–1.2; $p = .56$) ***Completion imaging vs no completion imaging*** In multivariate models, completion imaging was not associated with improved primary graft patency at discharge (OR, 1.1; 95% CI 0.7–1.7; $p = .64$) or at 1 year (OR, 0.9; 95% CI 0.7–1.2; $p = .47$)
Gilbertson JJ	1991	Prospective single center study	20	Routine. Blinded comparison of DUS, angiography and angioscopy Criteria for revision: Residual valve cusp: Doubling of PSV or marked spectral broadening compared with adjacent graft. PSV < 40 cm/s or > 150 cm/s Unligated side branch: B-mode or color flow image directed away from lumen Anastomotic stenosis: High velocity jet or turbulence	unknown	***Residual cusps ($n = 9$)*** Angiography: (2/9) Angioscopy: (9/9) DUS: (1/9) ***Unligated side branch ($n = 32$)*** Angiography: (14/32) Angioscopy: (21/32) DUS: (4/32) ***Anastomotic stenosis ($n = 0$)*** Angiography: (4/0), FP rate 20% Angioscopy: (0/0) DUS: (2/0), FP rate 10% Denominator = confirmed on exploration

Table 2 (continued)

Lower limb revascularisations						
First author	**Year**	**Study design**	**No procedures**	**Imaging criteria (selective or routine)/revision criteria**	**Revision rate**	**Graft thrombosis/revision**
Descriptive studies						
Bandyk DF	1994 *(series from 1990–1993)*	Prospective single center study	368 in total, of which 135 were bypasses	Routine *Completion arteriography was also performed in 81% of cases (110/135)* Criteria for revision: Severe (PSV > 180 cm/s with broadening or PSVR 2.5 to 4) or high grade (PSV > 300 cm/s or PSVR > 4) stenosis velocity spectra in the presence of anatomic lesion on DUS	14.1% (19/135)	Within 30 days Combined graft thrombosis: 0.7% (1/135) Combined secondary intervention: *2.2%* (3/135) *Due to a lesion and low graft flow* Combined assisted patency: 100% (135/135) *All of the four cases had residual lesions on completion DUS. 60% (3/5) unrepaired vein graft lesions required revision. No patients with a normal completion scan required a secondary procedure during a minimum of 2-month follow-up* *Completion angiography did not demonstrate any additional significant lesions*

Table 2 (continued)

First author	Year	Study design	No procedures	Imaging criteria (selective or routine)/revision criteria	Revision rate	Graft thrombosis/revision
Lower limb revascularisations						
Bandyk DF	1996 *(series from 1991–1995)*	Prospective single center study	275	Routine Criteria for revision: Severe (PSV > 180 cm/s with broadening or PSVR 2.5 to 4) or high grade (PSV > 300 cm/s or PSVR > 4) stenosis velocity spectra in the presence of vessel lumen defect or narrowing Lesions associated with low graft flow Segments with borderline stenosis (125–180 cm/s) were rescanned after additional papaverine administration—if PSV increased to > 200 cm/s in a normal diameter vein or anastomosis revision was performed When increased velocities (> 180 cm/s) were measured in outflow tibial arteries but the velocity ratio was less than < 2.5, an angiogram was performed confirm patency beyond distal anastomosis	15.6% (43/275)	<u>Within 30 days</u> *Graft thrombosis* Overall: 1.1% (3/275) Unrepaired flow abnormality (PSV < 180 cm/s): 4% (1/25) *Secondary intervention* Unrepaired flow abnormality (PSV < 180 cm/s): 16% (4/25) *Assisted patency* Overall: 100% (275/275) *Mortality:* Overall: 1.1% 3/275 <u>Between 30 and 90 days</u> *Graft thrombosis* Normal imaging*: 0.4% (1/235) Unrepaired flow abnormality (PSV < 180 cm/s): 4% (1/25) *Secondary intervention* Normal imaging*: 2.6% (26/235) Unrepaired flow abnormality (PSV < 180 cm/s): 36% (9/25) Abnormal imaging after repair: 40% (6/15) *Overall graft thrombosis/secondary intervention in normal imaging vs* Unrepaired *flow abnormality; $p < 0.001$* *60% 15/25 uncorrected abnormalities had thrombosis or re-intervention in first 3 months* **202 without repair, 33 with repair*

Table 2 (continued)

Lower limb revascularisations						
First author	**Year**	**Study design**	**No procedures**	**Imaging criteria (selective or routine)/revision criteria**	**Revision rate**	**Graft thrombosis/revision**
Johnson BL	2000 *(series from 1991–1998)*	Retrospective single center study		Routine Criteria for revision: Same criteria as Bandyk (1996). However, low flow and unrepaired graft lesions were managed with specified antithrombotic regimen or adjunctive procedure Normal graft flow (> 45 cm/s, low PVR defined as antegrade flow throughout pulsed cycle)- dextran + aspirin (325 mg/day) Low flow and low PVR- heparin + dextran + aspirin Low flow and high PVR- adjunct procedure (e.g., arteriovenous fistula or jump graft to another outflow artery) if possible. If not treated as low flow + low PVR Low flow graft stenosis (> 200 cm/s at site of stenosis- repair stenosis + heparin + dextran + aspirin	15.3% (96/626)* *Revision* of 99 graft *segments* for stenosis and 5 *adjunct procedures* to improve graft flow * **104 defects in 96 bypasses*	Within 30 days (secondary intervention rate) Combined: 4.2% (26/626) Normal flow: 1.1% (5/464) Normal flow (revised graft): 1.5% (1/67) Residual flow abnormality (revised graft): 34.5%(10/29) Unrepaired flow abnormality): 13.2% (7/53) Low flow (but no stenosis): 23.1% (3/13) Between 30 and 90 days (secondary intervention rate) Combined: 4.3% (27/626) Normal flow: 1.3% (6/464) Normal flow (revised graft): 1.5% (1/67) Residual flow abnormality (revised graft): 10.3% (3/29) Unrepaired flow abnormality: 24.5% (13/53) Low flow (but no stenosis): 15.4% (2/13) Total (within 90 days) (secondary intervention rate) Combined: 8% (51/626) Normal flow: 2.4% (11/464) Normal flow (revised graft): 3%(2/67) Residual flow abnormality (revised graft): 44.8% (13/29) Unrepaired flow abnormality: 37.7% (20/53) Low flow (but no stenosis): 38.5% (5/13)

Table 2 (continued)

Lower limb revascularisations						
First author	**Year**	**Study design**	**No procedures**	**Imaging criteria (selective or routine)/revision criteria**	**Revision rate**	**Graft thrombosis/revision**
MacKenzie KS	1999	Retrospective single center study	78	Selective Criteria for revision: Surgeons discretion	15.3% (12/78)	Within 30 days (n = 76): *Secondary intervention rate/ primary patency/secondary patency* Normal flow: 1.3%/100%/*N.A* *Revised graft: 8.3%/100%/*N.A* Unrepaired flow abnormality: 11.1%/83%/*unknown* Between 30 days and an average intermediate follow-up of 7.4 months (n = 72) *Secondary intervention rate / primary patency/secondary patency* Normal flow: 1.3%/93%/97% Revised graft: 8.3%/91%/*100%* Unrepaired flow abnormality: 11.1%/53.1%/71.1% *Statistical significant difference in patency rates when comparing unrepaired flow abnormality to normal flow ($p < 0.001$) or to repaired group ($p < 0.001$)* **Repeat scan normal at completion in all 12 cases*

and cases in which no intraoperative imaging was used [15]. Conversely, Wallaert and colleagues demonstrated higher rates of stroke/mortality in cases in which completion imaging was used as compared to cases in which no imaging was used (2.6% with imaging, 1.3% with no imaging; $p<0.001$) [14]. This difference was still statistically significant after risk adjustment [odds-ratio (OR), 1.9; 95% CI 1.2–2.7; p=0.002] [14].

Comparing outcomes from IODUS with other completion imaging modalities

Knappich et al. provide an analysis of 142,074 CEAs from the German statutory nationwide quality assurance database [13]. Within this large cohort, 66.9% (95,044) underwent completion imaging using IODUS, angiogram, flowmetry or other. In their results, they provide subgroup analysis demonstrating that utilisation of either intraoperative angiography (RR 0.8 (CI 0.71–0.9) $p<0.001$) or IODUS (RR 0.74 (CI 0.63–0.88) $p=0.001$) is associated with lower rates of stroke/mortality. Their analysis seems to show a slightly stronger affect for IODUS as compared to angiography.

Another study by Rockman and colleagues provides analysis from 9278 CEAs from the New York Carotid Artery Surgery (NYCAS) study [15]. Amongst these cases, completion imaging was performed in 3318 cases. In the majority of cases, imaging merely consisted of continuous wave Doppler assessment (70.3%; 2331/3318), followed by IODUS (17.6%; 585/3318), angiogram (5.4%; 178/3318), or a combination of angiogram ± Doppler or IODUS (5.9%; 196/3318). Stroke/mortality rates for each modality were not statistically significant (angiogram: 5.2%, Doppler: 4.3%, IODUS: 4.3%; *p* value not given).

A smaller prospective study of 53 patients compared the ability to detect abnormalities with audible handheld Doppler assessment, digital subtraction angiography (DSA) and IODUS colour flow [16]. In this cohort, 6 patients (11.3%) required revision due to significant abnormalities. IODUS detected all six defects requiring revision, whilst audible Doppler assessment detected only 1 and DSA 4 [16].

Primary revision surgery based on IODUS findings and 30-day stroke/mortality risk

Eight of the 16 studies presented data on stroke/mortality rates. The largest of these was a retrospective analysis of the Vascular Study Group of New England (VSGNE) Registry performed by Wallaert and colleagues [14]. In this studyWO completion imaging was performed in 2033 CEAs. The mainstay imaging modality of choice was IODUS (94% of cases; 1919/2033). They found the combined stroke/mortality rate was significantly higher in revised group as compared to cases not requiring revision (3.9% (7/178) v 1.7% (102/5937); $p=0.028$). However, this was not statically significant after risk adjustment (OR 2.1 (CI 0.9–5.0); $p=0.076$). Data regarding follow-up imaging for these two groups was not available for comparison.

The remaining 7 studies were either of too small sample size or did not include meaningful statistical comparisons of revised vs non-revised groups [7, 8, 11, 12, 17, 18]. Cumulatively, the stroke rates in these studies was 1% (1 of 101) in cases requiring revision and 1.2% (24 of 2026) in cases not requiring revision based on completion imaging.

Follow-up of revised cases

Six studies included data on follow-up imaging of revised cases [6, 8, 11, 12, 17, 18]. Cumulatively in these studies, abnormalities were detected in 7.6% of revised cases (6 of these 79 cases) and 2.6% (37/1448) of unrevised cases. However, meaningful comparison and interpretation of this data is challenging due to variable follow-up periods (2 weeks to 24 months), variable or unclear criteria for stenosis assessment, lack of risk adjustment and variable surgical techniques (e.g., patch plasty, primary closure, eversion). Of the 6 abnormalities described, 2 were of asymptomatic occlusions and 4 of stenosis.

Follow-up of 'non-significant' findings detected on IODUS

Six studies included descriptive analysis of stroke rates for cases in which abnormal completion imaging results were not considered significant and thus not revised [7, 8, 11, 17–19]. Cumulatively for these studies, stroke rates were 1.6% (18/1108) in cases with normal completion studies as compared to 2.5% (6/238) in cases with abnormal completion imaging.

Similarly, 5 studies included descriptive analysis of abnormalities detected on follow-up imaging [7, 8, 11, 17, 18]. Cumulatively for these studies, abnormalities on follow-up scans were detected in 1.2% (12/968) in cases with normal completion imaging as compared to 10.3% (19/185) in cases with abnormal completion imaging.

Lower extremity bypass surgery

Study characteristics and designs

Six studies investigating the role of IODUS completion imaging in LEB were included. All studies considered infra-inguinal bypass procedures with vein conduit. Three of these studies are sequential publications from the University of South Florida group [10, 20, 21]. It is not made explicitly clear from the manuscripts whether each builds upon the previously published series, but this is implicitly suggested by the overlapping periods of data collection. Of the other studies, one compared completion imaging vs no completion imaging [22] and the other compared the accuracy of angiography, IODUS and angioscopy as completion imaging modalities [23]. IODUS was performed routinely in 4 of 6 [10, 20, 21, 23] studies and selectively in 2 of 5 [22, 24]. The decision to use selective IODUS was left to the discretion of individual surgeons. However, when used selectively, IODUS was performed mostly when the outflow artery was a tibial or tibioperoneal trunk [22]. Four out of 6 studies provided the revision rate, which ranged between 10 and 27% [10, 20–22].

Two studies did not include their criteria for intraoperative revision, which was left to the discretion of the operating surgeon [22, 24]. In the remaining studies criteria for defining severe flow abnormalities were based on peak systolic velocity reading of > 180 cm/s, grading of residual lesions (velocity ratio of > 2.5 was considered significant), and qualitative arterial waveform features including spectral broadening and absence of diastolic flow. If abnormalities were found, the hemodynamic response to flow augmentation was either evaluated by transverse imaging or rescanned after the administration of papaverine. Three studies assessed flow abnormalities with no identifiable cause on B-mode ultrasound followed by on table angiography before any revision [10, 20, 21]. In addition, if high velocities were identified in the outflow tibial arteries, with a velocity ratio of less than 2.5, then angiography was performed [10, 21].

Comparing outcomes from completion imaging vs no completion imaging

Only one study compared primary graft patency following infra-inguinal lower extremity bypass (LEB) between cases in which completion imaging was used vs those in which it was not [22]. In this retrospective analysis of registry data, completion imaging was used by 67.3% ($n = 1368/2032$) of vascular surgeons, with 67% using it selectively (< 80% of LEBs) and 33% routinely (≥ 80% of LEBs). The most commonly used imaging modality was angiography (89%, $n = 1217/1368$) followed by IODUS (11%, $n = 151/1368$). They authors found no association between using completion imaging and improved primary graft patency at discharge (OR, 1.1; $p = 0.64$) or at 1 year (OR, 0.9; $p = 0.47$), with similar results in bypass procedures performed with or without completion imaging. However, number of patients who had IODUS performed were comparatively much smaller ($n = 151$) as compared to patients who had angiography ($n = 1217$). Similarly, no effect was found between the surgeons' strategy to perform completion imaging selectively or routinely on bypass graft patency at discharge (RR, 0.8; $p = 0.31$) or at 1 year (RR, 1.1; $p = 0.56$).

Comparing IODUS with other completion imaging modalities

Only one study compared IODUS against other modalities in lower extremity bypass procedures. However, this paper considered diagnostic accuracy and not clinical outcomes such as primary patency. Gilbertson conducted a prospective analysis of 20 femoral-infragenicular bypass procedures using in situ saphenous vein grafts [23]. They compared the ability to detect three specific abnormalities (patent vein side branches, residual valve cups and anastomotic stenoses > 30%) with angiography, angioscopy and IODUS. Within this cohort, 63 critical graft defects were identified by at least one of the imaging modalities and 41 of these were confirmed by direct inspection. Their results suggest that sensitivity of angioscopy (66% $n = 21/32$) and angiography (44%, $n = 14/32$) is higher than IODUS (12%, $n = 4/32$) for detecting patent vein branches ($p < 0.01$). For the detection of residual valve cups, angioscopy was the most sensitive (100%, $n = 9/9$), followed by angiography (22%, $n = 2/9$) and IODUS (11%, $n = 1/9$). They detected no anastomotic stenoses but false-positive rates were highest for angiography (20%), followed by IODUS (10%) and angioscopy (0%).

Follow-up of revised cases and those with 'non-significant' findings detected on IODUS

Johnson et al. [21] retrospectively identified 626 infrainguinal vein bypass procedures, where IODUS was used as the completion imaging. Of these, 15% ($n = 96/626$) were found to be abnormal, leading to the revision of 99 graft segments. The most commonly identified problem on imaging was the result of incomplete valve lysis (63%, 31/49). They found an improvement in the velocity spectra of 71% of segments and residual moderate stenosis in 29% of segments following graft revision. They found a significantly higher revision rate (27%, $p < 0.01$) with the use of alternative vein grafts as well as an increase in the frequency of unrepaired graft defects ($p < 0.05$). Johnson et al. found that secondary intervention rates within the first 90 days were highest for cases were there was an unrepaired flow abnormality as compared to those with a normal flow profile (37.7% vs 2.4%). Interestingly, in cases, where repair was performed, outcomes were considerably better if normal flow profile was established compared to if residual flow abnormality was detected (3% vs 44.8%) [21].

Another retrospective study by Bandyk et al. [20], considered 275 infrainguinal vein bypasses assessed using colour IODUS. A total of 50 (16%) abnormalities were detected in 43 grafts and necessitated revision. The revision rate was lowest for reversed saphenous vein bypasses (7%, $p < 0.02$) compared to other grafting techniques.

Revision rate for popliteal and tibial bypasses were similar (14% vs 17%). Combined graft thrombosis and secondary revision rates at 90 days in those cases with normal completion imaging as compared to those with unrepaired flow abnormalities was significantly lower (graft thrombosis 0.4% vs 4%, secondary revision 2.6% vs 36%; combined $p < 0.001$). Overall, 15 out of 25 (60%) cases with uncorrected flow abnormalities had thrombosis or re-intervention in the first 3 months.

In a single centre retrospective study by MacKenzie et al. of 78 cases, secondary intervention rates at 30 days were lowest for cases with normal completion imaging (1.3%), followed by revised cases (8.3%) and unrepaired flow abnormalities (11.1%) [24]. They detected a statistically significant difference in patency rates when comparing unrepaired flow abnormality to normal flow ($p < 0.001$) or to repaired group ($p < 0.001$).

Discussion

In this systematic review, we have summarised current evidence relating to the use of IODUS for CEA and LEB.

Carotid artery endarterectomy

For completion assessment of CEA, there is conflicting evidence regarding the benefits of completion imaging from analysis of registry data [13–15]. However, the largest of these studies (over 140,000 cases) reports a modest reduction in adjusted risk of stroke/mortality when using IODUS selectively (RR 0.74, CI 0.63–0.88, $p = 0.001$) [13]. The results also suggest that outcomes when using IODUS are at least as good as intraoperative angiography. An opposing result reported by Wallaert and colleagues, suggests a higher stroke rate when using completion imaging (risk adjusted OR 1.9, CI 1.2–2.7, $p = 0.002$). However, when comparing different practice patterns, they found that the lowest rates were seen in cases, where completion imaging was used selectively (routine 2.4%, selective 1.2%, rare 1.7%; $p = 0.048$). This suggests that selective practice may be the most effective strategy, although the criteria for selecting cases was not explored in any of the studies. Wallaert and colleagues also noted that the rate of restenosis at 1-year follow-up was highest for cases, where completion imaging was rarely used (routine 1.1%, selective 1.1%, rare 2.8%; $p = 0.09$) [14]. This may be due to the failure to detect residual defects which may progress during the follow-up period. Data from other studies suggests that 'non-significant' residual defects detected on IODUS are associated with higher rates of restenosis during the follow-up (range 2.1% to 20%) [7, 8, 17–19]. These finding would suggests that although revision surgery can improve outcome, it is certainly not without risk and not all abnormalities detected on IODUS necessitate surgical revision. Isolated high velocities in the absence of other concerning waveform features, such as waveform broadening, or B-mode abnormalities may be related to vessel spasm [6]. If acted upon, these may add risk of complication. Parsa et al., have proposed protocolised imaging and interpretation guidance for both carotid and lower limb completion imaging [25].

Lower extremity bypass surgery

There is paucity of evidence when considering the benefit of IODUS on patency rates following LEB. This may be because of perceived challenges in scanning smaller calibre vessels in a larger deeper surgical field. In the single study addressing IODUS, it was only used in 11% of cases [22], limiting its relevance.

A single paper comparing IODUS with other completion modalities. This study, by Gilbertson et al., compared angioscopy, angiography and IODUS and concluded that angioscopy and angiography were superior to IODUS in detecting residual cusps and un-ligated side branches. However, this study is also limited by its small sample size of 20 and was conducted almost 30 years ago.

Johnson and colleagues suggests that most benefit from IODUS scanning may be gained for in-situ and non-reversed translocated bypasses, as they have a significantly higher rate of lesions requiring revision [21]. Their results also report a 90-day secondary re-intervention rate of 37.7% in grafts with residual flow abnormalities. In comparison, grafts with normal flow, either without or following revision, revision rates of 2.4 and 3% respective, were reported. MacKenzie and colleagues report similarly, but with lower rates of secondary intervention in grafts with un-corrected flow abnormalities (11.1% within 7 months). This may have bearing on optimal post-operative surveillance strategy.

Limitations

None of the studies were of randomised controlled trial design. There was also considerable heterogeneity between studies in terms of intervention, outcome measures and follow-up. Therefore, it was not possible to perform a meta-analysis.

Future work

There is a need for well-designed prospective, multicentre randomised controlled trials to evaluate the effectiveness of IODUS in comparison to other modalities in reducing stroke/mortality outcomes in CEA procedures and primary patency in LEB. Further data are also required to determine the natural progression of different defects detected on IODUS to achieve evidence-based consensus on criteria for revision surgery.

Conclusion

IODUS is a sensitive method to detect defects in both CEA and LEB. However, there is a need for more robust prospective studies to determine the best scanning strategy, criteria for intervention and the impact on clinical outcomes.

Acknowledgements
None.

Authors' contributions
Conception: PN, UJ. Data collection: PN, BK. Writing of manuscript: PN, BK, VS, MA, SP, UJ. All authors read and approved the final manuscript.

Author details
[1] Imperial Vascular Unit, Imperial College Healthcare NHS Trust, London, UK. [2] Department of General Surgery, Kingston Hospital, London, UK. [3] St Marys Hospital, Level 2, Patterson Building, Paddington W21NY, UK.

References

1. Conte MS, Bandyk DF, Clowes AW, Moneta GL, Seely L, Lorenz TJ et al (2006) Results of PREVENT III: a multicenter, randomized trial of edifoligide for the prevention of vein graft failure in lower extremity bypass surgery. J Vasc Surg 43(4):742–751 (**discussion 751**)
2. Rothwell PM, Eliasziw M, Gutnikov SA, Fox AJ, Taylor DW, Mayberg MR et al (2003) Analysis of pooled data from the randomised controlled trials of endarterectomy for symptomatic carotid stenosis. Lancet 361(9352):107–116
3. Stept LL, Flinn WR, McCarthy WJ, Bartlett ST, Bergan JJ, Yao JST (1987) Technical defects as a cause of early graft failure after femorodistal bypass. Arch Surg 122(5):599
4. Walsh DB, Zwolak RM, McDaniel MD, Schneider JR, Cronenwett JL (1990) Intragraft drug infusion as an adjunct to balloon catheter thrombectomy for salvage of thrombosed infragenicular vein grafts: a preliminary report. J Vasc Surg 11(6):753–759 (**discussion 760**)
5. Wölfle KD, Bruijnen H, Mayer B, Loeprecht H (1994) Follow-up of infrainguinal bypass operations: value of the peak systolic velocity and arm-ankle index for evaluation of femorodistal reconstructions. Vasa 23(4):349–356
6. Mays BW, Towne JB, Seabrook GR, Cambria RA, Jean-Claude J (2000) Intraoperative carotid evaluation. Arch Surg 135(5):525–528 (**discussion 528-9**)
7. Kinney EV, Seabrook GR, Kinney LY, Bandyk DF, Towne JB (1993) The importance of intraoperative detection of residual flow abnormalities after carotid artery endarterectomy. J Vasc Surg 17(5):912–922 (**discussion 922-3**)
8. Panneton JM, Berger MW, Lewis BD, Hallett JW, Bower TC, Gloviczki P et al (2001) Intraoperative duplex ultrasound during carotid endarterectomy. Vasc Surg 35(1):1–9
9. Steinmetz OK, MacKenzie K, Nault P, Singher F, Dumaine J (1998) Intraoperative duplex scanning for carotid endarterectomy. Eur J Vasc Endovasc Surg 16(2):153–158
10. Bandyk DF, Mills JL, Gahtan V, Esses GE (1994) Intraoperative duplex scanning of arterial reconstructions: fate of repaired and unrepaired defects. J Vasc Surg 20(3):426–432 (**discussion 432-3**)
11. Yuan JY, Durward QJ, Pary JK, Vasgaard JE, Coggins PK (2014) Use of intraoperative duplex ultrasonography for identification and patch repair of kinking stenosis after carotid endarterectomy: a single-surgeon retrospective experience. World Neurosurg 81(2):334–343
12. Ascher E, Markevich N, Kallakuri S, Schutzer RW, Hingorani AP (2004) Intraoperative carotid artery duplex scanning in a modern series of 650 consecutive primary endarterectomy procedures. J Vasc Surg 39(2):416–420
13. Knappich C, Kuehnl A, Tsantilas P, Schmid S, Breitkreuz T, Kallmayer M et al (2017) Intraoperative completion studies, local anesthesia, and antiplatelet medication are associated with lower risk in carotid endarterectomy. Stroke 48(4):955–962
14. Wallaert JB, Goodney PP, Vignati JJ, Stone DH, Nolan BW, Bertges DJ, et al. Completion imaging after carotid endarterectomy in the Vascular Study Group of New England. J Vasc Surg. 2011;54(2):376–85, 385.e1–3.
15. Rockman CB, Halm EA (2007) Intraoperative imaging: does it really improve perioperative outcomes of carotid endarterectomy? Semin Vasc Surg 20(4):236–243
16. Lingenfelter KA, Fuller BC, Sullivan TM (1995) Intraoperative assessment of carotid endarterectomy: a comparison of techniques. Ann Vasc Surg 9(3):235–240
17. Dorffner R, Metz VM, Trattnig S, Eibenberger K, Dock W, Hörmann M et al (1997) Intraoperative and early postoperative colour Doppler sonography after carotid artery reconstruction: follow-up of technical defects. Neuroradiology 39(2):117–121
18. Baker WH, Koustas G, Burke K, Littooy FN, Greisler HP (1994) Intraoperative duplex scanning and late carotid artery stenosis. J Vasc Surg 19(5):829–832 (**discussion 832-3**)
19. Lane RJ, Ackroyd N, Appleberg M, Graham J (1987) The application of operative ultrasound immediately following carotid endarterectomy. World J Surg 11(5):593–597
20. Bandyk D, Johnson B, Gupta A, Esses G (1996) Nature and management of duplex abnormalities encountered during infrainguinal vein bypass grafting. J Vasc Surg 24(3):430–438
21. Johnson BL, Bandyk DF, Back MR, Avino AJ, Roth SM (2000) Intraoperative duplex monitoring of infrainguinal vein bypass procedures. J Vasc Surg 31(4):678–690
22. Tan T-W, Rybin D, Kalish JA, Doros G, Hamburg N, Schanzer A et al (2014) Routine use of completion imaging after infrainguinal bypass is not associated with higher bypass graft patency. J Vasc Surg 60(3):678-685.e2
23. Gilbertson JJ, Walsh DB, Zwolak RM, Waters MA, Musson A, Magnant JG et al (1992) A blinded comparison of angiography, angioscopy, and duplex scanning in the intraoperative evaluation of in situ saphenous vein bypass grafts. J Vasc Surg 15(1):121–127 (**discussion 127-9**)
24. MacKenzie KS, Hill AB, Steinmetz OK (1999) The predictive value of intraoperative duplex for early vein graft patency in lower extremity revascularization. Ann Vasc Surg 13(3):275–283
25. Parsa P, Hodgkiss-Harlow K, Bandyk DF (2013) Interpretation of intraoperative arterial duplex ultrasound testing. Semin Vasc Surg 26(2–3):105–110

12

Descriptive analysis of a comparison between lung ultrasound and chest radiography in patients suspected of COVID-19

Giovanni Volpicelli[1*], Luciano Cardinale[2], Thomas Fraccalini[1], Marco Calandri[2], Clara Piatti[2], Carlotta Geninatti[2] and Giuseppe Stranieri[2]

Abstract

Background: Lung ultrasound (LUS) and chest radiography (CXR) are the most used chest imaging tools in the early diagnosis of COVID-19 associated pneumonia. However, the relationship between LUS and CXR is not clearly defined. The aim of our study was to describe the comparison between LUS interpretation and CXR readings in the first approach to patients suspected of COVID-19.

Methods: In the time of the first COVID-19 pandemic surge, we prospectively evaluated adult patients presenting to an emergency department complaining of symptoms raising suspicion of COVID-19. Patients were studied by LUS and only those performing also CXR were analyzed. All the patients performed viral reverse transcriptase-polymerase chain reaction (RT-PCR). LUS studies were classified in 4 categories of probabilities, based on the presence of typical or alternative signs of COVID-19-associated interstitial pneumonia. Accordingly, the CXR readings were retrospectively adapted by 2 experts in 4 categories following the standard language that describes the computed tomography (CT) findings. Patients were divided in two groups, based on the agreement of the LUS and CXR categories. Results were also compared to RT-PCR and, when available, to CT studies.

Results: We analyzed 139 cases (55 women, mean age 59.1 ± 15.5 years old). The LUS vs CXR results disagreed in 60 (43.2%) cases. RT-PCR was positive in 88 (63.3%) cases. In 45 cases, a CT scan was also performed and only 4 disagreed with LUS interpretation versus 24 in the comparison between CT and CXR. In 18 cases, LUS detected signs of COVID-19 pneumonia (high and intermediate probabilities) while CXR reading was negative; in 14 of these cases, a CT scan or a RT-PCR-positive result confirmed the LUS interpretation. In 6 cases, LUS detected signs of alternative diagnoses to COVID-19 pneumonia while CXR was negative; in 4 of these cases, CT scan confirmed atypical findings.

Conclusion: Our study demonstrated a strong disagreement between LUS interpretation and CXR reading in the early approach to patients suspected of COVID-19. Comparison with CT studies and RT-PCR results seems to confirm the superiority of LUS over a second retrospective reading of CXR.

Introduction

The COVID-19 pandemic poses unprecedented challenges to the health care systems even in the most advanced and rich countries. During the pandemic surge, there is the need to isolate new cases and diagnose promptly interstitial pneumonia, the most common complication of the SARS-CoV-2 infection [1]. Chest imaging plays a crucial role in the frontline. Among the chest imaging tools of common use, chest computed tomography scan (CT) represents the gold standard for diagnosing pneumonia. In recent studies, CT showed to be highly sensitive in revealing the early signs of interstitial pneumonia even on asymptomatic COVID-19 patients and on

*Correspondence: giovi.volpicelli@gmail.com
[1] Department of Emergency Medicine, San Luigi Gonzaga University Hospital, Torino, Italy
Full list of author information is available at the end of the article

patients with initial negative reverse transcriptase-polymerase chain reaction (RT-PCR) swab test [2, 3]. However, a systematic application of CT during the pandemic surge is not feasible for many reasons, including the biological and economic cost, the unavailability in scarce resource areas and the increase in the risk of in-hospital cross-infections when infected patients are moved to the radiology facilities. The recommendation to limit the use of CT studies in the time of a pandemic surge is also supported by societal guidelines [4, 5]. Lung ultrasound (LUS) and chest radiography (CXR) are valid alternatives to be applied in the frontline [1, 6–14]. Particularly, LUS demonstrated highly feasible and sensitive for COVID-19 pneumonia, with a specificity that increases during the peaks of prevalence [15]. The correct application of LUS depends also on the consideration of different degrees of likelihood for COVID-19 pneumonia and the combination of LUS patterns with the patient's clinical phenotype at presentation to the emergency department (ED) [1, 7, 14]. Instead, the application of CXR in the first diagnosis of COVID-19 pneumonia is limited by a low sensitivity, even if this latter seems to improve in cases with a longer duration of symptoms [10, 16].

To the best of our knowledge, there are no studies comparing LUS and CXR in the first diagnosis of COVID-19 pneumonia, when a systematic classification in patterns of probability is applied. The main aim of our study was to describe the agreement between LUS interpretation and CXR reading in symptomatic patients suspected of COVID-19 who presented to the ED during the peak of COVID-19 pandemic in the spring 2020. A second aim was to describe the combination with the results of CT scan and RT-PCR, in cases showing LUS/CXR disagreement.

Methods

This was a monocenter observational descriptive study performed at San Luigi Gonzaga University Hospital in Torino, Italy. We received the ethical approval from the local ethical committee. During the first surge of the COVID-19 pandemic, from March 10 to May 15, adult patients (≥ 18 years old) presenting to the ED complaining of symptoms raising suspicion of SARS-CoV-2 infection and studied by LUS at presentation, were enrolled. Clinical suspicion was based on the following symptoms: at least one major criteria between fever > 37.5° C, cough, dyspnea, anosmia and/or ageusia; or at least two minor criteria between sore throat, bilateral conjunctivitis, deep weakness, rhinorrhea, headache, diffuse muscle-skeletal pain, gastrointestinal symptoms (diarrhea, nausea, vomit); (2) age ≥ 18-year-old. Symptoms were to last for at least 3 days in the absence of an alternative more probable diagnosis. Exclusion criteria were: (1) a previous diagnosis of COVID-19 pneumonia; (2) a previous pneumonectomy, pleurodesis or history of fibrothorax.

All patients were prospectively studied by bedside LUS at presentation for signs of COVID-19 pneumonia. Decision about performing a CXR study was taken by the physician in charge, blinded to the LUS evaluation and for clinical reasons independent from the study protocol. Only patients who performed both LUS and CXR were analyzed. Performance of a CT scan was decided by the physician in charge for clinical reasons independent from the study protocol, after having considered both the results of LUS and CXR. All the enrolled patients were submitted to RT-PCR swab test immediately after presentation.

Clinical characteristics

The clinical characteristics at presentation were simplified by considering respiratory symptoms and the clinical history. We identified 3 different clinical phenotypes based on pre-existing chronic cardiac or respiratory diseases that may entail the possibility of confounding ultrasound and radiologic signs (*mixed phenotype*), and on the presence (*severe phenotype*) or absence (*mild phenotype*) of signs and/or symptoms of respiratory failure. The list of significant chronic conditions included: severe chronic obstructive pulmonary disease, pulmonary fibrosis, lung cancer, heart failure, or cor pulmonale. Respiratory failure was determined according to the presence of dyspnea, either objective or self-reported to the attending physician at admission, and/or desaturation defined as either a $PaO_2/FiO_2 < 300$ mmHg or $Sat.O_2/FiO_2 < 357$.

Lung ultrasound

For many years, LUS has become a routine diagnostic tool in our institution. The exam was performed by experienced operators with documented previous experience in bedside LUS in the diagnosis of common lung pathologies seen in emergency and critical care. The operator assigned the LUS pattern at patient's presentation being aware of symptoms but blinded to any other exam and diagnostic tool. Further details about the technique are reported in previous publications [1, 7]. An Esaote MyLab and a Mindray TE7 equipped with convex transducers (3.5–6.0 MHz) were used. The focus was placed at the height of the pleural line. The depth of the image was set at 8–10 cm (according to patient's size). The gain was regulated to maintain the homogeneity of the echoic image on the whole screen, including the bottom edge of the lung image. Patients were examined in the supine and lateral decubitus. We performed 5 scans per side by recording as many clips of a duration of 10 secs, in the following areas and the following probe orientation: anterior chest in longitudinal, lateral chest in longitudinal, lateral base in oblique, posterior paravertebral in longitudinal, posterior sub-scapular in oblique. We considered the presence of some basic LUS signs: A-lines; multiple B-lines, either separated, coalescent or "light beam" [6, 17]; regular or irregular pleural line; peripheral consolidations; large consolidation with air bronchogram; pleural effusion. The combination and distribution of the LUS signs were analyzed to assign to each exam one of 4 LUS patterns that express different levels of likelihood for COVID-19 pneumonia in the time of a high pandemic prevalence of the disease:

- *High probability* LUS pattern (HighLUS), typical of COVID-19 pneumonia showing bilateral and multifocal clusters of separated and coalescent B-lines, large echoic bands (light beams), multifocal small peripheral consolidations, alternating regular and irregular pleural line, with or without large consolidations; these clusters should appear in patchy distribution, alternating abruptly with normal A-lines patterns ("spared areas");
- *Intermediate probability* LUS pattern (IntLUS), less typical pattern of COVID-19 pneumonia, which includes unilateral isolated clusters of B-lines and light beam or focal multiple B-lines, with or without small peripheral consolidations;
- *Alternative probability* LUS pattern (AltLUS), a condition more consistent with other diagnosis than COVID-19 pneumonia, such as an isolated large consolidation with dynamic air bronchograms (suggesting bacterial pneumonia) or without bronchograms (suggesting obstructive atelectasis), a large pleural effusion (either hydrostatic or inflammatory), diffuse homogeneously distributed B-lines (suggesting cardiogenic edema or diffuse fibrosis);
- *Low probability* LUS pattern (LowLUS), a normal or near-normal LUS pattern characterized by bilateral A-lines with respiratory sliding without significant B-lines.

Chest radiography

All radiological studies were acquired as a digital radiograph in the bedside antero-posterior view using portable x-ray units (GE OPTIMA XR 200amx, General Electric Healthcare, Milwaukee WI, US) in the isolation wards following local protocols (95 kV, 1,6 mAs, no grid). The CXR images were retrospectively reviewed independently by two radiologists with long-standing experience on thoracic imaging. In case of disagreement in the reading, a consensus was reached after discussion. The findings considered were presence of few basic signs and their distribution in the two lungs. We used a standard definition of CXR alterations, according to the language approved by the Fleischner Society [18]: *ground glass opacities* (GGO), extensive blurred lung opacities, with indistinct margins of blood vessels; *reticular alterations*, visualized as a net image, formed by summation of several small linear opacities; *consolidations*, homogeneous increase in parenchymal attenuation that obscures the visualization of walls of vessels and airways. The distribution of CXR signs of interstitial pneumonia and the presence of additional signs atypical of COVID-19 pneumonia, were used to define 4 classes similar to those used to standardize CT readings [19]:

- *Typical* appearance in the presence of bilateral distribution of GGO and reticular alterations, with or without presence of limited consolidations;
- *Indeterminate* appearance when opacities were limited and monolateral or smooth and not well defined;
- *Atypical* appearance when signs alternative to COVID-19 pneumonia were predominant or isolated, like a large effusion, a large lobar consolidation with evidence of well-defined air bronchograms, clear signs of atelectasis;
- *Negative* when the CXR did not demonstrate any significant alteration.

Computed tomography

Patients with clinical indication to CT scan were moved to the radiology unit to perform the study. A multidetector CT (GE OPTIMA 660 General Electric Healthcare, Milwaukee WI, USA) was used. The patients were in supine and head-first position and received scanning with breath held. Parameters used were: 10 0 kV; 100, mAs real-time adaptive control; layer thickness 1–2.5 mm; pitch, 1–1.5; matrix, 512 × 512. No contrast was administered. All images were transmitted to the post-processing workstation and reconstructed using high-resolution and conventional algorithms. Each study was read and interpreted by two experts with long-standing experience in chest imaging. Interpretation of CT scans was performed by radiologists not involved in CXR readings, blind to the results of LUS and CXR. Signs and nomenclature of CT scan were those recommended and reported in the Radiological Society of North America Expert Consensus document [19]. Each CT scan was assigned to one of the 4 imaging classification recommended in the consensus document:

- *Typical* appearance, in the presence of peripheral, bilateral, multifocal GGO with or without consolidation or visible lines ("crazy-paving");

- *Indeterminate* appearance, in the presence of multifocal perihilar or unilateral GGO with or without consolidation, or very small GGO non-rounded or non-peripheral;
- *Atypical* appearance, in the presence of isolated lobar or segmental consolidation without GGO, or discrete small nodules, or lung cavitation, or smooth interlobular septal thickening with large pleural effusion;
- *Negative*, in case of no CT features suggesting pneumonia.

Statistical analysis

Patients were grouped according to agreement or disagreement between LUS interpretation and CXR reading, following the reciprocal classification in the four categories. Continuous variables are expressed as mean with SD. Categorical variables were expressed as numbers and percentages. The normality of distribution for continuous numeric data was assessed with Shapiro–Wilk test. Non-continuous non-normally distributed variables were analyzed using Chi-Squared test or Fisher's test in case of small numbers. Mann–Whitney test was used to compare continuous non-normally distributed variables. Unpaired T-Test in case of continuous normally distributed variables. P values below 0.05 were considered statistically significant. Statistical analysis was performed using MedCalc statistical software.

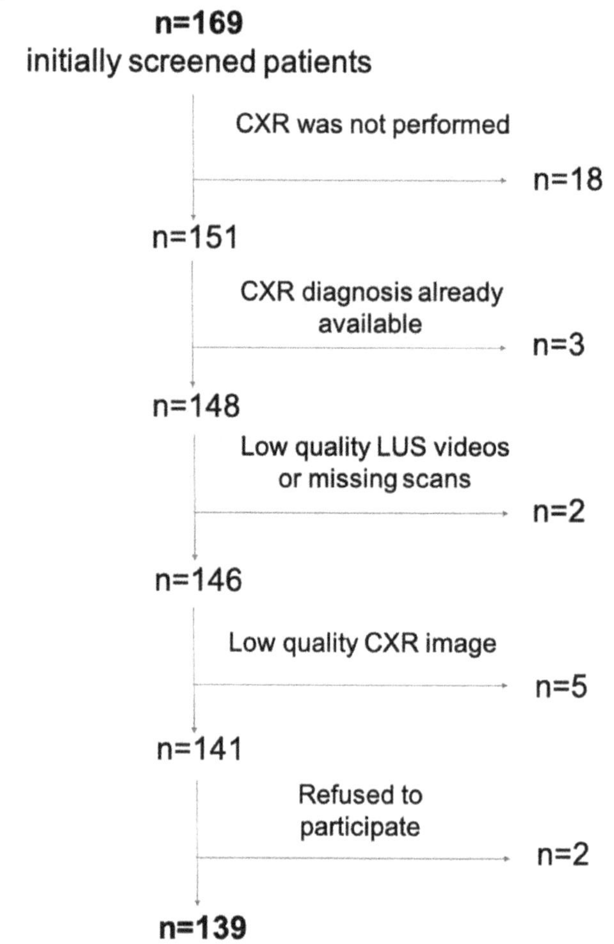

Fig. 1 The flow chart of patients enrolled in the study

Results

Out of 169 patients enrolled in the study, 139 (55 women and 84 men) with a mean age 59.1 ± 15.5 years old performed both CXR and LUS and were examined. The patient's flow chart is represented in Fig. 1. RT-PCR confirmed the SARS-CoV-2 infection in 88 cases (63.3%). Mean number of days from onset of symptoms in the overall population was 7.05 ± 5.6 days. In 45 patients, a thoracic CT study was performed. All the CXR and CT studies were performed within 2 h from the LUS exam. After having assigned each CXR reading and LUS pattern interpretation to the four appearance and probability classes, patients were divided in two groups: 79 (56.8%) patients with agreement (Fig. 2) and 60 (43.2%) with disagreement of CXR vs LUS. Table 1 reports the patient's characteristics in the two subgroups. No statistically significant difference was found between the two groups, apart from the age that resulted higher in the group with LUS vs CXR disagreement (62.8 ± 14.2 vs 56.4 ± 17.6; $p = 0.022$).

When the two LUS classifications HighLUS and IntLUS are mixed together and matched with both CXR *typical* and *indeterminate*, the number of cases showing disagreement was reduced to 46 (33.1%). In the 79 patients showing agreement between LUS pattern and CXR reading, the LUS diagnoses were: 28 LowLUS, 39 HighLUS, 5 IntLUS and 7 AltLUS. Table 2 reports the assignments of LUS patterns together with CXR and CT readings and results of RT-PCR in the subgroup with disagreement.

CT scans: out of the 45 CT studies, 24 disagreed with CXR reading and 4 with LUS interpretation. The 4 cases showing CT vs LUS disagreement, were: one case of *negative* CT that was interpreted AltLUS and *typical* CXR; one case of *typical* CT that was interpreted LowLUS and *negative* CXR; one case of *indeterminate* CT that was interpreted AltLUS and *typical* CXR; one case of *atypical* CT that was interpreted IntLUS but confirmed *atypical* at CXR.

HighLUS and IntLUS with negative CXR: in 18 cases HighLUS ($n = 8$) and IntLUS ($n = 10$) corresponded to *negative* CXR readings (Figs. 3 and 4). Out of the 8 disagreement HighLUS cases, in one case, a CT study was performed that confirmed the *typical* appearance. All the other 7 cases were confirmed by positivity of RT-PCR. Out of the 10 IntLUS cases, in 3 cases, a CT study

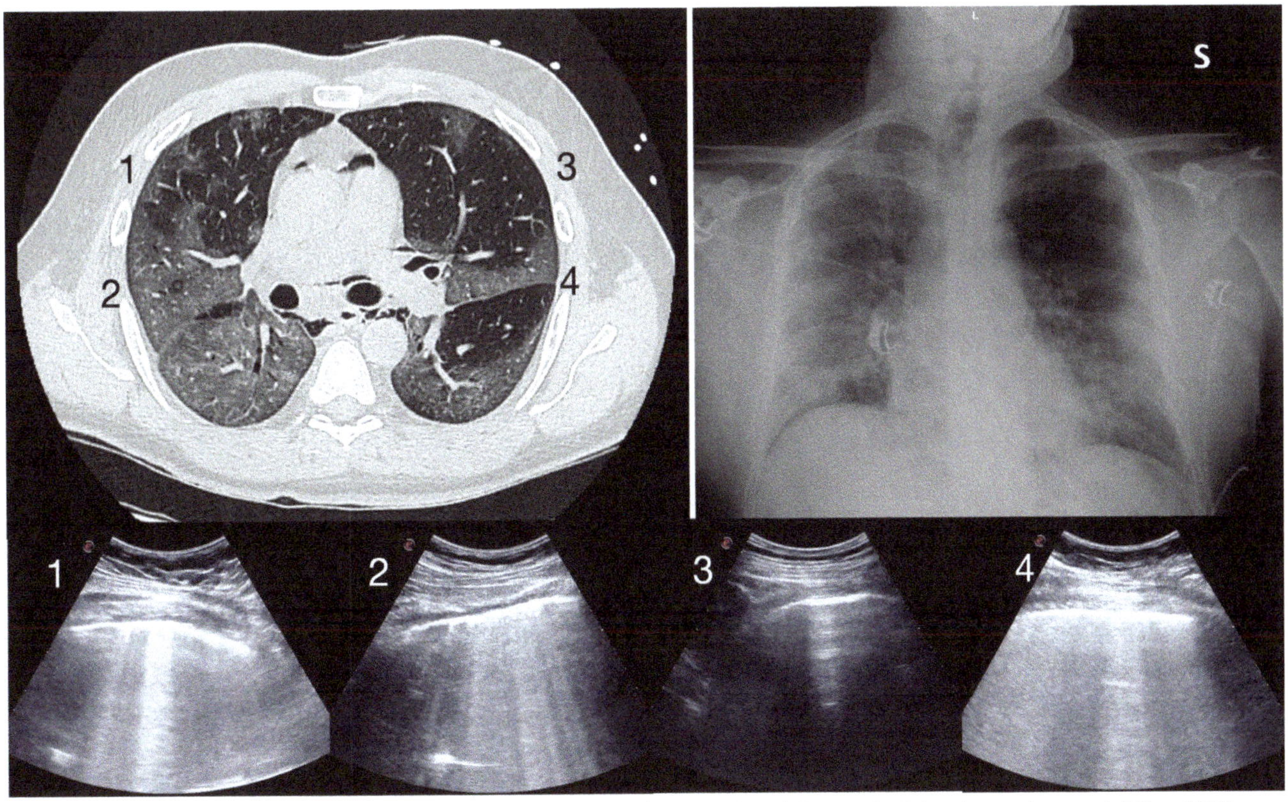

Fig. 2 The case of an otherwise healthy 46-year-old man complaining of fever, cough and dyspnea for 7 days (*severe phenotype*). LUS and CXR were in agreement. LUS showed a *high probability pattern* for COVID-19 pneumonia. The LUS scans reported in the bottom panel show a patchy and bilateral distribution of clusters of B-lines and light beam (1, 2, 4), alternating with normal A-lines pattern (3). CXR in the upper right panel was read *typical* for the presence of bilateral GGO and reticular alterations. The corresponding CT scan in the upper left panel shows multiple GGO alterations that were considered *typical appearance*. The points numbered in the CT image correspond to the 4 LUS scans. RT-PCR was positive. Unfortunately, the patient died of COVID-19 after 20 days from admission. *LUS* Lung Ultrasound, *CXR* Chest Radiography, *COVID-19* Corona Virus Disease 2019, *GGO* Ground Glass Opacity, *CT* Computed Tomography, *RT-PCR* Reverse Transcriptase-Polymerase Chain Reaction

Table 1 Patients' characteristics according to agreement between CXR readings and LUS patterns

	Concordant cases ($n=79$)	Discordant cases ($n=60$)	P
Age (mean ± SD, years)	56.4 ± 17.6	62.8 ± 14.2	0.022
Female sex (*n*)	37 (46.8%)	18 (30.0%)	0.055
Days symptoms onset (mean ± SD)	7.53 ± 5.7	6.43 ± 5.5	0.256
Mild phenotype (*n*)	35 (44.3%)	32 (53.3%)	0.309
Severe phenotype (*n*)	35 (44.3%)	19 (31.7%)	0.161
Mixed phenotype (*n*)	9 (11.4%)	9 (15.0%)	0.613

confirmed an *indeterminate* appearance and in other 3 cases, the RT-PCR was positive. In the remaining 4 cases, RT-PCR resulted negative.

LowLUS: in 6 cases showing disagreement, LowLUS corresponded to *indeterminate* CXR ($n=3$) and *atypical* CXR ($n=3$). Two of these patients performed CT scan that confirmed a *negative* appearance. One other was confirmed negative by the RT-PCR. The other 3 cases, of which one with *atypical* CXR and two *indeterminate* CXR, resulted RT-PCR-positive.

AltLUS: in 6 cases showing disagreement, AltLUS corresponded to *negative* CXR and in 4 of these cases, the CT study showed *atypical* appearance, confirming the LUS interpretation. In the remaining 2 cases, RT-PCR resulted positive in one and negative in the other. In 5 cases, AltLUS corresponded to *typical* CXR, but RT-PCR resulted negative in all and in two cases CT scan confirmed the *atypical* appearance (Fig. 5). In two cases, AltLUS corresponded to *indeterminate* CXR with a positive RT-PCR in one and a confirmation of *atypical* CT in the other.

Discussion

Our study demonstrated a high rate of disagreement between LUS interpretation and CXR reading when the symptomatic patients are examined in the ED for suspected COVID-19 pneumonia during the pandemic

Table 2 Distribution of LUS patterns, CXR readings (*n*), CT findings (*n*) and RT-PCR results (*n*) in 60 cases with disagreement between LUS and CXR, out of 139 patients suspected of COVID-19

LUS pattern	CXR positive	CXR negative	CXR indeterm	CXR atypical	CT typical	CT negative	CT indeterm	CT atypical	RT-PCR positive	RT-PCR negative
HighLUS ($n = 27$)	–	8	12	7	11	0	0	0	24	3
IntLUS ($n = 14$)	2	10	–	2	0	0	3	1	8	6
AltLUS ($n = 13$)	5	6	2	–	0	1	1	6	2	11
LowLUS ($n = 6$)	0	–	3	3	0	2	0	0	3	3

LUS Lung Ultrasound, *CXR* Chest X-Ray, *CT* Computed Tomography of the chest, *RT-PCR* Reverse Transcriptase-Polymerase Chain reaction, *COVID-19* Corona Virus Disease 2019, *HighLUS* High Probability Lung Ultrasound, *LowLUS* Low Probability Lung Ultrasound, *IntLUS* Intermediate Probability Lung Ultrasound, *AltLUS* Alternative Probability Lung Ultrasound, *Indeterm* indeterminate

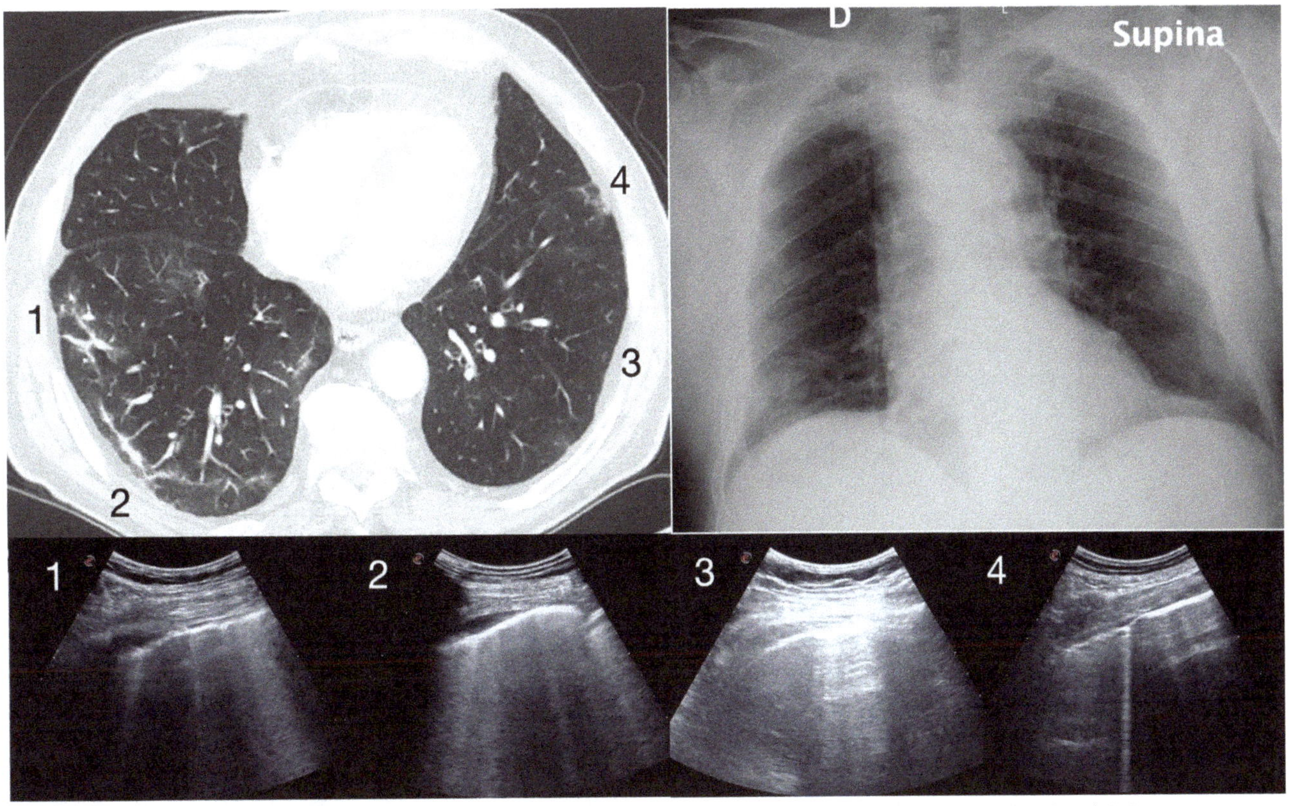

Fig. 3 The case of an otherwise healthy 77-year-old man complaining of fever and cough for 7 days (*mild phenotype*). LUS and CXR were in disagreement. LUS showed a *high probability pattern* for COVID-19 pneumonia. The LUS scans reported in the bottom show the patchy and bilateral distribution of clusters of B-lines and light beam (1, 2, 4) with some irregularity of the pleural line (1, 4), alternating with normal A-lines pattern (3). CXR in the upper right panel was read *negative*. Corresponding CT scan in the upper left panel shows bilateral GGO and was considered *typical appearance*. The points numbered in the CT image correspond to the 4 LUS scans. Viral RT-PCR was positive. *LUS* Lung Ultrasound, *CXR* Chest Radiography, *COVID-19* Corona Virus Disease 2019, *GGO* Ground Glass Opacity, *CT* Computed Tomography, *RT-PCR* Reverse Transcriptase-Polymerase Chain Reaction

surge. Disagreement between LUS and CXR was irrespective of the main patient's characteristics, including sex, days of symptoms onset and clinical phenotype. The group with disagreement resulted only significantly slightly older.

The high rate of disagreement may be due to the classification in 4 different LUS patterns of probability. However, the LUS probability approach demonstrated highly practical when suspected cases are examined in the ED and helps to allocate the patients during the pandemic surge [1, 14]. Indeed, quite a similar classification is recommended for CT readings in COVID-19 pneumonia [19]. The LUS classification includes the possibility of interpreting an intermediate likelihood for COVID-19 pneumonia, corresponding to the "*indeterminate*" classification of the CT language. Like for CT, the LUS *intermediate* probability is assigned in cases of unilateral and mostly isolated interstitial signs. Indeed, to compare LUS probability patterns and CXR readings, it was necessary to introduce the possibility of an "*indeterminate*" reading also for the interpretation of the CXR exams, which may have increased LUS vs CXR disagreement. However, even mixing together *typical* and *indeterminate* CXR readings and *high* and *intermediate* probability LUS interpretation, the rate of disagreement still remained high.

Age may have a role, as an older age may imply an increase in confounding sonographic and radiologic signs. Indeed, the age of the group of disagreement cases was slightly but significantly older than in the other group. However, in other studies, CXR showed a low sensitivity in the early diagnosis of COVID-19 pneumonia irrespective of patient's age, whereas sensitivity improved when symptoms had started from a longer time [16].

Based on our data, it is reasonable to hypothesize that LUS is a more powerful tool in the early diagnosis of COVID-19 pneumonia and that the high rate of disagreement is justified by a difference in diagnostic accuracy between LUS and CXR. This hypothesis is supported also by a more detailed analysis of our disagreement cases, based on the comparison with CT studies and results of the viral swab test. Our study was not specifically designed to investigate a systematic

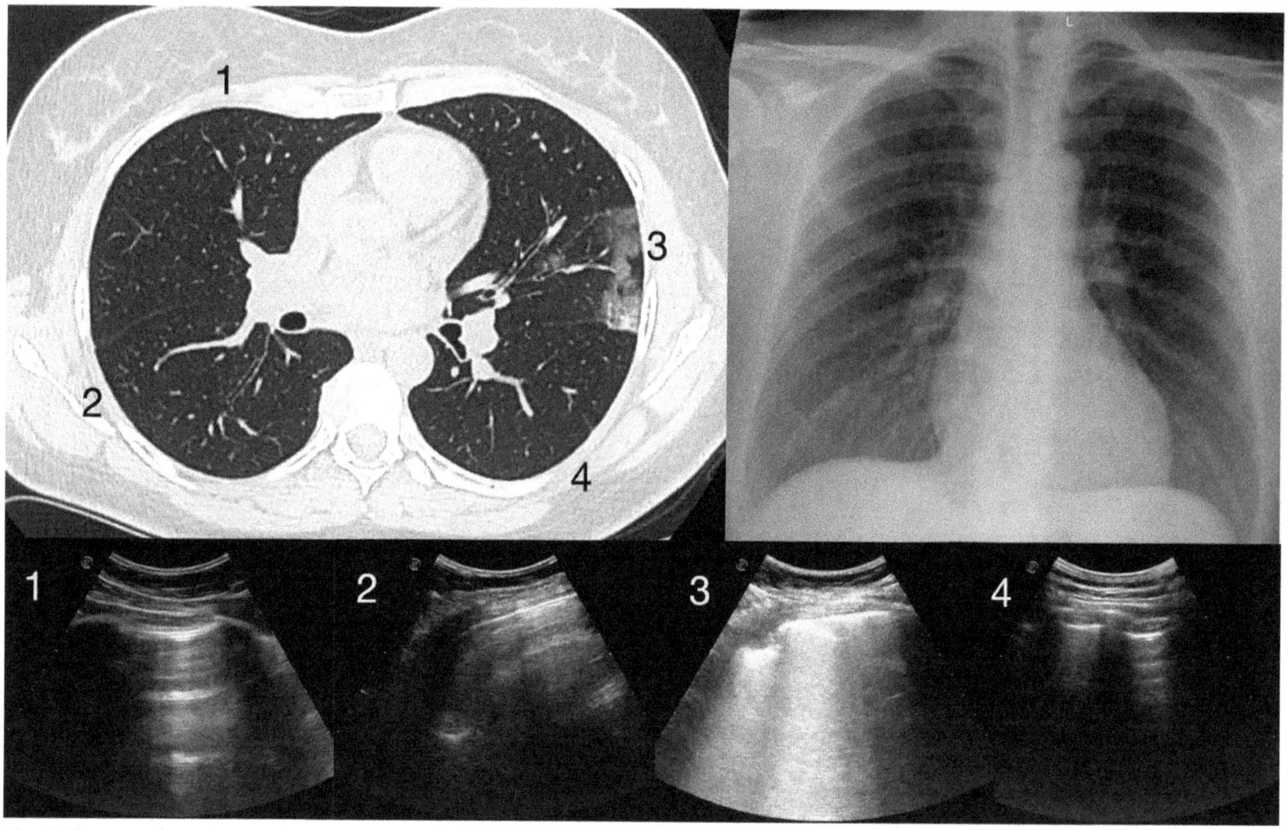

Fig. 4 The case of an otherwise healthy 44-year-old woman complaining of malaise, anosmia, fever and cough for 4 days (*mild phenotype*). LUS and CXR were in disagreement. LUS showed an *intermediate probability pattern* for COVID-19 pneumonia. One of the LUS scans reported in the bottom shows an isolated area with B-lines, light beam and a peripheral consolidation (3). The other LUS scans show A-lines (1, 2, 4). CXR in the upper right panel was read *negative*. Corresponding CT scan in the upper left panel shows a limited peripheral area with GGO and a consolidation and was considered *indeterminate appearance*. The points numbered in the CT scan correspond to the 4 LUS scans. Viral RT-PCR was positive. *LUS* Lung Ultrasound, *CXR* Chest Radiography, *COVID-19* Corona Virus Disease 2019, *GGO* Ground Glass Opacity, *CT* Computed Tomography, *RT-PCR* Reverse Transcriptase-Polymerase Chain Reaction

comparison between CT scan and LUS, but the subgroup of patients submitted to all the three imaging tools showed the striking superiority of LUS to CXR, based on a higher rate of agreement between CT vs LUS interpretation than CT vs CXR reading. When a CT scan was not performed, the results of RT-PCR demonstrated a high rate of confirmation of the LUS classification. Of course, this latter result should be considered cautiously as the viral test is useful to confirm the SARS-CoV-2 infection but not necessarily this latter condition is complicated by pneumonia. Thus, a negative chest imaging test may easily be coupled with a positive RT-PCR in case of SARS-CoV-2 infection not complicated by pneumonia. On the other side, it is also well known that the molecular RT-PCR is limited by quite a low sensitivity, especially when performed early in the first approach to suspected cases [20, 21]. It is common experience that hospitalized patients with a typical clinical picture and suggestive computed tomography (CT) pattern but repeatedly negative RT-PCR, have been considered and treated as COVID-19 pneumonia, particularly in the peak of the COVID-19 surge [2].

Other studies compared LUS and CXR in COVID-19, demonstrating a higher sensitivity of LUS [22, 23]. These studies used a binary classification of the interpretation of LUS based on the presence of generic artifactual abnormalities that, in our opinion, does not adapt to the real practice. Indeed, cases of COVID-19 pneumonia are characterized by non-specific ultrasound signs that can only allow assignment of degrees of probability after the analysis of their distribution. Thus, we strongly suggest comparing abilities of LUS and CXR in the definition of degrees of probability, more than assigning binary diagnoses of positive or negative COVID-19 [1, 7]. Moreover, there is a misconception on the utility of chest imaging that cannot be evaluated for the ability in allowing a definitive diagnosis of COVID-19 infection [24]. The role of chest imaging tools is limited to the diagnosis of pneumonia, which not necessarily complicates COVID-19

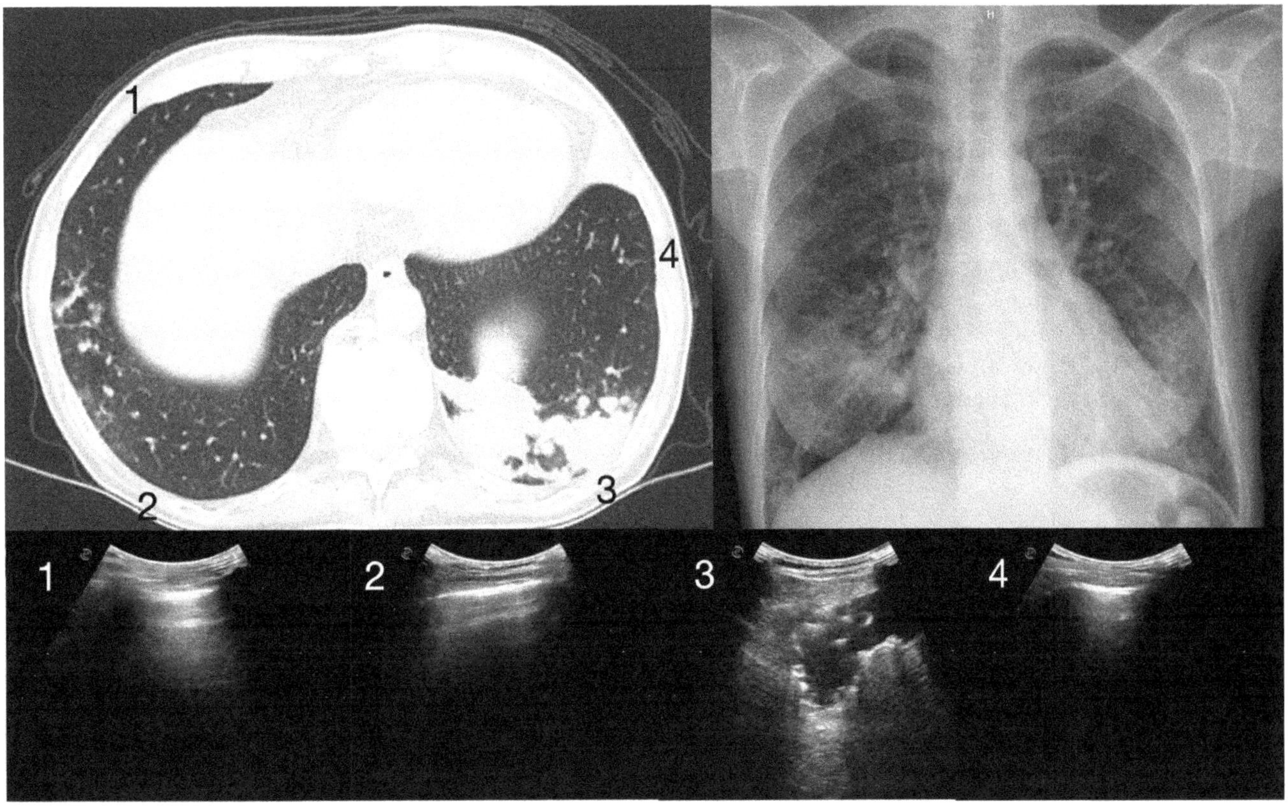

Fig. 5 The case of a 48-year-old woman with a history of HCV related chronic hepatitis, complaining of fever and cough for two weeks (*mild phenotype*). LUS and CXR were in disagreement. LUS showed an *alternative pattern* to COVID-19 pneumonia. One of the LUS scans reported in the bottom shows a large lobar isolated consolidation with dynamic air bronchograms (3). The other LUS scans show A-lines (1, 2, 4). CXR in the upper right panel was read *typical* of COVID-19 pneumonia due to bilateral reticular alterations and GGO. Corresponding CT scan in the upper left panel shows a large consolidation with air bronchograms without significant GGO alterations and was confirmed *atypical appearance* (bacterial pneumonia) The points numbered in the CT scan correspond to the 4 LUS scans. Viral RT-PCR was negative. The patient recovered after antibiotic treatment. *LUS* Lung Ultrasound, *CXR* Chest Radiography, *COVID-19* Corona Virus Disease 2019, *GGO* Ground Glass Opacity, *CT* Computed Tomography, *RT-PCR* Reverse Transcriptase-Polymerase Chain Reaction

and, when confirmed, not always is caused by SARS-CoV-2. Only a combination of chest imaging, clinical data, RT-PCR and follow-up should guide patient's management and safe assignment of differential diagnoses.

Limitations

In our study, the CXR reading was performed retrospectively by expert radiologists. We did not consider the original reading performed in the ED by the radiologist in charge, which would had been more realistic of what happens in the early approach to patients during the surge. However, for intuitive reasons, the CXR readings on the field could not adhere to a strict standardization and the language used could not facilitate a systematic comparison with CT and LUS interpretations.

Another limitation of our study, was the lack of a systematic comparison with CT. Indeed, CT represents the gold standard in the diagnosis of COVID-19 pneumonia. Notwithstanding, the systematic application of CT studies is not ethical in the time of a COVID-19 pandemic surge, due mainly to the problem of overexposure of personnel outside the dedicated hospital areas and lack of clinical utility during the early management of the vast majority of COVID-19 cases [5]. We used the result of RT-PCR to select patients with and without infection. However, the diagnosis of pneumonia is independent from RT-PCR as COVID-19 not necessarily involves the lung and patients with pneumonia may present with negative RT-PCR. Thus, the results of our study should be read as purely descriptive in a moment of extremely high COVID-19 prevalence, and cannot be used for a definitive statistical diagnostic analysis.

A further limitation may be considered the application of bedside CXR antero-posterior projections. It is well known the limitation of this view in the evaluation of the pulmonary parenchyma. However, due to the necessity of limiting the possibility of hospital cross-infections, the bedside CXR is the standard of care in the time of the COVID-19 pandemic surge.

Finally, the study was conducted in a single center where LUS is used as a standard bedside diagnostic tool from many years. In other centers, the quality of LUS performance may vary depending on the level of experience of the operators.

Conclusion

Our descriptive study showed a high rate of disagreement between LUS and CXR performed during the early evaluation of patients suspected of COVID-19. The results of this study support the idea that LUS is superior to CXR in the first approach to COVID-19.

Abbreviations

COVID-19: Corona Virus Disease 2019; SARS-CoV-2: Severe Acute Respiratory Syndrome Corona Virus-2; CT: Computed Tomography; GGO: Ground Glass Opacity; LUS: Lung Ultrasound; ED: Emergency Department; CXR: Chest Radiography; RT-PCR: Reverse Transcriptase-Polymerase Chain Reaction; PaO_2: Partial Pressure of Oxygen in arterial blood; Sat.O_2: Oxygen Saturation; FiO_2: Fraction of inspired Oxygen; HighLUS: High Probability Lung Ultrasound pattern; IntLUS: Intermediate Probability Lung Ultrasound pattern; AltLUS: Alternative Probability Lung Ultrasound pattern; LowLUS: Low Probability Lung Ultrasound pattern; kV: kilovoltage; mAs: milliampere-second; SD: Standard Deviation.

Acknowledgements

We are deeply thankful to all the Doctors, Nurses and Healthcare Personnel, who have been risking their lives to assist and cure these patients and collaborated to the acquisition of LUS scans. We also are thankful to the personnel of the Radiology Department who collaborated to CXR and CT acquisition.

Authors' contributions

All the authors of the article are responsible for concept and writing. GV and LC designed the study. GV and TF were operators and responsible for the LUS studies. LC, MC, CP, CG, GS were responsible for CXR readings and CT interpretation. GV and MC performed the data analysis and statistical calculations. GV, LC, MC collaborated to the writing process. All the authors approved the final draft. All authors read and approved the final manuscript.

Author details

[1] Department of Emergency Medicine, San Luigi Gonzaga University Hospital, Torino, Italy. [2] Department of Oncology, Radiology Unit, San Luigi Gonzaga University Hospital, Torino, Italy.

References

1. Volpicelli G, Lamorte A, Villén T (2020) What's new in lung ultrasound during the COVID-19 pandemic. Intensive Care Med 46:1445–1448.
2. Ai T, Yang Z, Hou H, Zhan C, Chen C, Lv W, Tao Q, Sun Z, Xia L (2020) Correlation of chest CT and RT-PCR testing for coronavirus disease 2019 (COVID-19) in China: A Report of 1014 Cases. Radiology 296:E32–E40.
3. Han R, Huang L, Jiang H, Dong J, Peng H, Zhang D (2020) Early clinical and CT manifestations of coronavirus disease 2019 (COVID-19) Pneumonia. AJR Am J Roentgenol 215:338–343.
4. Hope MD, Raptis CA, Shah A, Hammer MM, Henry TS, six signatories (2020) A role for CT in COVID-19? What data really tell us so far. Lancet 395:1189–1190
5. Revel MP, Parkar AP, Prosch H, Silva M, Sverzellati N, Gleeson F, Brady A; European Society of Radiology (ESR) and the European Society of Thoracic Imaging (ESTI) (2020) COVID-19 patients and the radiology department - advice from the European Society of Radiology (ESR) and the European Society of Thoracic Imaging (ESTI). Eur Radiol 30:4903–4909
6. Volpicelli G, Gargani L (2020) Sonographic signs and patterns of COVID-19 pneumonia. Ultrasound J 12:22. htps://doi.org/10.1186/s13089-020-00171-w
7. Millington SJ, Koenig S, Mayo P, Volpicelli G (2021) Lung ultrasound for patients with coronavirus disease 2019 pulmonary disease. Chest 159:205–211
8. Zieleskiewicz L, Markarian T, Lopez A, Taguet C, Mohammedi N, Boucekine M, Baumstarck K, Besch G, Mathon G, Duclos G, Bouvet L, Michelet P, Allaouchiche B, Chaumoître K, Di Bisceglie M, Leone M; AZUREA Network (2020) Comparative study of lung ultrasound and chest computed tomography scan in the assessment of severity of confirmed COVID-19 pneumonia. Intensive Care Med 46:1707–1713
9. Pivetta E, Goffi A, Tizzani M, Locatelli SM, Porrino G, Losano I, Leone D, Calzolari G, Vesan M, Steri F, Ardito A, Capuano M, Maria G, Giulia S, Dutto S, Avolio M, Cavallo R, Bartalucci A, Paglieri C, Morello F, Richiardi L, Maule M, Lupia E (2020) Lung ultrasound for the diagnosis of SARS-CoV-2 pneumonia in the emergency department. Ann Emerg Med. https://doi.org/10.1016/j.annemergmed.2020.10.008
10. Ippolito D, Pecorelli A, Maino C, Capodaglio C, Mariani I, Giandola T, Gandola D, Bianco I, Ragusi M, Talei Franzesi C, Corso R, Sironi S (2020) Diagnostic impact of bedside chest X-ray features of 2019 novel coronavirus in the routine admission at the emergency department: case series from Lombardy region. Eur J Radiol. https://doi.org/10.1016/j.ejrad.2020.109092.
11. Pakray A, Walker D, Figacz A, Kilanowski S, Rhodes C, Doshi S, Coffey M (2020) Imaging evaluation of COVID-19 in the emergency department. Emergency Radiol 27:579–588
12. Schiaffino S, Tritella S, Cozzi A, Carriero S, Blandi L, Ferraris L, Sardanelli F (2020) Diagnostic performance of chest X-ray for COVID-19 pneumonia during the SARS-CoV-2 pandemic in Lombardy, Italy. J Thorac Imaging 35:W105–W106
13. Vespro V, Andrisani MC, Fusco S, Di Meglio L, Plensich G, Scarabelli A, Stellato E, Ierardi AM, Scudeller L, Coppola A, Gori A, Pesenti A, Grasselli G, Aliberti S, Blasi F, Villa C, Ippolito S, Pirrò B, Damiani G, Galli M, Rizzardini G, Catena E, Orlandi MA, Magnani S, Cipolla G, Ianniello AA, Petrillo M, Xhepa G, Scamporrino A, Cazzulani A, Carrafiello G (2020) Chest X-ray findings in a large cohort of 1117 patients with SARS-CoV-2 infection: a multicenter study during COVID-19 outbreak in Italy. Intern Emerg Med. https://doi.org/10.1007/s11739-020-02561-3.
14. Volpicelli G, Gargani L, Perlini S, Spinelli S, Barbieri G, Lanotte A, Casasola GG, Nogué Bou R, Lamorte A, Agricola E, Villén T, Deol PS, Nazerian P, Corradi F, Stefanone V, Fraga DN, Navalesi P, Ferre R, Boero E, Martinelli G, Cristoni L, Perani C, Vetrugno L, McDermott C, Miralles-Aguiar F, Secco G, Zattera C, Salinaro F, Grignaschi A, Boccatonda A, Giostra F, Nogué Infante M, Covella M, Ingallina G, Burkert J, Frumento P, Forfori F, Ghiadoni L, on behalf of the International Multicenter Study on LUS in COVID-19 (2021) Lung ultrasound for the early diagnosis of COVID-19 pneumonia: an international multicenter study. Intensive Care Med **(in press)**
15. Gargani L, Soliman-Aboumarie H, Volpicelli G, Corradi F, Pastore MC, Cameli M (2020) Why, when, and how to use lung ultrasound during the COVID-19 pandemic: enthusiasm and caution. Eur Heart J Cardiovasc Imaging 21:941–948
16. Vancheri SG, Savietto G, Ballati F, Maggi A, Canino C, Bortolotto C, Valentini A, Dore R, Stella GM, Corsico AG, Iotti GA, Mojoli F, Perlini S, Bruno R, Preda L (2020) Radiographic findings in 240 patients with COVID-19 pneumonia: time-dependence after the onset of symptoms. Eur Radiol 30:6161–6169
17. Volpicelli G, Elbarbary M, Blaivas M, Lichtenstein DA, Mathis G, Kirkpatrick AW, Melniker L, Gargani L, Noble VE, Via G, Dean A, Tsung JW, Soldati G, Copetti R, Bouhemad B, Reissig A, Agricola E, Rouby JJ, Arbelot C, Liteplo A, Sargsyan A, Silva F, Hoppmann R, Breitkreutz R, Seibel A, Neri L, Storti E, Petrovic T; International Liaison Committee on Lung Ultrasound (ILC-LUS) for International Consensus Conference on Lung Ultrasound (ICC-LUS) (2012) International evidence-based recommendations for point-of-care lung ultrasound. Intensive Care Med 38:577–591
18. Hansell DM, Bankier AA, MacMahon H, McLoud TC, Muller NL, Remy J (2008) Fleischner Society: glossary of terms for thoracic imaging. Radiology 246:697–722
19. Simpson S, Kay FU, Abbara S, Bhalla S, Chung JH, Chung M, Henry TS, Kanne JP, Kligerman S, Ko JP, Litt H (2020) Radiological Society of North America Expert Consensus Statement on Reporting Chest CT Findings Related to COVID-19. Endorsed by the Society of Thoracic Radiology, the American College of Radiology, and RSNA. J Thorac Imaging 35:219–227

20. Li Y, Yao L, Li J, Chen L, Song Y, Cai Z, Yang C (2020) Stability issues of RT-PCR testing of SARS-CoV-2 for hospitalized patients clinically diagnosed with COVID-19. J Med Virol 92:903–908
21. Arevalo-Rodriguez I, Buitrago-Garcia D, Simancas-Racines D, Zambrano-Achig P, Del Campo R, Ciapponi A, Sued O, Martínez-García L, Rutjes A, Low N, Bossuyt PM, Perez-Molina JA, Zamora J (2020) False-negative results of initial RT-PCR assays for COVID-19: a systematic review. https://www.medrxiv.org/content/10.1101/2020.04.16.20066787v1
22. Shumilov E, Hosseini ASA, Petzold G, Treiber H, Lotz J, Ellenrieder V, Kunsch S, Neesse A (2020) Comparison of Chest Ultrasound and Standard X-Ray Imaging in COVID-19 Patients. Ultrasound Int Open 6:E36–E40. https://doi.org/10.1055/a-1217-1603.
23. Pare JR, Camelo I, Mayo KC, Leo MM, Dugas JN, Nelson KP, Baker WE, Shareef F, Mitchell PM, Schechter-Perkins EM (2020) Point-of-care lung ultrasound is more sensitive than chest radiograph for evaluation of COVID-19. West J Emerg Med 21:771–778
24. Islam N, Salameh JP, Leeflang MM, Hooft L, McGrath TA, van der Pol CB, Frank RA, Kazi S, Prager R, Hare SS, Dennie C, Spijker R, Deeks JJ, Dinnes J, Jenniskens K, Korevaar DA, Cohen JF, Van den Bruel A, Takwoingi Y, van de Wijgert J, Wang J, McInnes MD; Cochrane COVID-19 Diagnostic Test Accuracy Group (2020) Thoracic imaging tests for the diagnosis of COVID-19. Cochrane Database Syst Rev. https://doi.org/10.1002/14651858.CD013639.pub3

B-line quantification: comparing learners novice to lung ultrasound assisted by machine artificial intelligence technology to expert review

Frances M. Russell[1*], Robert R. Ehrman[2], Allen Barton[3], Elisa Sarmiento[1], Jakob E. Ottenhoff[2] and Benjamin K. Nti[1]

Abstract

Background: The goal of this study was to assess the ability of machine artificial intelligence (AI) to quantitatively assess lung ultrasound (LUS) B-line presence using images obtained by learners novice to LUS in patients with acute heart failure (AHF), compared to expert interpretation.

Methods: This was a prospective, multicenter observational study conducted at two urban academic institutions. Learners novice to LUS completed a 30-min training session on lung image acquisition which included lecture and hands-on patient scanning. Learners independently acquired images on patients with suspected AHF. Automatic B-line quantification was obtained offline after completion of the study. Machine AI counted the maximum number of B-lines visualized during a clip. The criterion standard for B-line counts was semi-quantitative analysis by a blinded point-of-care LUS expert reviewer. Image quality was blindly determined by an expert reviewer. A second expert reviewer blindly determined B-line counts and image quality. Intraclass correlation was used to determine agreement between machine AI and expert, and expert to expert.

Results: Fifty-one novice learners completed 87 scans on 29 patients. We analyzed data from 611 lung zones. The overall intraclass correlation for agreement between novice learner images post-processed with AI technology and expert review was 0.56 (confidence interval [CI] 0.51–0.62), and 0.82 (CI 0.73–0.91) between experts. Median image quality was 4 (on a 5-point scale), and correlation between experts for quality assessment was 0.65 (CI 0.48–0.82).

Conclusion: After a short training session, novice learners were able to obtain high-quality images. When the AI deep learning algorithm was applied to those images, it quantified B-lines with moderate-to-fair correlation as compared to semi-quantitative analysis by expert review. This data shows promise, but further development is needed before widespread clinical use.

Keywords: Artificial intelligence, Point-of-care ultrasound, Lung ultrasound, Acute heart failure, Novice learner

Introduction

Lung ultrasound (LUS) for the evaluation of pulmonary edema in acute heart failure (AHF) has become standard care in many emergency departments (ED) and intensive care settings [1]. Ultrasound can be used by practitioners across a broad range of expertise to evaluate the lungs for the presence of B-lines, indicating pulmonary edema or

*Correspondence: framruss@iu.edu
[1] Department of Emergency Medicine, Indiana University School of Medicine, 720 Eskenazi Ave, FOB 3rd Floor, Indianapolis, IN 46202, USA
Full list of author information is available at the end of the article

loss of lung aeration [2]. Presence of B-lines is highly specific for the presence of interstitial and alveolar fluid. In the evaluation of a patient with dyspnea, this can rapidly alter the differential as well as dictate initial management [3]. Delays in recognizing pulmonary congestion can delay initiation of appropriate treatments and increase the likelihood of adverse events.

The workup of AHF has traditionally centered on identifying radiographic and physical exam findings consistent with fluid overload such as pretibial edema, rales, hepatojugular reflux, and pulmonary edema on chest X-ray. The most recent 2019 guidelines from the American College of Cardiology continue to emphasize estimation of fluid status and therapy centered on decongestion in AHF [4]. However, even in AHF without total body fluid overload (e.g., Sympathetic Crashing Acute Pulmonary Edema), identifying pulmonary edema is critical in expediting diagnosis and management [5]. LUS has consistently been shown to identify extravascular lung water with greater accuracy than chest X-ray and has the advantage of being performed rapidly and repeatedly at the bedside [6, 7]. However, LUS relies heavily on clinician competence in obtaining and interpreting images. The use of artificial intelligence (AI) software packages embedded in ultrasound systems to identify and quantify B-lines has the potential to offer these same benefits to novice learners without extensive ultrasound training.

While automated LUS image analysis has been described [8, 9], no prior study has investigated how existing AI B-Line quantification packages perform when used in this putatively beneficial scenario. Therefore, the goal of this study was to compare B-line quantification from an AI software package to those of an expert reviewer, using images acquired by novice learners on ED patients with AHF. Secondarily, we assessed image quality.

Methods

Study design and patient selection

This was a prospective observational study performed from December 2018 to March 2020 at two urban academic EDs, each of which supports a 3-year Emergency Medicine (EM) residency and serves as a site for medical student EM rotations. The study was approved by the institutional review board at each site (protocol #1809442708).

Patients > 18 years-of-age who were able to provide written informed consent were eligible for inclusion when the following criteria were met: subjective report of dyspnea at rest or with minimal exertion, a clinical diagnosis of AHF by the treating provider, and clinical signs of volume overload (pulmonary edema on chest X-ray, jugular venous distension, pulmonary rales/crackles on chest auscultation, or bilateral lower extremity edema). Patients with a temperature > 38.6° Celsius, history of interstitial lung disease, or suspected acute lung injury/acute respiratory distress syndrome were excluded. Demographics, past medical history, New York Heart Association (NYHA) symptom classification, and B-type natriuretic peptide level were collected for each patient. Study data were collected and managed using REDCap electronic data capture tools.

Novice learner training and lung ultrasound protocol

Novice learners consisted of medical students and EM residents. In order to be able to enroll patients in the study, novice learners first participated in a 30-min training session lead by a study investigator at each site that consisted of a brief lecture covering the etiology and appearance of B-lines on LUS as well as image acquisition technique. After the initial lecture, novice learners completed proctored hands-on scanning of patients with pulmonary edema. Each participating learner completed a data collection form recording their level of training, total number of US examinations of any modality performed, and total number of LUS examinations performed previously.

LUS examinations were performed in accordance with a previously published protocols [10]. Briefly, patients were scanned supine with head-of-bed elevation as close to 45 degrees as their comfort would allow. All exams were performed using a GE Venue ultrasound system (GE Healthcare, Milwaukee, WI) with a curvilinear probe in the "Lung" setting. Depth was set to 18 cm, and the probe was placed in a horizonal orientation (indicator to patient's right side) in 4 zones per hemi-thorax. Tissue harmonics and compounding were turned off, speckle reduction minimal, and the focal zone was defaulted to just deep to one centimeter to be close to the pleural line. For each lung zone, a 6-s video clip was stored. Novice learners were aware of the study purposes and were not blinded to patient physical appearance. The same patient could be scanned by more than one learner (if the patient was willing), but only one learner was present at a time when serial examinations were performed.

B-line quantification

B-line counts by novice learners were obtained by using the "Auto B-Line" AI feature on the US system. This feature was turned off during image acquisition and the counts were obtained offline once the examination was completed. This was to allow later blinded quantification by an expert. The AI settings were configured to a "scan across rib spaces" setting, which automatically counts B-lines in the central two-thirds of the image rather than across the entire screen. The software package counts the maximum number of B-lines visualized during the clip in integers from 0 to 5, or ≥ 5 if there are more than 5 discrete B-lines or confluence of B-lines occupying > 50% of the pleural line (Fig. 1). Clips where no pleural line was visible on the LUS image were excluded from analysis. Clips where bowel or rib was imaged, and no pleural line was seen, were excluded from AI analysis but were included in the image quality analysis.

The criterion standard for B-line counts was manual counts performed by a point-of-care ultrasound expert physician reviewer with extensive experience in LUS research. They were blinded to AI counts and patient information. De-identified clips were exported from the US system and interpreted offline, using the same counting method. The expert reviewer determined image quality using a 5-point scale (1: pleural line not in view, 2: small part of pleural line in view with technical flaws, 3: moderate amount of pleural line in view with technical flaws, 4: pleural line in full view with small technical flaws, 5: pleural line in view with excellent image quality). A score > 3 was pre-determined to be good image quality. A randomized subset of LUS videos were assessed for B-line quantification and image quality by a second expert reviewer, with extensive LUS experience, to assess for expert agreement. This second expert was not involved in the study design or training. They were blinded to clinical data, site, and expert and AI quantification.

Statistical analysis

We reported frequencies and percentages for categorical variables and median (minimum–maximum) for continuous variables. Data were compared using the Wilcoxon test and Spearman's correlation for determining interclass correlation. We performed all statistical analysis using SAS, Version 9.4 (SAS Institute, Cary, NC). On individual scans, machine AI was considered to be in agreement with the expert if counts were within 1 B-line. Intraclass correlation (ICC) coefficients were used to determine agreement between experts for B-line quantification and image quality.

Results

Eighty-seven LUS examinations (696 lung zones) were performed on 29 individual patients. Out of 696 lung zones assessed, 611 (88%) images were used in the B-line quantification analysis. To be eligible for the B-line quantification analysis, the images had to show a pleural line interface. Thus, 85 images were excluded: 4 images were either not saved properly or not acquired, and 81 images did not include a pleural interface. For example, if the image only included a heart in view it was excluded from analysis, which is common in left zone 2. Additionally, if

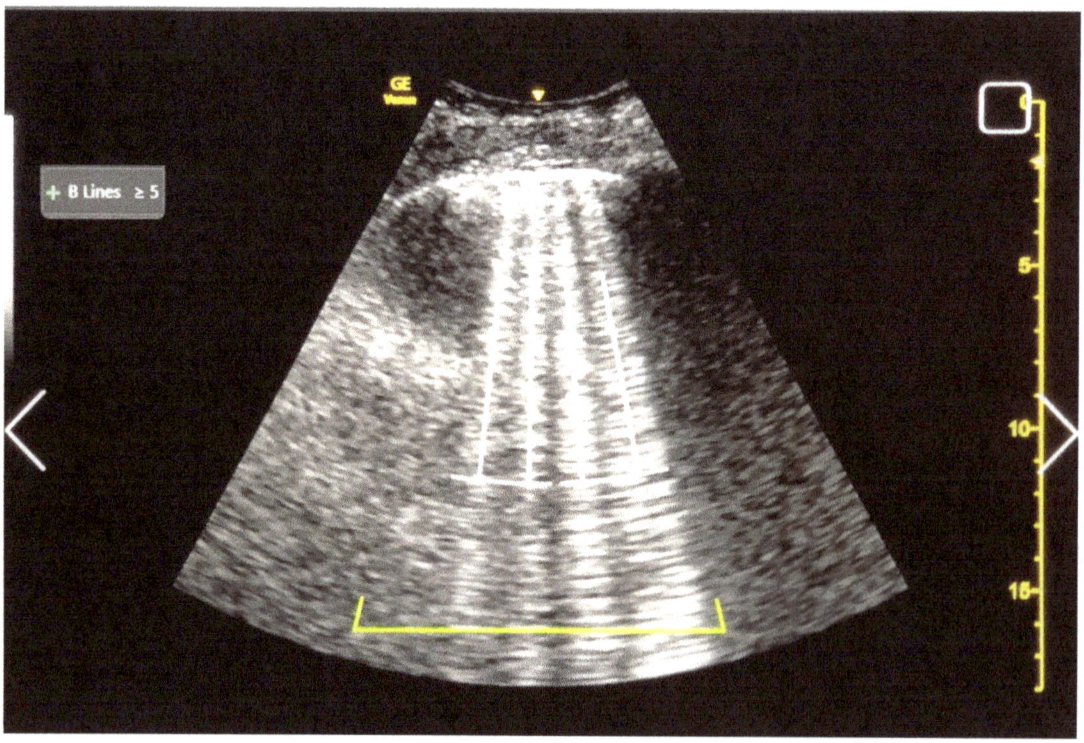

Fig. 1 Lung ultrasound image of B-lines using machine AI for quantification. This image shows the zone analyzed (green line at bottom) and demonstrates ≥ 5 B-lines

the patient had a large pleural effusion and or pneumonia these scans were excluded from analysis. If the learner only captured bowel or ribs these images were also excluded from quantification analysis ($n=28$).

Out of 696 lung zones assessed, 639 (92%) were analyzed for image quality. The 28 videos, where images were inadequately acquired (i.e., only bowel or rib was visualized), were excluded from quantification analysis, but included in the image quality analysis.

The median age of included patients was 65, 55% of patients were male, and the median body mass index was 28.2. Twenty-two (76%) patients had a history of heart failure, 14 with a history of systolic heart failure, and 8 with diastolic heart failure. A majority of patients were NYHA class 2. Median initial B-type natriuretic peptide level was 576. Sixteen (55%) patients were admitted to a medical floor with cardiac monitoring, 4 (13%) were admitted to the intensive care unit and 5 (17%) were discharged from the emergency department. See Table 1 for patient demographics.

There were 51 learners that completed the LUS examinations: 18 were medical students, 21 interns, and 12 residents. The level of ultrasound experience varied with the median number of prior LUS ranging from 1 to 10 overall. See Table 2 for learner demographics.

Of the 611 lung zones analyzed, 281 (46%) had 0–2 B-lines, 105 (17%) had 3–4 B-lines, and 225 (37%) had 5 or greater B-lines. Intraclass correlation between ultrasound machine AI and expert read was 0.56 (0.51–0.62) overall. See Table 3 for correlation by zone, and median read by machine AI and expert by lung zone. Correlation was highest in the lateral zones (right zone 3, 4 and left zone 3), and lowest in the left anterior lung zones.

Overall image quality was a median of 4, range 1 to 5, with all zones having a median of 4 or 5; see Table 4. ICC between machine AI and expert based on image quality was 0.58 (confidence interval [CI] 0.52–0.64) for scans with a quality rating of 4 or 5, and 0.41 (CI 0.37–0.53) for scans with a quality rating of 1 through 3, see Table 5. ICC between faculty experts after blinded review of 33% of images was 0.82 (CI 0.73–0.91) for B-line quantification and 0.65 (CI 0.48–0.82) for image quality.

Table 1 Patient demographics, $n=29$, n (%)

Age, median (Min.–Max.)	65.0 (31–90)
Gender, male	16 (55.2)
Race	
Black	12 (41.4)
Hispanic	1 3.5)
White	16 (55.2)
Height in cm, median (Min.–Max.)	170.2 (149.9–193.0)
BMI, median (Min.–Max.)	28.2 (18.8–58.4)
Heart failure history	
New onset	7 (24.1)
Systolic HF	14 (48.3)
Diastolic (HFpEF)	8 (27.6)
NYHA, symptom classification	
Class 1	1 (14.4)
Class 2	17 (58.6)
Class 3	7 (24.1)
Class 4	4 (13.8)
Initial BNP level, median (Min.–Max.)	576.0 (26.0–5,000.0)
Disposition from ED	
Admit (non ICU)	16 (55.17)
ICU	4 (13.79)
Observation	4 (13.79)
Discharge	5 (17.24)

BMI body mass index, *ICU* intensive care unit, *HF* heart failure, *HFpEF* heart failure with preserved ejection fraction

Table 3 ICC between machine AI and expert, $n=611$

Zone	GE machine, median (Min.–Max.)	Expert, median (Min.–Max.)	Spearman correlation (95% CI)
Right zone 1	5.0 (0.0–5.0)	3.0 (0.0–5.0)	0.57 (0.42–0.70)
Right zone 2	4.0 (0.0–5.0)	3.0 (0.0–5.0)	0.46 (0.27–0.62)
Right zone 3	5.0 (0.0–5.0)	2.5 (0.0–5.0)	0.65 (0.51–0.76)
Right zone 4	5.0 (0.0–5.0)	4.0 (0.0–5.0)	0.77 (0.66–0.85)
Left zone 1	4.0 (0.0–5.0)	3.0 (0.0–5.0)	0.40 (0.21–0.57)
Left zone 2	4.0 (0.0–5.0)	2.0 (0.0–5.0)	0.32 (0.05–0.55)
Left zone 3	4.0 (0.0–5.0)	2.5 (0.0–5.0)	0.60 (0.44–0.72)
Left zone 4	5.0 (0.0–5.0)	5.0 (0.0–5.0)	0.54 (0.35–0.69)
Overall ICC	–	–	0.56 (0.51–0.62)

Intraclass correlation between machine AI and expert by zone and overall. Data are based off of 611 images

Table 2 Learner demographics, $n=51$

	MS4 $n=18$	Intern $n=21$	Resident $n=12$
Level of US experience	Some (none–moderate)	Some (some–large)	Large (moderate–large)
LUS prior	1–10 (0–25)	11–25 (0–50)	25–50 (25- > 100)

Table 4 Image quality by zone and overall, $n = 639$

Zone	Median (Min.–Max.)
Right zone 1	5.0 (3.0–5.0)
Right zone 2	4.0 (1.0–5.0)
Right zone 3	4.0 (1.0–5.0)
Right zone 4	4.0 (1.0–5.0)
Left zone 1	5.0 (2.0–5.0)
Left zone 2	4.0 (1.0–5.0)
Left zone 3	4.0 (1.0–5.0)
Left zone 4	4.0 (1.0–5.0)
Overall image quality	4.0 (1.0–5.0)

Image quality by zone and overall. Data are based off of 639 images

Table 5 ICC between machine AI and expert by image quality, $n = 611$

Zone	Overall image quality (1–3) Spearman correlation (95% CI)	Overall image quality (4–5) Spearman correlation (95% CI)
Right zone 1	0.68 (-0.16–0.95)	0.58 (0.41–0.71)
Right zone 2	0.17 (-0.31–0.58)	0.56 (0.36–0.71)
Right zone 3	0.55 (0.24–0.76)	0.62 (0.42–0.76)
Right zone 4	0.53 (0.11–0.79)	0.67 (0.49–0.80)
Left zone 1	0.06 (-0.51–0.59)	0.48 (0.27–0.64)
Left zone 2	0.50 (-0.19–0.86)	0.27 (-0.04–0.54)
Left zone 3	0.41 (0.04–0.68)	0.51 (0.29–0.69)
Left zone 4	0.22 (-0.22–0.59)	0.63 (0.42–0.78)
Overall correlation	0.41 (0.37–0.53)	0.58 (0.52–0.64)

Intraclass correlation between machine AI and expert by image for each zone and overall. Data are based off of 611 images

Discussion

LUS B-line quantification is a useful tool for diagnosis, prognosis, and monitoring response to treatment in patients with AHF [10–13]. European Society of Cardiology expert consensus guidelines support the use of LUS in the management of AHF [14]. LUS image acquisition and interpretation is highly dependent on the skill of the operator. Machine AI with technology to automatically quantify B-lines has the potential to decrease inter-operator variability and if this technology works it could allow novice learners the ability to count B-lines and incorporate findings into their clinical decisions in patients with AHF.

The results of our study suggest that after limited training, learners with some to no prior LUS experience were able to generate high-quality images. Machine AI was able to quantify B-lines using these images with fair correlation when compared to an expert reviewer. This data suggests that further AI technology development is necessary to improve the algorithm to achieve good correlation. If successful, this has great implications clinically as a clinician or even a non-clinician could track treatment progress in patients with AHF to determine response to treatment, guide additional therapy, and determine when a patient is decongested and ready for hospital discharge [2].

Overall machine AI tended to overcount the number of B-lines when compared to the expert in every lung zone expect left zone 4, where median counts were equal. Interestingly, the lateral zones had higher correlation with expert reads than the anterior lung zones. Anterior lung zones are generally easier to acquire compared to the lateral lung zones which require the probe be positioned in an oblique manner to stay within the rib space, which can be challenging for a novice learner to orient the probe. In addition, lateral lung zone image acquisition is difficult in obese patients.

The left anterior lung zones 1 and 2 had the lowest correlation 0.40 and 0.32, respectively. These zones also had the lowest number of assessments as the heart commonly sits in view and can make it tough to view the pleural line. If any portion of the pleural line was obtained these images were included in analysis. It is possible that the machine AI overcounted B-lines in these zones secondary to cardiac motion.

We found that after a 30-min training session, learners both novice and those with limited LUS experience were able to obtain high-quality images on the vast majority of patients. However, it is important to note that 28 (4%) images were inadequately acquired, where the learner was unable to obtain pleural line. In these instances, it was common for the learner to image below the diaphragm or over a rib. Bowel gas can appear similar to lung artifacts on US and could easily be confused by a novice learner. Additionally, rib with shadow can appear similar to pleural line, especially when viewing in a horizontal orientation. While this may have been expected in novice learners, the proportion of these inadequate images was quite low supporting that a brief training is sufficient. The importance of image quality is demonstrated by the fact that correlation between AI and expert counts increased as image quality improved—from 0.41 with lower quality images to 0.58 with higher-quality images (rated as a 4 or 5).

To our knowledge, this was the largest study assessing novice learners' ability to use machine AI to objectively quantify LUS B-lines. Prior literature has found that machine-assisted quantification of LUS artifacts generally performs well, but studies are small. Corradi et al. [15] evaluated 32 patients with suspected community-acquired pneumonia, comparing quantitative ultrasound to chest X-ray and computed tomography as the gold standard. They found quantitative ultrasound to have high sensitivity, specificity, and diagnostic accuracy, outperforming chest X-ray and visual ultrasonography for the diagnosis of community-acquired pneumonia. Although this was a small study, evaluating pneumonia and not B-line quantification, they were able to show machine AI's ability to accurately detect lung artifacts.

Brusasco et al. [8] studied 12 intensive care unit patients with acute respiratory distress, comparing an automated quantitative scoring system for B-lines with semi-quantitative measurements of extravascular lung water using thermo-dilution. They found computer-aided B-line quantification on LUS had a strong correlation with extravascular lung water ($R^2 = 0.57$). This was a pilot study limited by a small sample size and single sonographer. Additionally, the B-line analysis was performed in post-processing, limiting the real-time application of the technology.

Corradi et al. [16] assessed computer-assisted LUS B-line quantification in 48 ventilated cardiac surgery patients, compared to pulmonary capillary wedge pressure or extravascular lung water assessments using thermo-dilution. They found high correlations between quantitative LUS and pulmonary congestion. This study differs from ours in that it included ventilated cardiac patients, different standards were used for comparison, and all images were obtained by the same operator.

The data from these studies and our study suggest that use of AI software to identify clinically useful LUS artifacts—including B-line quantification—shows promise, but further development is needed before widespread use. Future studies should be aimed at further refining this technology and prospectively assessing a larger number of patients and novice learners in diverse clinical environments, with careful attention to the impact of image quality on algorithm performance.

There are several limitations to consider. This was overall a relatively small study, although there were a large number of learners. Previously published methods of LUS B-line assessment have used differing protocols and semi-quantitative methods [17]. For this study, we used an 8-zone protocol and compared an automatic quantitative method to a semi-quantitative method by one expert. Our criterion standard was expert review using a semi-quantitative method. While this is currently used in clinical practice and has a high correlation with extravascular lung water (EVLW) [18], the true quantity of EVLW present remains unknown as there was no direct measurement thereof. In addition, we found high correlation between experts.

The machine AI software only has the ability to count 0–4 and ≥ 5 B-lines within one lung zone. Semi-quantitative methods typically use a scale of 0 through 10, or 0 through 20. From a clinical standpoint, a count of ≥ 5 B-lines within a lung zone by the US machine would be significant for a large amount of extravascular lung water, and thus clinically significant pulmonary edema. Finally, patients were scanned by multiple learners, but each set of LUS images was treated as independent in our analysis, thereby ignoring potential within-subject correlation for B-line counts. Image acquisition technique (probe location on chest wall, angle of insonation, timing during the respiratory cycle) has a substantial impact on image quality and thus B-line counts. Given the varied experience level of each learner and the fact that they scanned independently, we felt that, overall, between-learner variability in image acquisition technique would minimize the impact of the within-subject B-line correlation.

Conclusion

After a limited structured training learners with no to little prior experience performing LUS were able to obtain high-quality images. However, B-line quantification of these images using a deep learning AI algorithm found only moderate-to-fair correlation when compared to semi-quantitative analysis by an expert. This data shows promise, but further development is needed before widespread clinical use.

Abbreviations

LUS: Lung ultrasound; AHF: Acute heart failure; ED: Emergency departments; AI: Artificial intelligence; EM: Emergency medicine; NYHA: New York Heart Association; ICC: Intraclass correlation; CI: Confidence interval.

Acknowledgements

Not applicable.

Authors' contributions

FMR was responsible for conceptualization, data curation, writing, editing, project administration. RRE was responsible for data curation, writing, editing. ES was responsible for data analysis and writing. BN, AB and JEO were responsible for data curation, writing, editing. All authors read and approved the final manuscript.

Author details

[1]Department of Emergency Medicine, Indiana University School of Medicine, 720 Eskenazi Ave, FOB 3rd Floor, Indianapolis, IN 46202, USA. [2]Department of Emergency Medicine, Wayne State University School of Medicine, 4021 St Antoine Ave, Suite 6G, Detroit, MI 48201, USA. [3]Boone County Emergency Physicians, Zionsville, IN 46077, USA.

References

1. Lee F (2016) Lung ultrasound—a primary survey of the acutely dyspneic patient. J Intensive Care 4(1):57
2. Russell FM, Ferre RR, Ehrman RR, Noble V, Gargani L, Collins SP, Levy PD, Fabre KL, Eckert GJ, Pang PS (2020) What are the minimum requirements to establish proficiency in lung ultrasound training for quantifying B-lines? ESC Heart Failure 7(5):2941–2947

3. Volpicelli G, Mussa A, Garofalo G, Cardinale L, Casoli G, Perotto F, Fava C, Frascisco M (2006) Bedside lung ultrasound in the assessment of alveolar-interstitial syndrome. Am J Emer Med 24(6):689–696
4. Hollenberg SM, Warner Stevenson L, Ahmad T, Amin VJ, Bozkurt B, Butler J, Davis LL, Drazner MH, Kirkpatrick JN, Peterson PN, Reed BN, Roy CL, Storrow AB (2019) 2019 ACC Expert consensus decision pathway on risk assessment, management, and clinical trajectory of patients hospitalized with heart failure: a report of the American College of Cardiology solution set oversight committee. J Am Coll Cardiol 74(15):1966–2011
5. Agrawal N, Kumar A, Aggarwal P, Jamshed N (2016) Sympathetic crashing acute pulmonary edema. Indian J Crit Care Med 20(12):719–723
6. Lichtenstein D, Goldstein I, Mourgeon E, Cluzel P, Grenier P, Rouby JJ (2004) Comparative diagnostic performances of auscultation, chest radiography and lung ultrasonography in acute respiratory distress syndrome. Anesthesiology 100:9–15
7. Pivetta E, Goffi A, Lupia E, Tizzani M, Porrino G, Ferreri E, SIMEU Group for Lung Ultrasound in the Emergency Department in Piedmont (2015) Lung ultrasound-implemented diagnosis of acute decompensated heart failure in the ED: A SIMEU multicentre study. Chest 148(1):202–210
8. Brusasco C, Santori G, Bruzzo E, Trò R, Robba C, Tavazzi G, Guarracino F, Forfori F, Boccacci P (2019) Corradi F (2019) Quantitative lung ultrasonography: a putative new algorithm for automatic detection and quantification of B-lines. Crit Care 23:288
9. Correa M, Zimic M, Barrientos F, Barrientos R, Román-Gonzalez A, Pajuelo MJ, Anticona C, Mayta H, Alva A, Solis-Vasquez L, Figueroa DA, Chavez MA, Lavarello R, Castañeda B et al (2018) Automatic classification of pediatric pneumonia based on lung ultrasound pattern recognition. PLoS ONE 13(12):e0206410
10. Russell FM, Ehrman RR, Ferre R, Gargani L, Noble V, Rupp J, Collins SP, Hunter B, Lane KA, Levy P, Li X, O'Connor C, Pang PS (2019) Design and rationale of the B-lines lung ultrasound guided emergency department management of acute heart failure (BLUSHED-AHF) pilot trial. Heart Lung 48(3):186–192
11. Russell FM, Ehrman RR, Cosby K, Ansari A, Tseeng S, Christain E, Bailitz J (2015) Diagnosing acute heart failure in patients with undifferentiated dyspnea: a lung and cardiac ultrasound (LuCUS) protocol. Acad Emerg Med 22(2):182–191
12. Gargani L, Pang PS, Frassi F, Miglioranza MH, Dini FL, Landi P, Picano E (2015) Persistent pulmonary congestion before discharge predicts rehospitalization in heart failure: a lung ultrasound study. Cardiovasc Ultrasound 13:40
13. Coiro S, Rossignol P, Ambrosio G, Carluccio E, Alunni G, Murrone A, Tritto I, Zannad F, Girerd N (2015) Prognostic value of residual pulmonary congestion at discharge assessed by lung ultrasound imaging in heart failure. Eur J Heart Fail 17(11):1172–1181
14. Price S, Platz E, Cullen L, Tavazzi G, Christ M, Cowie MR, Acute Heart Failure Study Group of the European Society of Cardiology Acute Cardiovascular Care Association (2017) Acute Heart Failure Study Group of the European Society of Cardiology Acute Cardiovascular Care Association. Expert consensus document: Echocardiography and lung ultrasonography for the assessment and management of acute heart failure. Nat Rev Cardiol 14(7):427–440
15. Corradi F, Brusasco C, Garlaschi A, Paparo F, Ball L, Santori G, Pelosi P, Altomonte F, Vezzani A, Brusasco V (2015) Quantitative analysis of lung ultrasonography for the detection of community-acquired pneumonia: a pilot study. Biomed Res Int 2015:868707
16. Corradi F, Brusasco C, Vezzani A, Santori G, Manca T, Ball L, Nicolini F, Gherli T, Brusasco V (2016) Computer-aided quantitative ultrasonography for detection of pulmonary edema in mechanically ventilated cardiac surgery patients. Chest 150(3):640–651
17. Volpicelli G, Elbarbary M, Blaivas M, Lichtenstein DA, Mathis G, Kirkpatrick AW, International Liaison Committee on Lung Ultrasound (ILC-LUS) for International Consensus Conference on Lung Ultrasound (ICC-LUS) (2012) International evidence-based recommendations for point-of-care lung ultrasound. Intensive Care Med 38(4):577–591
18. Maw AM, Hassanin A, Ho PM, McInnes MDF, Moss A, Juarez-Colunga E, Soni NJ, Miglioranza MH, Platz E, DeSanto K, Sertich AP, Salame G, Daugherty SL (2019) Diagnostic accuracy of point-of-care lung ultrasonography and chest radiography in adults with symptoms suggestive of acute decompensated heart failure: a systematic review and meta-analysis. JAMA Netw Open 2(3):e190703

14

Results from a Spanish national survey on the application of ultrasound in pulmonology services

Cristina Ramos-Hernández[1*], Maribel Botana-Rial[1], Rosa Cordovilla-Pérez[2], Manuel Núñez-Delgado[1] and Alberto Fernández-Villar[1]

Abstract

Background: This was an observational, cross-sectional, and multicentre study carried out from October to December 2020, through a survey sent to Spanish Society of Pulmonology and Thoracic Surgery members in public hospitals with different levels of complexity. Our objective was to complete a national analysis of clinical practice, organisation, infrastructure, the services portfolio, teaching, and research activity related to ultrasound.

Results: Data from 104 hospitals were analysed. Ultrasound was used in 56.7% of cases, both in the area of bronchopleural techniques and on conventional wards, with no differences between centres. Lung ultrasound (LUS) was performed more often in the procedures area in intermediate-complexity centres compared to high- and low-complexity centres (36% vs. 31% and 6.25%, respectively). More high-complexity centres had three or more ultrasound scanners than intermediate-complexity centres (38% vs. 16%); 43% of low-complexity centres shared their ultrasound equipment with other specialties. Fewer than 6% of centres did not have an ultrasound machine. LUS was most often used during the treatment of pleural effusion (91.3%), in the differential diagnosis of dyspnoea (51.9%), and to rule out iatrogenic pneumothorax (50.9%). Only 5.7% of the centres had a pulmonologist specialised in LUS. Finally, fewer than 35% of the hospitals were teaching centres and fewer than 18% participated in research projects.

Conclusions: The use and availability of LUS has grown in pulmonology services, however, still relatively few pulmonologists are specialised in its use. Moreover, teaching and research activity in this field is scarce. Strategies are necessary to improve physicians' skill at using LUS and to promote its use, with the ultimate goal of improving healthcare activity.

Keywords: Ultrasound, LUS, Pulmonology, Survey

Introduction

The use of ultrasound in pulmonology services is evident, not only because of the increase in its indications but also because of the number of specialists who have incorporated it into their daily clinical practice. Although, ultrasound initially started to be used as a guide during pleural procedures [1], over time it has proven useful in the assessment of the lung parenchyma, diaphragm, and chest wall, and it has became a basic first-line tool to establish a differential diagnosis in patients with dyspnoea [2, 3]. The use of ultrasound by pulmonologists has also extended to the evaluation of the lower limbs [4], vocal chords [5], and even for performing echocardiography [6] at the patient's bedside to obtain data that may be useful in the diagnosis of pulmonary pathologies. Lung ultrasound (LUS) is a technique performed in bronchopleural procedures units and in intermediate

*Correspondence: cristina.ramos.hernandez@sergas.es
[1] Department of Pneumology, Hospital Alvaro Cunqueiro, Neumo Vigo I + I. Institute of Health Research Galicia South (IISGS), Xerencia de Xestión integrada de Vigo, C/Clara Campoamor 341, 36312 Vigo, Pontevedra, Spain
Full list of author information is available at the end of the article

respiratory care units, but its use in conventional hospital floor settings or in pneumology consultations is not as well established.

It is important to understand the degree to which ultrasound is used in the field of pulmonology at the national level to help researchers to detect potential difficulties in further developing this technique and to create recommendations or training programs that target the fields that need them the most, which helps physicians to achieve higher quality care. Thus, we carried out this study to evaluate the current situation in clinical settings and to address the issues set out above. Our main objective was to describe current clinical care practices regarding the use of ultrasound and to collect data related to its use in pulmonology services, organisational and infrastructural factors, the portfolio of services available, and ultrasound teaching and research activity.

Methods

Design

From October to December 2020, we carried out a cross-sectional, national level, multicentre study through a survey sent to every member of the Spanish Society of Pulmonology and Thoracic Surgery (SEPAR) working in hospitals with different levels of complexity. The latter factor was evaluated considering the criteria used in other national studies [7]. High-complexity centres were considered as those with a large technological endowment, more than 500 beds, and 160–300 medical intern residents (MIRs); intermediate-complexity centres were those with 200–500 beds and more than 50 MIRs; and low-complexity centres had fewer than 200 hospital beds and/or fewer than 50 MIRs.

Every pulmonologist and MIR in this specialty who were SEPAR members and who may be involved in the routine use of LUS (in hospital wards, consultations, intermediate respiratory care units, or bronchopleural procedures area) were sent the study survey. Privately managed centres and those located outside the national territory were excluded. When responses were obtained from several professionals from the same centre, the answers from the first participant were recorded.

Using a methodology similar to one our group has previously employed in a similar study [7], SEPAR members were contacted with the questionnaire by email and asked to complete it using an online platform. The survey included a total of 21 items, four of them designed to assess technological resources and the organisation and infrastructure available for LUS (Table 1), 12 items aimed to assess the portfolio of services available using this technique (Table 2), and five items were used to understand the centre's involvement in teaching, training, and research related to ultrasound (Table 3).

Statistical analysis

Qualitative variables were expressed as absolute frequencies and percentages. Comparisons between study groups were made according to the level of care provided at the hospital centre and the association between qualitative variables was evaluated with Chi-squared tests (χ^2). The outcomes from all the statistical comparisons were considered significant when the probability of error was less than 5%. The data processing and analysis was carried out using SPSS software (v21, IBM Corp., Armonk, NY, USA).

Ethical factors

Due to the nature of this study, neither informed consent nor approval by the Research Ethics Committee was required. The collection, treatment, and conservation of the data was carried out anonymously in accordance with the current provisions of the General Data Protection Regulation (EU Regulation 2016-679 of the European Parliament and Council, of April 27, 2016) and Spanish regulations on the protection of personal data.

Results

Sample description

A total of 155 health professionals belonging to 109 hospital centres responded to the survey. The results from three centres were excluded, because they were not located in the national territory and two other centres were excluded, because they were privately managed. Thus, data from 104 publicly managed hospitals were analysed in this work, of which 58 (55.8%) were highly complex centres, 30 (28.8%) were of intermediate complexity, and 16 (15.4%) were low-complexity centres.

Results related to organisation and infrastructure

We found significant differences in the availability of ultrasound machines depending on the complexity of the care provided at the centre. The pneumology service in high-complexity centres more often had at least 3 ultrasound scanners compared to low-complexity centres (37.9% vs. 0%; $p = 0.008$), with the latter being more likely to share an ultrasound system with other services (43.7% vs. 13.3% vs. 3.4%, respectively; $p = 0.0001$). We found no differences between the different levels of care in terms of the availability of different types of transducers; 35.5% of the centres surveyed had 3 types of transducer (convex, linear, and sector), 41.3% had linear and convex transducers, and 20% only had one type, usually a convex transducer (66.6%). LUS was routinely used (in 56.7% of cases) both in the bronchopleural procedures area and in the hospital ward, with no differences between the centre types. However, high- and intermediate-complexity

Table 1 Organisational and infrastructural factors related to the use of ultrasound

Organisation and infrastructure	Total $N = 104$	High-complexity centre $N = 58$	Intermediate-complexity centre $N = 30$	Low-complexity centre $N = 16$
Availability of ultrasound scanners				
Two exclusive-use ultrasound scanners are available in the pneumology service	24/104 (23.0%)	17/58 (29.3%)	5/30 (16.6%)	2/16 (12.5%)
Three or more exclusive-use ultrasound scanners are available in the pneumology service	27/104 (25.9%)	22/58 (37.9%)[a]	5/30 (16.6%)	0/16 (0%)
An ultrasound system is shared with other services	13/104 (12.5%)	2/58 (3.4%)[a]	4/30 (13.3%)[b]	7/16 (43.7%)
Only one ultrasound machine is available in the pulmonology service	34/104 (32.6%)	14/58 (2.1%)	14/30 (46.6%)	6/16 (37.5%)
No ultrasound scanner is available in the pulmonology service	6/104 (5.7%)	2/58 (3.4%)	2/30 (6.6%)	1/16 (6.25%)
Probe availability				
A linear, convex, and sector probe is available	37/104 (35.5%)	23/58 (39.6%)	9/30 (30%)	5/16 (31.2%)
A linear and convex probe is available	43/104 (41.3%)	26/58 (44.8%)	11/30 (36.6%)	6/16 (37.5%)
Only one probe is available	21/104 (20.1%)	9/58 (15.5%)	8/30 (26.6%)	4/16 (25%)
Linear	3/21	1/9	–	2/4
Convex	13/21	4/9	7/8	2/4
Microconvex	2/21	2/9	–	–
Sectorial	3/21	2/9	1/8	–
New applications				
Elastography is available	14/104 (13.4%)	9/58 (15.5%)	3/30 (10%)	2/16 (12.5%)
Elastography type				
Strain	6/104 (5.7%)	4/58 (6.8%)	1/30 (3.3%)	1/16 (6.2%)
SWE	0/104 (0%)	0/58 (0%)	0/30 (0%)	0/16 (0%)
Both	8/104 (7.6%)	5/58 (6.89%)	2/30 (6.6%)	1/16 (6.2%)
Elastography probe				
Linear	2/104 (1.9%)	1/58 (1.7%)	0/30 (0%)	1/16 (6.2%)
Convex	5/104 (4.8)	3/58 (5.1%)	2/30 (6.6%)	0/16 (0%)
Both	7/104 (6.7%)	5/58 (8.6%)	1/30 (3.6%)	1/16 (6.2%)
EBUS elastography is available	13/104 (12.5%)	11/58 (18.9%)	1/30 (3.3%)	1/16 (6.25%)
Dedicated LUS staff				
LUS is performed only in the bronchopleural procedures area	30/104 (28.8%)	18/58 (31.0%)	11/30 (36.6%)[b]	1/16 (6.25%)
LUS is performed in the bronchopleural procedures area and in the hospital ward on a routine basis	59/104 (56.7%)	32/58 (55.1%)	17/30 (56.6%)	10/16 (62.5%)
A person specialised in performing LUS is available	6/104 (5.7%)	4/58 (6.8%)	0/30 (0%)	2/16 (12.5%)

Data expressed as absolute frequencies (%)

SWE shear wave, *LUS* lung ultrasound, *EBUS* endobronchial ultrasound

[a] $p < 0.05$ high-complexity compared to low-complexity centres

[b] $p < 0.05$ intermediate-complexity compared to low-complexity centres

care centres more often performed LUS exclusively in the bronchopleural procedures area compared to low-complexity centres (31% vs. 6.25%, $p = 0.09$ and 36.6% vs. 6.25%, $p = 0.04$, respectively). New ultrasonography techniques such as elastography were available in 13.4% of the centres, regardless of the level of care provided (Table 1, Fig. 1).

Results related to the ultrasound service portfolio

LUS was most often used to evaluate pleural effusion (91.3%), to determine a differential diagnosis between pulmonary pathologies (51.9%), and to rule out iatrogenic pneumothorax after completing a broncho-pleural procedure (50.9%). The least common uses for LUS were for the evaluation of vocal cord dysfunction (3.8%) and the use of elastography to study masses (7.6%) and pleural effusions (5.7%). We only found significant differences for this item regarding the use of LUS for the diagnosis and/or follow-up of interstitial lung diseases (ILD) in low- vs. medium-complexity centres (31.2% vs. 3.3%, $p = 0.02$), and when performing lower limb (LL) ultrasound for suspected thromboembolic disease, which more often

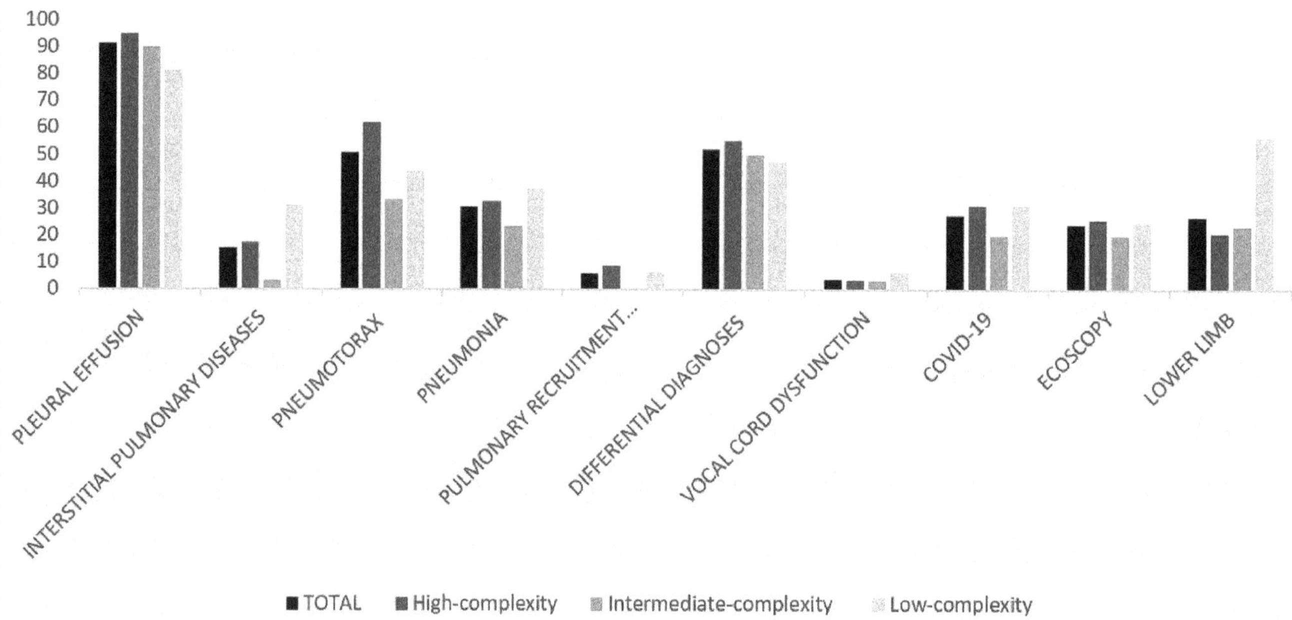

Fig. 1 Factors related to the portfolio of ultrasound services available

presented at low-complexity centres compared to intermediate (56.2% vs. 23.3%, $p=0.05$) or high-complexity centres (56.2% vs. 20.6%, $p=0.01$) (Table 2).

Results related to teaching, training, and research

Overall, 34.6% and 30.7% of the centres taught undergraduate and postgraduate courses related to LUS and physicians in up to 17.3% of the centres were undertaking research projects related to LUS. In this sense, we only found significant differences in the number of multicentre research projects related to TE carried out at high-complexity centres vs. low-complexity centres (25.8% vs. 0%, $p=0.05$).

Table 2 Factors related to the portfolio of ultrasound services available

SERVICES PORTFOLIO	Total $N=104$	High-complexity centre $N=58$	Intermediate-complexity centre $N=30$	Low-complexity centre $N=16$
LUS is routinely used to diagnose and manage **PLEURAL EFFUSION**	95/104 (91.3%)	55/58 (94.8%)	27/30 (89.9%)	13/16 (81.2%)
LUS is routinely used to diagnose and/or follow-up **INTERSTITIAL PULMONARY DISEASES**	16/104 (15.3%)	10/58 (17.2%)	1/30 (3.3%)[b]	5/16 (31.2%)
LUS is routinely used to rule out **IATROGENIC PNEUMOTORAX** after bronchopleural procedures	53/104 (50.9%)	36/58 (62.0%)	10/30 (33.3%)	7/16 (43.7%)
LUS is routinely used for the diagnosis and/or **follow-up of PNEUMONIA**	32/104 (30.7%)	19/58 (32.7%)	7/30 (23.3%)	6/16 (37.5)
LUS is routinely used to guide **PULMONARY RECRUITMENT MANEUVERS**	6/104 (5.9%)	5/58 (8.6%)	0 (0%)	1/16 (6.25%)
LUS is routinely used to resolve **DIFFERENTIAL DIAGNOSES** between different pulmonary pathologies	54/104 (51.9%)	32/58 (55.1%)	15/30 (49.9%)	7/16 (43.7%)
LUS is routinely used to assess **VOCAL CORD DYSFUNCTION**	4/104 (3.8%)	2/58 (3.4%)	1/30 (3.3%)	1/16 (6.25%)
LUS is routinely used to diagnose and follow-up patients with **COVID-19**	29/104 (27.8%)	18/58 (31.0%)	6/30 (20%)	5/16 (31.2%)
ECOSCOPY is used for LVEF estimation, to measure cavities, for pericardial assessment, and to calculate the TAPSE	25/104 (24.0%)	15/58 (25.8%)	6/30 (20%)	4/16 (25%)
LL ultrasound is routinely performed when thromboembolic disease is suspected	28/104 (26.9%)	12/58 (20.6%)[a]	7/30 (23.3%)[b]	9/16 (56.2%)
ELASTOGRAPHY is used to assess masses	8/104 (7.6%)	7/58 (12.1%)	0 (0%)	1/16 (6.2%)
ELASTOGRAPHY is used to assess pleural effusions	6/104 (5.7%)	4/58 (6.8%)	1/30 (3.3%)	1/16 (6.2%)

LL lower limb, *COVID-19* coronavirus SARS-CoV2, *LVEF* left ventricular ejection fraction, *TAPSE* tricuspid annular plane systolic excursión

[a] $p<0.05$ high-complexity compared to low-complexity centres

[b] $p<0.05$ intermediate-complexity compared to low-complexity centres

Discussion

This is the first study at a state level to assess the degree to which LUS is used by pulmonologist in Spain. Our data showed that LUS is widely used to study the pathologies for which it was first developed, but that training in new indications (for which never exceeded 65%) is required.

The assessment of pleural effusions showed the most consolidated use of LUS (91.3%), with the use of ultrasound improving the results obtained in this healthcare field compared to previous years. After the safety alert issued by the United Kingdom in 2008 [8] when a series of iatrogenic complications caused by the insertion of chest drains was identified, in 2010, the British Thoracic Society (BTS) recommended performing all pleural procedures with ultrasound guidance [9]. Nonetheless, a 2014 survey completed by 500 pulmonologists [10] found that up to 35% of LUSs used to guide these procedures were not yet performed by personnel specialised in pulmonology, and in a 2016 survey carried out among resident pulmonology and internal medicine physicians, only 44% said they routinely used LUS to perform thoracentesis [11].

In other recently introduced examinations, such as the diagnosis and follow-up of SARS-CoV2 pneumonia, LUS was used by 27.8% of the centres in this study, with no difference between the complexity of the centres. These results are lower than those obtained by the Academy of Thoracic Ultrasound [12] in Italy, who reported that 60.2% and 63.4% of their survey respondents used LUS for diagnosing and following up this pathology, respectively. However, this study was subject to selection bias, because the study cohort comprised clinicians with a special interest in LUS. Moreover, up to 14.6% of respondents started using LUS because of the COVID19 pandemic, thanks to the increased availability of equipment and training (through webinars, video tutorials, and local teaching programs) at the time. Thus, these two factors were key pillars in the development of this technique.

A 2018 study from Italy which attempted to clarify the main difficulties in establishing the regular use of LUS, found that a lack of ultrasound scanners (52%) and a deficit in training (22%) were the main barriers to more common use of the technique [13]. However, current accessibility to ultrasound scanners in our specific environment should favour the adequate development of this technique given that only 5.7% of the centres we surveyed did not have access to this equipment. Notwithstanding, this current work highlighted the need to improve the provision of global training in ultrasound, especially for new diagnostic techniques and for the evaluation of the heart, lower limbs, and vocal cords. Both in the Italian study and in the present one carried out in Spain, the most explored pathology by LUS was pleural effusion; however, in the Italian group, there is evidence of a higher degree of development of LUS for evaluation of pneumonia (55% vs. 30.7%), which could be justified by the inclusion, in the Italian survey, of personnel belonging not only to pulmonology but also to internal medicine or intensive care [13].

The continuous development of new and more complex ultrasound modalities, such as elastography [14, 15], means that more focussed training will be required to ensure adequate implementation of these techniques in clinical practice. Although the use of LUS appears in the postgraduate training program in pulmonology, the learning curve necessary to identify different pathologies is not well accounted for in this program. Proficiency in LUS is often developed at the bedside in clinical environments while supervised by a more experienced operator, or in specific training courses with simulation systems to acquire theoretical–practical knowledge [16]. LUS is not associated with any complications from the ultrasound technique, but clinical decisions made based on LUS mean that it is vital to professionally train operators to achieve high levels of diagnostic precision. Thus, to regulate and ensure training in LUS, the BTS published five levels of training in four main modalities, emergencies, basic, advanced, and expert [17], ranging from an initial degree as an observer to an expert level with permission to supervise and train other professionals. All pulmonologists in training must reach the basic level and can go on to complete the advanced levels, while the expert level would be assigned to people specifically specialised in ultrasound; in our sample this corresponded to only 5.7% of the population (Table 1).

Regarding organisational and infrastructural factors, with respect to low-complexity hospitals, LUS tended to be performed only in the bronchopleural procedures area in high and intermediate-complexity centres (6.15% vs. 31% and 36.6%, respectively). However, of note, a significantly wider range of techniques, such as the evaluation of DVT, were carried out in low-complexity centres (56.2% vs. 20.6% and 23.3%, respectively), perhaps because more complex centres are more subspecialised.

Only 20.1% of the surveyed centres taught accredited courses, with this figure being slightly higher than for high-complexity centres. Regarding research, there were very few institutional or multicentre projects being carried out in relation to ultrasound. Thus, we consider this as another objective for improvement, because such research translates into improvement of the quality of care, which is both a corporate and healthcare provision goal.

The limitations of this current study included the low percentage of professionals included that belonged to

Table 3 Factors related to teaching, training, and research in ultrasound

Teaching, training, and research	Total $N = 104$	High-complexity centre $N = 58$	Intermediate-complexity centre $N = 30$	Low-complexity centre $N = 16$
Accredited courses in pleural pathology are taught	21/104 (20.1%)	16/58 (27.5%)	4/30 (13.3%)	1/16 (6.2%)
Undergraduate teaching related to LUS is provided	36/104 (34.6%)	24/58 (41.3%)	9/30 (30%)	3/16 (18.7%)
Postgraduate teaching related to thoracic ultrasound is provided	32/104 (30.7%)	21/58 (36.2%)	9/30 (30%)	2/16 (12.5%)
Researchers working on their own thoracic ultrasound projects are present	18/104 (17.3%)	14/58 (24.1%)	3/30 (10%)	1/16 (6.2%)
There is participation in multicentre projects related to thoracic ultrasound	18/104 (17.3%)	15/58 (25.8%)[a]	3/30 (10%)	0/16 (0%)

[a] $p < 0.05$ high-complexity compared to low-complexity centres

low-complexity centres, the lack of stratification by autonomous communities, which prevented us from performing an analysis of variability between territories, and that possible areas of development of LUS, such as consultations or critical units, have not been included. However, in our opinion, the analysed sample was sufficient to reflect how LUS is currently used in Spain and allowed us to establish recommendations for the better management of these processes. At the national level, other research groups have developed surveys to investigate the use of LUS in other prevalent pathologies, such as COPD [18], for the management of pleural effusion [7, 11] or in palliative care units [19]. We believe this type of analysis is required to develop new strategic lines of research through scientific societies, because ultrasound could be used to internally evaluate the quality of healthcare provision in different services, develop guidelines to improve the quality of care, promote the development of training, and to facilitate comparative studies between different hospitals.

Conclusions

Ultrasound is a tool whose use has increased in recent years, not only in bronchopleural procedure units, but also in the context of conventional ward hospitalisation, intermediate care units, and consultations. In parallel, the availability of ultrasound machines in pneumology services has also increased as a result of the clear advantages of this technique, which is why it seems necessary to gradually implement ultrasound as the fifth pillar of the physical examination of every type of pulmonary pathology. Nonetheless, this implies that pulmonologists must complete training to acquire advanced knowledge in this technique.

Abbreviations

BTS: British Thoracic Society; COVID-19: Coronavirus disease; DVT: Deep vein thrombosis; EBUS: Endobronchial ultrasound; EU: Europe; ILD: Interstitial lung disease; LVEF: Left ventricular ejection fraction; LL: Lower limb; LUS: Lung ultrasound; MIRs: Medical intern residents; SEPAR: Spanish Society of Pulmonology and Thoracic Surgery; SWE: Shear wave; TAPSE: Tricuspid annular plane systolic excursion.

Acknowledgements

SEPAR integrated research programs (PII) in interventional pulmonology. SEPAR techniques and transplantation area.

Authors' contributions

CR-H: conceptualization, methodology, software, validation, formal analysis, writing—original draft and project administration, and final approval of the version to be submitted; MB-R: methodology, validation, formal analysis, writing—review and editing, supervision, and final approval of the version to be submitted; RC-P: resources, software, data curation, and final approval of the version to be submitted, MN-D: data curation and final approval of the version to be submitted; AF-V: investigation, validation, supervision, and final approval of the version to be submitted. All authors read and approved the final manuscript.

Author details

[1]Department of Pneumology, Hospital Alvaro Cunqueiro, Neumo Vigo I + I. Institute of Health Research Galicia South (IISGS), Xerencia de Xestión integrada de Vigo, C/Clara Campoamor 341, 36312 Vigo, Pontevedra, Spain. [2]Department of Pneumology, University Hospital of Salamcanca, P.º de San Vicente, 182, 37007 Salamanca, Spain.

References

1. Villena Garrido V, Cases Viedma E, Fernández Villar A, de Pablo GA, Pérez Rodríguez E, Porcel Pérez JM et al (2014) Normativa sobre el diagnóstico y tratamiento del derrame pleural. Actualización Arch Bronconeumol 50(6):235–249
2. Pallarés JPC. Manual de procedimientos SEPAR: Ecografía torácica. www.separ.es. Accessed 10 Jan 2021
3. Lichtenstein DA (2015) BLUE-protocol and FALLS-protocol: two applications of lung ultrasound in the critically ill. Chest 147(6):1659–1670
4. Kearon C, Ginsberg JS, Hirsh J (1998) The role of venous ultrasonography in the diagnosis of suspected deep venous thrombosis and pulmonary embolism. Ann Intern Med 129(12):1044–1049
5. Kumar A, Sinha C, Singh AK, Bhadani UK (2017) Vocal cord dysfunction: ultrasonography-aided diagnosis during routine airway examination. Saudi J Anaesth 11(3):370–371
6. Labovitz AJ, Noble VE, Bierig M, Goldstein SA, Jones R, Kort S et al (2010) Focused cardiac ultrasound in the emergent setting: a consensus statement of the American society of echocardiography and American college of emergency physicians. J Am Soc Echocardiogr 23(12):1225–1230
7. Botana-Rial M, Núñez-Delgado M, Leiro-Fernández V, Fernández-Villar A (2019) Resultados de una encuesta nacional sobre la situación actual del manejo del derrame pleural. Arch Bronconeumol 55(5):274–276
8. Lamont T, Surkitt-Parr M, Scarpello J, Durand M, Hooper C, Maskell N (2009) Safety alerts insertion of chest drains: summary of a safety report from the National Patient Safety Agency. BMJ 339:b4923
9. Havelock T, Teoh R, Laws D, Gleeson F, on behalf of the BTS (2010) Pleural disease guideline group. Pleural procedures and thoracic ultrasound: British thoracic society pleural disease guideline 2010. Thorax 65(Suppl 2):61-i76
10. De Lucas Ramos P, Rodríguez-Moro JM. Libro Blanco. La Neumología en España. Respira. Fundación Española del Pulmón. SEPAR; 2015. 11
11. Porcel JM, Cases-Viedma E, Bielsa S (2016) Una encuesta a médicos residentes sobre la realización de toracocentesis diagnósticas y terapéuticas: ¿una laguna en la formación? Rev Clin Esp 216(9):474–480
12. Zanforlin A, Tursi F (2021) How is COVID-19 changing lung ultrasound? A survey by the thoracic ultrasound academy. J Ultrasound Med 40(2):417–418
13. Zanforlin A, Tursi F, Marchetti G, Pellegrino G, Vigo B, Smargiassi A et al (2020) Clinical use and barriers of thoracic ultrasound: a survey of Italian pulmonologists. Respiration 99(2):171–176
14. Zhou B, Bartholmai BJ, Kalra S, Osborn TG, Zhang X (2019) Lung US surface wave elastography in interstitial lung disease staging. Radiology 291(2):479–484
15. Jiang B, Li X, Yin Y, Zhang Q, Zang T, Song W et al (2019) Ultrasound elastography: a novel tool for the differential diagnosis of pleural effusion. Eur Respir J 54(2):1802018
16. Laursen CB, Clive A, Hallifax R, Pietersen PI, Asciak R, Davidsen JR et al (2020) European respiratory society statement on thoracic ultrasound. Eur Respir J. https://doi.org/10.1183/13993003.01519-2020
17. Stanton AE, Edey A, Evison M, Forrest I, Hippolyte S, Kastelik J et al (2020) British thoracic society training standards for thoracic ultrasound (TUS). BMJ Open Resp Res 7:e000552
18. Calle Rubio M, Rodríguez Hermosa JL, Miravitlles M, López-Campos JL (2020) Conocimiento de la enfermedad pulmonar obstructiva crónica, presencia de síntomas respiratorios crónicos y uso de la espirometría en la población española: estudio CONOCEPOC 2019. Arch Bronconeumol S0300–2896(20):30271–30274
19. Barril S, Alonso A, Rodríguez-Portal JA, Viladot M, Giner J, Aparicio F et al (2018) Cuidados paliativos en la enfermedad pulmonar intersticial difusa: resultados de una encuesta de ámbito nacional. Arch Bronconeumol 54(3):123–127

Feasibility of using a handheld ultrasound device to detect and characterize shunt and deep vein thrombosis in patients with COVID-19: an observational study

Rajkumar Rajendram[1,2*†], Arif Hussain[3†], Naveed Mahmood[1,2] and Mubashar Kharal[1,2]

Abstract

Background: Coronavirus disease 2019 (COVID-19) causes an atypical acute respiratory distress syndrome associated with thromboembolism and high shunt fraction. Shunt may be intrapulmonary, or extrapulmonary. Handheld devices are increasingly being used for point-of-care ultrasound, but their use to characterize shunt has not been reported.

Objectives: Determine the feasibility of using handheld ultrasound to detect and characterize anatomical substrates of hypoxia and deep vein thrombosis (DVT) in patients with COVID-19 suspected to have severe shunt.

Methods: A handheld ultrasound device (iQ, Butterfly, USA) was used to perform lung ultrasound, vascular assessment for DVT, and limited transthoracic echocardiography (TTE) with color Doppler and saline microbubble contrast in patients with COVID-19 suspected to have severe shunt. Images were reassessed by an independent reviewer.

Results: After screening 40 patients, six patients who fulfilled the inclusion criteria were identified. Two were excluded because palliation had been initiated. So, four patients were studied. Interpretable images were obtained in all cases. Interobserver agreement was good. All patients had abnormal lung ultrasound (lung ultrasound score range 17–22). Identified lung pathology included interstitial syndrome with light beams and small peripheral consolidation (4), lobar consolidation (1), and pleural effusion (1). Abnormal echocardiographic findings included interatrial shunt (2), intrapulmonary shunt (1), and dilated right ventricle with tricuspid valve regurgitation (1). Significant DVT was not detected.

Conclusion: Use of handheld ultrasound to perform combined lung ultrasound, DVT ultrasound, and limited TTE with color Doppler and saline microbubble contrast is feasible, and may be able to characterize shunt in critically hypoxic patients. Serial studies could be used to monitor changes in shunt. Further studies are required to determine whether this can guide treatment to improve the outcomes of patients with refractory hypoxia.

Keywords: COVID-19, SARS-CoV-2, Point-of-care ultrasound, Lung ultrasound, Echocardiography, Deep vein ultrasound, Handheld ultrasound device, Shunt, Patent foramen ovale

Introduction

The acute respiratory distress syndrome (ARDS) caused by Coronavirus Disease 2019 (COVID-19) is atypical [1–3]. Indeed, two distinct patterns of COVID-19 pneumonia (type L, low elastance and type H, high elastance) have been described [2].

*Correspondence: rajkumarrajendram@doctors.org.uk
†Rajkumar Rajendram and Arif Hussain contributed equally to this study, and are joint first authors
[1] Department of Medicine, King Abdulaziz Medical City, King Abdulaziz International Medical Research Center, Ministry of National Guard - Health Affairs, Riyadh, Saudi Arabia
Full list of author information is available at the end of the article

The pathogenesis of COVID-19 involves pulmonary microvascular thrombosis, and venous thromboembolism is very common [3, 4]. While this should increase dead space, one series of critically ill patients with COVID-19 had a high mean right-to-left (RTL) shunt fraction (0.50 ± 0.11) despite relatively normal lung compliance (50.2 ± 14.3 ml/cmH_2O) [1]. The pathogenesis of the dead space and shunt in COVID-19 is likely to be multifactorial [5]. Shunt may be intrapulmonary (IPS; e.g., lobar collapse or consolidation, ARDS, pulmonary arteriovenous malformations, hepatopulmonary syndrome), or extrapulmonary (e.g., intracardiac shunts) [5, 6]. Indeed, one study using lung ultrasound enhanced with sulfur hexafluoride microbubble contrast (SonoVue), demonstrated the presence of partial, inhomogeneous, regions of intrapulmonary hyperperfusion in patients with COVID-19 pneumonia [3].

The cardiac dysfunction associated with COVID-19 may vary with the respiratory phenotype [7]. For example, the high airway pressures required to ventilate patients with phenotype H are likely to have a significant effect on right heart function [7]. In contrast, as patients with phenotype L have relatively preserved lung compliance, the airway pressures required to achieve the set tidal volumes during the mechanical ventilation should be low [7]. So, less right heart impairment is expected in patients with phenotype L COVID-19 pneumonia.

Precise measurement of dead space, IPS, extrapulmonary shunt, and right heart function requires left, and right heart catheterization. However, this is too invasive to be used for screening. An alternative strategy to assess left and right heart function and screen for RTL shunt could include transthoracic echocardiography (TTE).

In spontaneously breathing, breathless patients with phenotype L, TTE may demonstrate the consequences of increased respiratory effort on ventricular interdependence. Extremely negative intrathoracic pressures may reduce stroke volume if diastolic ventricular septal shift results in right ventricular (RV) overload and left ventricular (LV) hypodiastole. In patients with phenotype H receiving positive pressure mechanical ventilation, TTE may detect cardiac complications of ventilatory support. These include RV dysfunction (i.e., RV dilation, tricuspid regurgitation, reduced RV systolic function), and secondary LV dysfunction (i.e., acute cor pulmonale) [7, 8]. Moreover, it is important to recognize that ventilator-induced heart failure can occur in patients with previously normal cardiac function [9].

Furthermore, TTE with color Doppler, and saline microbubble contrast [10, 11], a minimally invasive test, can detect and quantify shunt, and distinguish IPS from intracardiac shunt [10, 11]. Lung ultrasound can detect pulmonary pathology that may increase IPS [12]. Vascular ultrasound can detect deep venous thrombosis (DVT), a precursor for pulmonary embolism (PE). While PE is not universally present in patients with DVT, in the presence of DVT, anticoagulation is indicated to prevent PE. The detection of DVT is therefore important in patients with severe hypoxia. Thus, combined lung ultrasound, DVT ultrasound, and limited TTE with color Doppler and saline microbubble contrast could detect and characterize the substrates for severe hypoxia.

A previous study demonstrating the feasibility of performing limited TTE, and lung ultrasound, in critically ill patients, used a cart-based system [13]. Handheld ultrasound devices have several advantages over cart-based systems [14–16], particularly in the context of COVID-19 [16]. Yet, despite their widespread use, it is not known whether the image quality obtained from handheld devices is adequate to determine the etiology of shunt.

Aim

Determine the feasibility of using a handheld ultrasound device to detect and characterize the substrates for hypoxia and DVT in patients with COVID-19 pneumonia suspected to have severe shunt.

Methods

Setting

This prospective, observational study was approved by the institutional review board of the King Abdullah International Medical Research Center, Riyadh, Saudi Arabia (Reference RC20/296/R). The need for formal patient consent was waived as written consent for critical care included use of ultrasound and TTE.

The study took place in sites designated as COVID-19 high dependency (HDU), and intensive care units (ICU) in a 1600-bed, tertiary-care hospital, Riyadh, Saudi Arabia.

Protocol

Inclusion criteria were participants aged over 18 years, admitted to HDU or ICU, with COVID-19, in whom significant shunt was suspected. Significant shunt was suspected if any of the following criteria were present [6]:

(1) Known anatomical substrate for shunt (e.g., patent foramen ovale; PFO).
(2) Acute stroke or systemic thromboembolism.
(3) Platypnea-orthodeoxia.
(4) $PaO_2/FiO_2 < 200$ (estimated shunt fraction > 0.2).
(5) The lung injury present on imaging did not fully account for hypoxia.
(6) Supplemental oxygen did not significantly improve hypoxia.
(7) Significant acute drop in the PaO_2/FiO_2 ratio.

Patients were excluded if palliation had been initiated, or was imminent.

Sample size calculation: with a prevalence of 20–30% in the general population, the most common cause of shunt is PFO [17, 18]. To identify five patients with an anatomical substrate for shunt it was estimated that at least 20 patients would have to be screened using the criteria above. To allow for exclusion of up to 50% of patients, it was decided that at least 40 patients should be screened for imaging with ultrasound. To identify suitable participants, patients' electronic medical records were screened by A.H. and R.R. between 01/07/20 and 08/07/20 whenever both were available (convenience sampling).

Lung ultrasound, DVT ultrasound, and limited TTE with color Doppler and bubble contrast were performed by A.H. and R.R. Both are intensivists, accredited in full or limited echocardiography and point-of-care ultrasonography, with more than 15 years of imaging experience and institutional privileges. The imaging protocols used in our study were similar to previously described protocols [13, 19–23].

Devices used for imaging

A handheld, application-based, ultrasound device (iQ, Butterfly, USA) with a compatible smartphone (iPhone 10S, Apple, USA) was used for imaging. A cart-based ultrasound machine (Vivid I, General Electric Healthcare, USA) was immediately available for comparative imaging in case diagnostic quality images could not be obtained with the handheld device.

Lung ultrasound

Lung ultrasound was performed with the patient semi-recumbent (15° head elevation), or prone. The pleura and lungs were imaged at points in six zones for each lung: anterior upper, anterior lower, lateral upper, lateral lower, posterior upper, and posterior lower [13, 24–26].

A normal lung pattern was defined by the presence of smooth, thin pleural line with normal lung sliding, A-lines (pleural reverberation artifacts), and less than three B-lines (hyperechoic, vertical artifacts arising from the pleural line, reaching the bottom of the screen, and possibly fading or obliterating A-lines, moving with lung sliding) [13, 21].

The presence of 3, or more, B-lines, in a single intercostal space, in a non-dependent region was considered abnormal (B-Pattern). This could indicate pulmonary edema, pneumonitis, atelectasis, or contusion according to clinical context, and distribution of LUS findings in other regions. Interstitial syndrome was defined as B-pattern involving 2, or more, regions of both lungs [13, 21].

Poorly echoic, or isoechoic tissue-like ("hepatized") areas (either peripheral and wedge-shaped, or more extended, deeper with sharp peripheral margins) identified consolidations (C-Pattern) [13, 21]. Alveolar consolidation was differentiated from atelectasis by the presence of dynamic air bronchograms. Fluid bronchograms, static air bronchograms or absent bronchograms characterized atelectasis. Color Doppler was not used to assess C-Patterned lung because the limited capability of the color Doppler on the handheld device is insufficient to detect very low velocity blood flow such as may be present in consolidated lung.

Pneumothorax was defined in the absence of lung sliding, B-lines, lung pulse, and C-Pattern and, the presence of lung point in more dorsal areas [13, 21]. Pleural effusion was defined as an anechoic space between the parietal and visceral pleura [21].

'Small peripheral consolidation' was diagnosed in the presence of a small, peripheral area of consolidated lung tissue surrounded by multiple B-lines, and an irregular or fragmented pleural line [13, 21]. Bilateral areas of B-patterned lung (i.e., interstitial syndrome), with multiple, patchy, small peripheral consolidations, alternating with large, well demarcated, "spared" areas have recently been described in patients with COVID-19 pneumonia [22, 27].

Vascular ultrasound assessment for deep vein thrombosis

Screening for DVT using 2-D imaging, color Doppler, and compression ultrasonography, was based on two-point protocols for assessment of lower limb veins (common femoral, and popliteal) [19]. However, as the risk of thrombosis in COVID-19 is extremely high [4], upper limb veins (jugular, and subclavian) were also assessed.

Limited TTE with color Doppler

The limited TTE examination generally followed the methods described for Focused Cardiac Ultrasound (FoCUS) [23]. This is a simplified, problem-oriented, mostly qualitative two-dimensional (2-D) TTE examination performed by clinicians. The study uses five echocardiographic windows (parasternal long-axis, parasternal short-axis, apical four-chamber, subcostal four-chamber, and inferior vena caval view) [23]. We also used color Doppler, to assess gross valve abnormalities, and screen for intracardiac shunt. The presence, or absence, of impaired left ventricular (LV) function, LV dilatation, right ventricular (RV) dilatation, impaired RV function, valve stenosis or regurgitation, intracardiac shunt, pericardial effusion, or hypovolemia were documented.

Assessment of shunt using intravenous saline microbubble contrast

Saline microbubble contrast echocardiography was performed to detect interatrial shunt, and IPS. Saline microbubble contrast (10 ml) was prepared by agitation of normal saline (9 ml) with air (1 ml) between two Luer lock syringes connected via a 3-way stopcock [6, 11]. After obtaining a clear 4-chamber view (subcostal or apical), the saline microbubble contrast was injected intravenously (i.v.). If present, a central venous catheter was used in preference to peripheral venous catheters.

The diagnosis of shunt was made if the contrast was visualized in the left heart after opacification of right heart. Intracardiac shunt was diagnosed if contrast appeared in the left heart within 3 cardiac cycles of entering the right heart [6, 11]. If contrast required 4–6 cardiac cycles to reach the left heart, IPS was suspected [6, 11]. Cardiac cycles were counted by contractions as electrocardiography was not available on the handheld device.

Shunt was graded by the maximum number of bubbles seen in a single chamber of the left heart on a single still frame [10]. Grade 1: < 5 bubbles; grade 2: 5 to 25 bubbles; grade 3: > 25 bubbles; and grade 4: opacification of chamber [10].

Various maneuvers increase the sensitivity of screening tests for intracardiac shunt [28]. If no shunt was detected after the first injection, it was repeated on release of a Valsalva maneuver (spontaneously breathing patients), or on release of an inspiratory hold (mechanically ventilated patients).

Safety of imaging procedures with saline microbubble contrast in critically ill patients

To detect complications, patients were monitored continuously with at least pulse oximetry, non-invasive blood pressure, and three-lead electrocardiography, during and after imaging procedures. Patients were reviewed 24 h post-imaging for evidence of complications that may have been related to imaging, or injection of saline microbubble contrast.

Reporting and re-assessment of images

Lung ultrasound, DVT ultrasound, and limited TTE findings were agreed by the imaging intensivists while scanning. Ultrasound findings were then documented on structured report forms. If any scans could not be performed, this, and the reason for not being able to complete the ultrasound examination, was also recorded. A lung ultrasound score [25, 26] was used to quantify the severity of abnormalities detected on lung ultrasound. Each of the 12 zones imaged was graded on a scale from 0–3 based on the presence or absence of various specific sonographic findings Thus, the highest possible score was 36.

An independent observer (N.M.), accredited in full TTE, with over 10 years of imaging experience, blinded to all patient data, reviewed the TTE images and reports offline, for quality, interpretability, and accuracy of diagnosis within 6 h of imaging.

Digital images of at least 5 cardiac cycles for each standard TTE view and at least 10 cardiac cycles for each saline microbubble contrast study were assessed offline after download to a desktop computer from the Butterfly Cloud (Butterfly, USA). If the TTE diagnosis differed substantially between the initial report, and the review, discussion between A.H., R.R., and N.M. was used to resolve the discrepancies.

Results

Forty patients were screened to identify six who fulfilled the inclusion criteria. Two were excluded as palliative management had been initiated. Four patients (mean age 64.25 years; 3 women; 2 mechanically ventilated via endotracheal tubes, 2 receiving high-flow nasal oxygen) were recruited because their PaO_2/FiO_2 ratios were under 200, and there was clinical suspicion that the lung injury seen on chest X-ray did not fully account for this hypoxia. All patients improved with supplemental oxygen, and prone positioning. None had platypnea-orthodeoxia, or acute systemic embolism, and none were known to have an anatomical substrate for shunt prior to the study.

Complete examinations with lung ultrasound, DVT ultrasound, and limited TTE with color Doppler and saline microbubble contrast were performed on all participants. The ultrasound findings are correlated with patients' respiratory support and outcomes in Table 1. While two patients subsequently died, there were no immediate or delayed respiratory or hemodynamic complications related to imaging, or injection of saline microbubble contrast.

Image quality was considered to be interpretable by all the study sonographers. Use of the Vivid I ultrasound machine was not required. There were no disagreements between the study sonographers in any of the ultrasound findings. As a result, all investigators considered that the objectives of the present study had been fulfilled, and further investigation was deemed unnecessary.

Lung pathology

Interstitial syndrome with 'light beams' and small peripheral consolidations was diagnosed in all patients. One patient had lobar consolidation with a moderate pleural effusion (Fig. 1). These abnormalities may represent the anatomical substrate for increased dead space and IPS.

Ultrasound assessment for deep vein thrombosis

Adequate views of internal jugular, subclavian, femoral and popliteal veins were obtained in all patients. However, 2-D imaging, color Doppler, and compression

Table 1 Correlation of respiratory support with findings on imaging and outcomes

Subject	1	2	3	4
Respiratory support	High-flow nasal canula		Mechanical ventilation VC (AC) via endotracheal tube	
FiO_2	0.6	0.7	1.0	1.0
Flow (l/min)	60	60	–	–
PEEP (cmH_2O)	–	–	10	10
Tidal volume set/achieved (ml)	–	–	370/374	330/265
Peak airway pressure (cmH_2O)	–	–	34	32
Dynamic compliance (ml/cmH2O)	–	–	15.6	12
SpO_2	88%	89%	98%	97%
PaO_2/FiO_2	111	61	64	82
Lung ultrasound score	22	20	17	20
Lung ultrasound findings	Interstitial syndrome with pleural line thickening and irregularities, in all 12 zones, with light beams, and bilateral patchy areas with small peripheral consolidations			
			Left lobar consolidation, and moderate left pleural effusion	Bibasal atelectasis
DVT ultrasound	Negative	Negative	Negative	Negative
Echocardiography	Normal	Normal	Dilated RV with impaired function	Normal
Saline microbubble contrast study	Negative	Grade 2 interatrial shunt	Grade 4 interatrial shunt	Grade 3 intrapulmonary shunt
Day of imaging (after admission)	Day 9	Day 8	Day 14	Day 14
COVID-19 phenotype			H (high elastance)	H (high elastance)
Outcome	Discharged home Day 17	Intubated Day 10, discharged home Day 39	Death Day 17	Death Day 16

Shunt grading: grade 1: < 5 bubbles; grade 2: 5 to 25 bubbles; grade 3: > 25 bubbles; and grade 4: opacification of chamber [10]. *DVT* deep vein thrombosis, *PEEP* positive end expiratory pressure, *RV* right ventricle, *VC (AC)* volume control (assist control). Phenotypes of COVID-19 have been described: L (low elastance) and H (high elastance)

ultrasonography did not demonstrate any significant thrombus.

Limited TTE with color Doppler

Hemodynamic state abnormalities were identified with limited TTE in only one participant. This mechanically ventilated patient had a dilated right ventricle (Fig. 2) with poor function due to acute cor pulmonale.

Defining the etiology of shunt using color Doppler and saline microbubble contrast

Adequate subcostal views were obtained in all patients. Adequate apical 4-chamber views were obtained in two patients. Application of color Doppler did not demonstrate intracardiac shunt in any of the patients. However, it is important to note that the capability of the color Doppler on the handheld device is limited.

The subcostal views were used for all i.v. saline microbubble contrast studies. In two patients, microbubbles were detected in the left heart within 3 cardiac cycles of opacification of the right heart. Of these patients, a mechanically ventilated patient with acute cor pulmonale had grade 4 interatrial shunt (Fig. 2c; Additional file 1: Video S1), and a spontaneously breathing patient on high-flow nasal canula had grade 2 interatrial shunt, but TTE was otherwise unremarkable. It is important to note that when grade 3 or 4 interatrial shunt is detected with contrast-enhanced echocardiography, co-existing IPS cannot be excluded.

In the other mechanically ventilated patient, > 25 microbubbles were detected (grade 3 shunt; Fig. 3; Additional file 2: Video S2) in the left heart 5 cardiac cycles after opacification of the right heart. This suggested IPS which may have been related to the presence of lobar consolidation (Fig. 1) in COVID-19 pneumonia [3]. A single injection of contrast was sufficient to demonstrate the shunt in these patients. These three patients did not require any maneuvers to increase the sensitivity of TTE for investigation of their RTL shunts.

After i.v. injection of saline microbubble contrast, no microbubbles were detected in the left heart of the other patient breathing spontaneously on high-flow nasal canula. This patient received a second i.v. injection of saline microbubble contrast on release of a Valsalva maneuver.

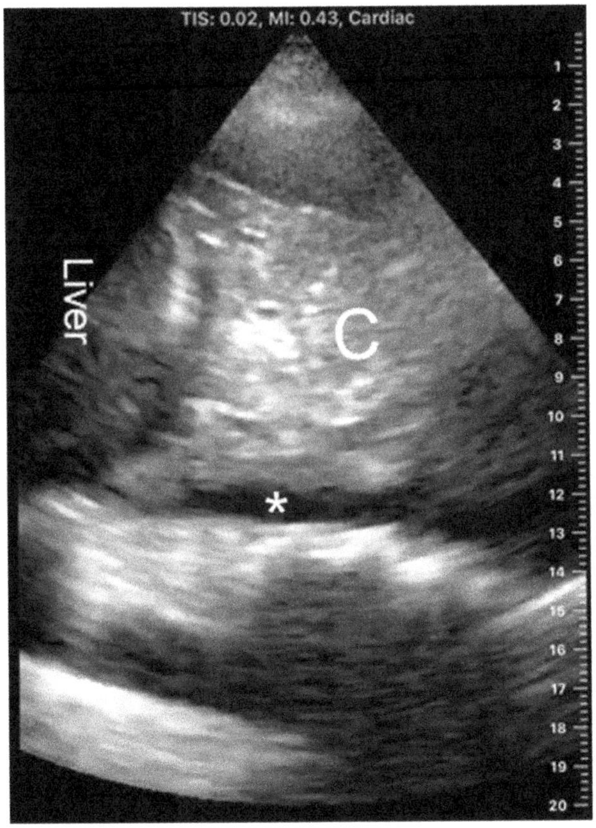

Fig. 1 Consolidated lung in a mechanically ventilated patient with intrapulmonary shunt. Consolidated lung in a mechanically ventilated patient with intrapulmonary shunt. Lung ultrasound demonstrating a large area of consolidated lung (C) surrounded by a moderate pleural effusion (*) in zone 6 of the right lung

As this was also negative, IPS could still contribute to the severe hypoxia in this patient.

The pathogenesis of COVID-19 is thought to involve pulmonary endothelialitis, microvascular thrombosis, and dysregulation of hypoxic pulmonary vasoconstriction [3, 4]. This may cause very small IPS which cannot be excluded by negative saline microbubble contrast-enhanced echocardiography. Thus, because the patient had severe interstitial syndrome (lung ultrasound score 22), the etiology of their hypoxia was considered to be related to increased dead space and IPS.

Discussion

The present study provides 'proof of concept' that combined lung ultrasound, DVT ultrasound, and limited TTE with saline microbubble contrast performed using handheld ultrasound may be able to define the etiology of hypoxia and shunt in patients with COVID-19 pneumonia.

Feasibility was demonstrated as interpretable images could be obtained in all participants and there was good inter-observer agreement. Importantly, no diagnostic errors in the reports were detected by an independent observer. Although one patient had grade 4 shunt, color Doppler failed to detect intracardiac shunt in any of our patients. Intravenous saline microbubble contrast was required to demonstrate this. The absence of any immediate, or delayed, complications following i.v. injection of saline microbubble contrast suggests that this procedure is safe in hypoxic, critically ill patients, but larger studies are required to confirm this.

Our observations confirm previous reports of lung ultrasound findings in COVID-19 pneumonia [12, 22, 27]. Our study also demonstrates that intrapulmonary, and interatrial shunt, and right ventricular dysfunction are present in select patients with COVID-19, and can be detected using a handheld ultrasound device.

Interatrial shunt is underdiagnosed in critically ill patients [11, 17, 18]. In a prospective study of 108 mechanically ventilated patients, using transesophageal echocardiography, patent foramen ovale (PFO) was detected in 27% overall [17]. However, when plateau pressure was over 26 cmH_2O, the prevalence of PFO was significantly higher (46%) [17].

Patients with RTL extrapulmonary shunt respond poorly to positive end expiratory pressure (PEEP), are ventilated longer, receive more treatments for refractory hypoxia, and have longer admissions in ICU [5, 11, 18]. There are no data from randomized controlled clinical trials to guide management of patients with extrapulmonary shunt. Indeed, the standard approach to the management of refractory hypoxia, which aims to reduce IPS, can exacerbate RTL extrapulmonary shunt, and may even worsen hypoxia [5, 11, 17]. So, pathophysiology-directed treatment should aim to reduce total shunt (i.e., IPS and extrapulmonary shunt) [29].

However, the demonstration of interatrial shunt in a patient with RV failure highlights the complex and poorly understood relationship between interatrial shunt and cardiac function in critically ill patients. Left-to-right interatrial shunt can cause pulmonary hypertension and RTL interatrial shunt can cause hypoxia and platypnea-orthodeoxia [6, 30]. Thus, indications for closure of PFO and atrial septal defects are well established [30]. While successful closure of interatrial defect is oft reported [6, 11, 30, 31], it is important to be aware that acute cor pulmonale may develop after shunt closure [6, 11, 31], and that closure is not always required because RTL shunt may improve spontaneously as the functional trigger resolves [11]. Furthermore, atrial septostomy may be performed to decompress the left atrium to treat LV failure [32], and to decompress the right atrium in patients with chronic RV failure and pulmonary hypertension [33].

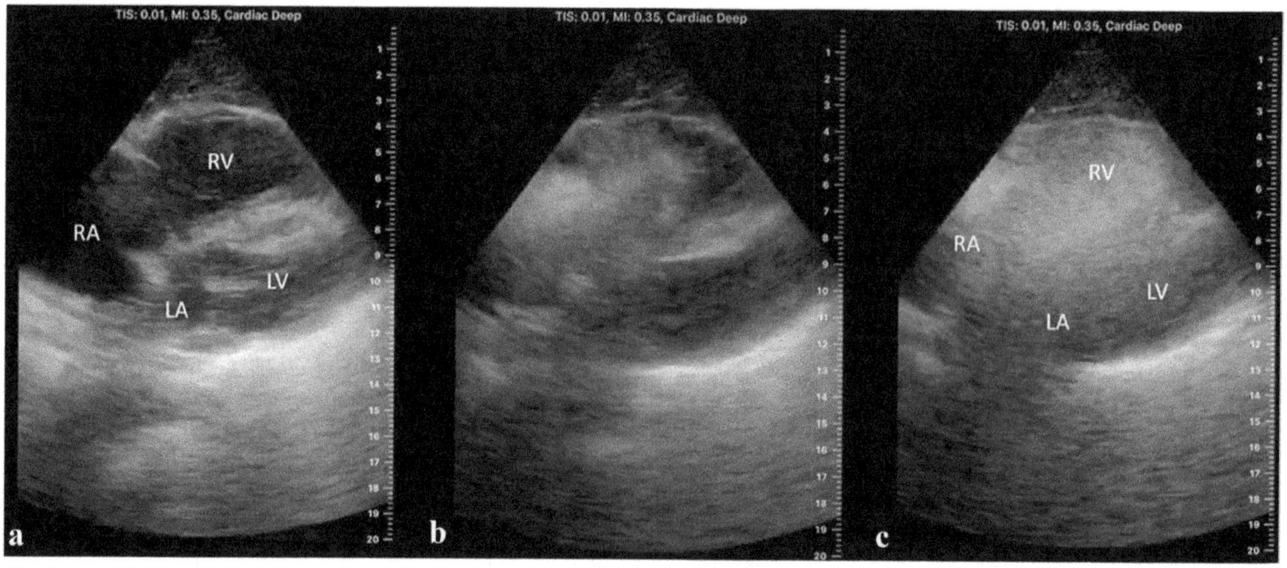

Fig. 2 Interatrial shunt in a mechanically ventilated patient with acute cor pulmonale. Interatrial shunt in a mechanically ventilated patient with acute cor pulmonale due to COVID-19. **a** Labeled 2-D subcostal 4-chamber transthoracic echocardiographic (TTE) view of the heart demonstrating dilatation of the right atrium (RA) and right ventricle (RV). LA, left atrium; LV, left ventricle. **b** 2-D subcostal 4-chamber TTE view of the heart after i.v. injection of saline microbubble contrast showing the arrival of the contrast in the RA and RV. **c** Labeled 2-D subcostal 4-chamber TTE view of the heart after i.v. injection of saline microbubble contrast demonstrating grade 4 shunt (opacification of left atrium). Bubbles appeared in the LA within 3 cardiac cycles of opacification of the RA demonstrating the presence of an interatrial shunt

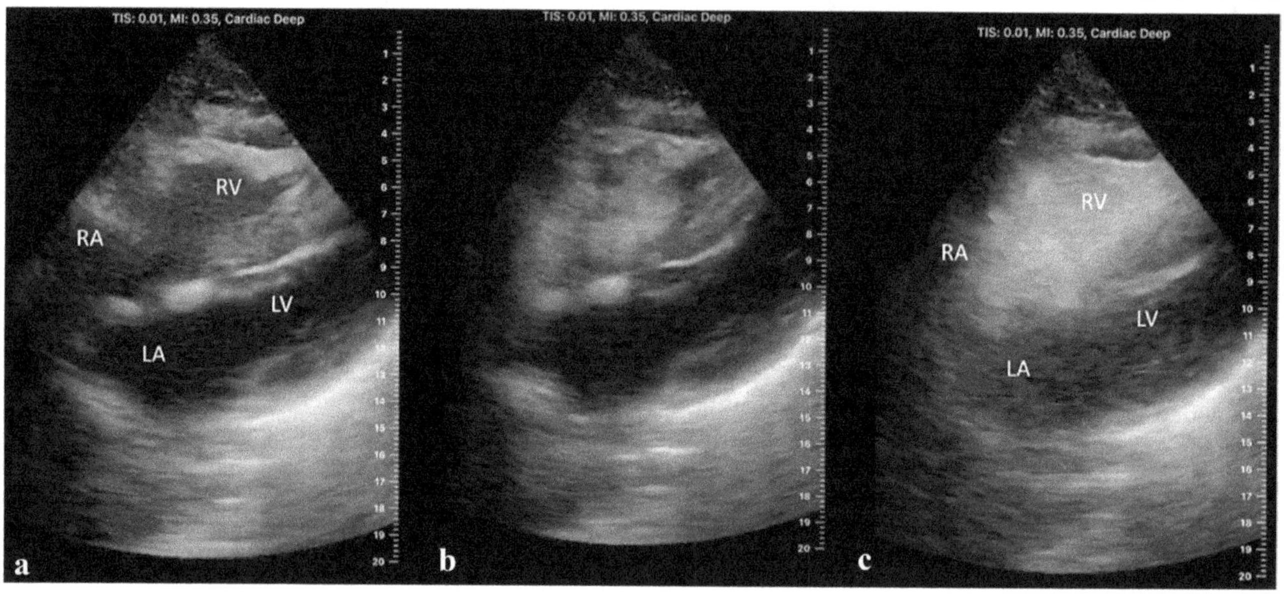

Fig. 3 Intrapulmonary shunt in a mechanically ventilated patient with consolidated lung. Intrapulmonary shunt in a mechanically ventilated patient with consolidated lung. a Labeled 2-D subcostal 4-chamber transthoracic echocardiographic (TTE) view of the heart. *RA* right atrium, *RV* right ventricle, *LA* left atrium, *LV* left ventricle. b 2-D subcostal 4-chamber echocardiographic view of the heart after i.v. injection of saline microbubble contrast showing the arrival of the contrast in the RA and RV. c Labeled 2-D subcostal 4-chamber echocardiographic view of the heart after i.v. injection of saline microbubble contrast demonstrating grade 3 shunt (> 25 bubbles). Bubbles appeared in the left ventricle 5 cardiac cycles after opacification of the right ventricle suggesting the presence of an intrapulmonary shunt

Thus, more data are required to define the most appropriate management strategies in hypoxic patients with interatrial shunt. As acute extrapulmonary shunt may be reversible, specific measures to identify, and where possible reduce or eliminate RTL extrapulmonary shunt may improve outcomes in select patients [5, 29].

Regardless, our observations suggest that combined lung ultrasound, DVT ultrasound, and limited TTE with saline microbubble contrast can define the etiology of shunt, and exclude DVT in hypoxic critically ill patients. When screening for the cause of hypoxia and shunt, these tools provide complementary data. The diagnostic information obtained can have an additive effect that provides new insights, improving decision-making.

Furthermore, our demonstration of the ease with which shunt can be detected could enhance the management of respiratory failure. Serial ultrasonography with handheld devices may allow monitoring of changes in lung pathology, shunt, and cardiac function after specific interventions, or with disease progression.

Further research is required to investigate the effects of specific causes of respiratory failure, and/or their treatment on total shunt (i.e., extrapulmonary shunt and IPS) [29, 34]. Our observations demonstrate that handheld ultrasound could facilitate such studies. Indeed, the COVID-19 pandemic offers a unique opportunity to advance the evidence base for critical care by studying patients with a unique etiology of respiratory failure [34]. Observations in COVID-19 may be relevant to other causes of respiratory disease [34].

Limitations of this study include the use of convenience rather than sequential sampling, which could cause inclusion bias. Our study only included select patients suspected to have severe shunt, and the detected shunts were relatively large. Further studies are required to determine whether handheld devices can detect small shunts in unselected critically ill patients.

Performance bias and overinterpretation by the investigators performing the ultrasound examinations was mitigated by a quality assurance check by an independent observer. This ensured that the images were interpretable, and that the correct diagnosis was made. No changes in diagnosis were made by the independent observer. The performance of imaging by experienced operators provides good internal validity. However, while this does limit external validity, intensivists with less imaging experience can ask a sufficiently experienced observer (e.g., cardiologist) to report their scans. Thus, this study provides a proof of concept.

Conclusion

Routine screening of patients with combined lung ultrasound DVT ultrasound, and limited TTE with saline microbubble contrast using handheld ultrasound is feasible, and may be able to define the etiology of hypoxia and shunt in critically ill patients. The authors recommend further studies to determine whether using handheld ultrasound to characterize shunt, and direct management could improve the outcomes of critically ill patients. Observations in COVID-19 may be relevant to other causes of respiratory disease [5, 29, 34]. However, to increase generalizability, future research should consider subgroup analyses to explore outcomes based on RTL shunt, and RV function, as well as lung mechanics [5, 29, 34].

Supplementary information

Additional file 1: Video S1. Intravenous microbubble contrast enhanced echocardiographic study suggesting intrapulmonary shunt. Labelled 2-D subcostal 4 chamber echocardiographic recording of the heart after i.v. injection of saline microbubble contrast demonstrating grade 3 shunt (> 25 bubbles). *RA* right atrium, *RV* right ventricle, *LA* left atrium, *LV* left ventricle. Bubbles appeared in the LA 5 cardiac cycles after opacification of the RA suggesting the presence of an intrapulmonary shunt.

Additional file 2: Video S2. Intravenous microbubble contrast enhanced echocardiographic study demonstrating interatrial shunt. Labelled 2-D subcostal 4 chamber transthoracic echocardiographic (TTE) recording of the heart after intravenous injection of saline microbubble contrast demonstrating grade 4 shunt (opacification of right atrium). Bubbles appeared in the left atrium (LA) within 3 cardiac cycles of opacification of the right atrium (RA) demonstrating the presence of an interatrial shunt. The RA and right ventricle (RV) are dilated and RV function is impaired. These findings are consistent with acute cor pulmonale. *LV* left ventricle.

Abbreviations

COVID-19: Coronavirus Disease 2019; DVT: Deep vein thrombosis; TTE: Transthoracic echocardiography; ARDS: Acute respiratory distress syndrome; RTL: Right-to-left; HDU: High dependency unit; ICU: Intensive care units; IPS: Intrapulmonary; PaO2: Arterial partial pressure of oxygen; FiO2: Inspired oxygen fraction; PE: Pulmonary embolism; PFO: Patent foramen ovale; 2-D: Two dimensional; LA: Left atrium; LV: Left ventricle; RA: Right atrium; RV: Right ventricle.

Acknowledgements

Not applicable

Authors' contributions

RR and AH developed the hypothesis. All authors were involved in literature search and refinement of the hypothesis. RR, AH and NM performed and interpreted imaging and collected data. RR prepared the initial draft of the manuscript. All authors read and approved the final manuscript.

Author details

[1] Department of Medicine, King Abdulaziz Medical City, King Abdulaziz International Medical Research Center, Ministry of National Guard - Health Affairs, Riyadh, Saudi Arabia. [2] College of Medicine, King Saud Bin Abdulaziz University for Health Sciences, Riyadh, Saudi Arabia. [3] Department of Cardiac Sciences, King Abdulaziz Medical City, King Abdulaziz International Medical Research Center, Ministry of National Guard - Health Affairs, Riyadh, Saudi Arabia.

References

1. Gattinoni L, Coppola S, Cressoni M et al (2020) Covid-19 does not lead to a "Typical" acute respiratory distress syndrome. Am J Respir Crit Care Med. https://doi.org/10.1164/rccm.202003-0817LE
2. Gattinoni L, Chiumello D, Caironi P et al (2020) COVID-19 pneumonia: different respiratory treatments for different phenotypes? Intensive Care Med. https://doi.org/10.1007/s00134-020-06033-2
3. Soldati G, Giannasi G, Smargiassi A et al (2020) Contrast-enhanced ultrasound in patients with COVID-19: pneumonia, acute respiratory distress syndrome, or something else? J ultrasound Med Off J Am Inst Ultrasound Med. https://doi.org/10.1002/jum.15338

4. Al-Ani F, Chehade S, Lazo-Langner A (2020) Thrombosis risk associated with COVID-19 infection. A scoping review. Thromb Res 192:152–160. https://doi.org/10.1016/j.thromres.2020.05.039
5. Rajendram R, Kharal GA, Mahmood N et al (2020) Intensive care medicine rethinking the respiratory paradigm of Covid-19: A ' hole ' in the argument. Intensive Care Med 46:1496–1497. https://doi.org/10.1007/s00134-020-06102-6
6. Agrawal A, Palkar A, Talwar A (2017) The multiple dimensions of Platypnea-Orthodeoxia syndrome: a review. Respir Med 129:31–38. https://doi.org/10.1016/j.rmed.2017.05.016
7. Guarracino F, Vetrugno L, Forfori F et al (2020) Lung, heart, vascular, and diaphragm ultrasound examination of COVID-19 patients: a comprehensive approach. J Cardiothorac Vasc Anesth. https://doi.org/10.1053/j.jvca.2020.06.013
8. Repessé X, Charron C, Vieillard-Baron A (2016) Assessment of the effects of inspiratory load on right ventricular function. Curr Opin Crit Care 22:254–259. https://doi.org/10.1097/MCC.0000000000000303
9. Mekontso Dessap A, Boissier F, Charron C et al (2016) Acute cor pulmonale during protective ventilation for acute respiratory distress syndrome: prevalence, predictors, and clinical impact. Intensive Care Med 42:862–870. https://doi.org/10.1007/s00134-015-4141-2
10. Rana BS, Thomas MR, Calvert PA et al (2010) Echocardiographic evaluation of patent foramen ovale prior to device closure. JACC Cardiovasc Imaging 3:749–760. https://doi.org/10.1016/j.jcmg.2010.01.007
11. Gallagher G, Joseph A, Rajendram R (2018) Platypnea-orthodeoxia: Patent foramen ovale unmasked by pulmonary emboli. Indian J Respir Care 7:50–52
12. Smith MJ, Hayward SA, Innes SM, Miller ASC (2020) Point-of-care lung ultrasound in patients with COVID-19—a narrative review. Anaesthesia. https://doi.org/10.1111/anae.15082
13. Haji K, Haji D, Canty DJ et al (2018) The feasibility and impact of routine combined limited transthoracic echocardiography and lung ultrasound on diagnosis and management of patients admitted to ICU: a prospective observational study. J Cardiothorac Vasc Anesth 32:354–360. https://doi.org/10.1053/j.jvca.2017.08.026
14. Clevert D-A, Schwarze V, Nyhsen C et al (2019) ESR statement on portable ultrasound devices. Insights Imaging 10:89. https://doi.org/10.1186/s13244-019-0775-x
15. Glogoza M, Urbach J, Rosborough TK et al (2020) Tablet vs station-based laptop ultrasound devices increases internal medicine resident point-of-care ultrasound performance: a prospective cohort study. Ultrasound J 12:18. https://doi.org/10.1186/s13089-020-00165-8
16. Gibson LE, Bittner EA, Chang MG (2020) Handheld ultrasound devices: an emerging technology to reduce viral spread during the Covid-19 pandemic. Am J Infect Control. https://doi.org/10.1016/j.ajic.2020.05.041
17. Vavlitou A, Minas G, Zannetos S et al (2016) Hemodynamic and respiratory factors that influence the opening of patent foramen ovale in mechanically ventilated patients. Hippokratia 20:209–213
18. Mekontso Dessap A, Boissier F, Leon R et al (2010) Prevalence and prognosis of shunting across patent foramen ovale during acute respiratory distress syndrome. Crit Care Med 38:1786–1792. https://doi.org/10.1097/CCM.0b013e3181eaa9c8
19. Lee JH, Lee SH, Yun SJ (2019) Comparison of 2-point and 3-point point-of-care ultrasound techniques for deep vein thrombosis at the emergency department: a meta-analysis. Medicine (Baltimore) 98:e15791. https://doi.org/10.1097/MD.0000000000015791
20. Price S, Via G, Sloth E et al (2008) Echocardiography practice, training and accreditation in the intensive care: document for the World Interactive Network Focused on Critical Ultrasound (WINFOCUS). Cardiovasc Ultrasound 6:49. https://doi.org/10.1186/1476-7120-6-49
21. Volpicelli G, Elbarbary M, Blaivas M et al (2012) International evidence-based recommendations for point-of-care lung ultrasound. Intensive Care Med 38:577–591. https://doi.org/10.1007/s00134-012-2513-4
22. Volpicelli G, Lamorte A, Villén T (2020) What's new in lung ultrasound during the COVID-19 pandemic. Intensive Care Med 46:1445–1448. https://doi.org/10.1007/s00134-020-06048-9
23. Via G, Hussain A, Wells M et al (2014) International evidence-based recommendations for focused cardiac ultrasound. J Am Soc Echocardiogr Off Publ Am Soc Echocardiogr 27:683.e1-683.e33. https://doi.org/10.1016/j.echo.2014.05.001
24. Lee FCY (2016) Lung ultrasound-a primary survey of the acutely dyspneic patient. J Intensive Care 4:57. https://doi.org/10.1186/s40560-016-0180-1
25. Mongodi S, Bouhemad B, Orlando A et al (2017) Modified lung ultrasound score for assessing and monitoring pulmonary aeration. Ultraschall Med 38:530–537. https://doi.org/10.1055/s-0042-120260
26. Rouby J-J, Arbelot C, Gao Y et al (2018) Training for lung ultrasound score measurement in critically Ill patients. Am J Respir Crit Care Med 198:398–401
27. Volpicelli G, Gargani L (2020) Sonographic signs and patterns of COVID-19 pneumonia. Ultrasound J 12:22. https://doi.org/10.1186/s13089-020-00171-w
28. Mongodi S, Via G, Riccardi M et al (2017) Patent foramen ovale diagnosis: the importance of provocative maneuvers. J Clin Ultrasound 45:58–61
29. Rajendram R, Kharal GA, Mahmood N, Kharal M (2020) Identifying phenotypes of COVID-19, defining their pathogenesis, and targeting treatments could improve outcomes. Respir Physiol Neurobiol 280:103477
30. Collado FMS, Poulin MF, Murphy JJ et al (2018) Patent foramen ovale closure for stroke prevention and other disorders. J Am Heart Assoc 7:1–22. https://doi.org/10.1161/JAHA.117.007146
31. Marples IL, Heap MJ, Suvarna SK, Mills GH (2000) Acute right-to-left inter-atrial shunt; an important cause of profound hypoxia. Br J Anaesth 85:921–925. https://doi.org/10.1093/bja/85.6.921
32. Guimaraes L, Del Val D, Bergeron S et al (2020) Interatrial shunting for treating acute and chronic left heart failure. Eur Cardiol 15:e18. https://doi.org/10.15420/ecr.2019.04
33. Kurzyna M, Dabrowski M, Bielecki D et al (2007) Atrial septostomy in treatment of end-stage right heart failure in patients with pulmonary hypertension. Chest 131:977–983. https://doi.org/10.1378/chest.06-1227
34. Rajendram R (2020) Building the house of CARDS by phenotyping on the fly. Eur Respir J. https://doi.org/10.1183/13993003.02429-2020

16

A case of intrathyroid parathyroid tumor that was difficult to diagnose by ultrasonography

Nobuyuki Takemoto[1*], Ai Koyanagi[2,3], Masanori Yasuda[4], Yuya Yamamoto[5] and Hiroshi Yamamoto[6]

Abstract

Background: With advances in diagnostic imaging such as ultrasonography (US), computed tomography (CT), and ^{99m}Tc-MIBI-sestamibi (MIBI) scintigraphy, localized diagnosis of hyperparathyroidism (pHPT) has become possible with considerable accuracy. However, even with the use of these imaging techniques, since intrathyroid parathyroid tumors exist as a mass within the thyroid, it is often difficult to distinguish from thyroid masses. Although there have been various reports on US images of intraparathyroid tumors, we experienced a case with US images that were distinct from previous reports. Herein we present a case of an intrathyroid parathyroid adenoma (IPA) that was difficult to diagnose, with a main focus on US images.

Case presentation: A 53-year-old man with a diagnosis of hyperparathyroidism was referred to our department in December 2018. Ultrasonography revealed a tumor that was located in the inferior pole of the right lobe of the thyroid gland and no parathyroid mass was observed. The tumor had an irregular round shape and showed heterogeneous hyperechogenicity with a defined margin, but within it, there were a few irregular and hypoechogenic area with unclear margins, while the tumor had a mosaic appearance at first glance. Although ^{99m}Tc-MIBI scintigraphy showed accumulation at the same location in delayed phase, it was difficult to determine the presence of a parathyroid tumor on the image. The patient underwent an operation on April 2019 and the tumor could not be identified on both naked eye and palpation. We used US intraoperatively to define the location and resected the tumor. A parathyroid adenoma was diagnosed by frozen section and the final diagnosis was an intrathyroid parathyroid adenoma.

Conclusion: We experienced an IPA presenting an US image that was atypical and has previously not been reported. IPA has no established US image to confirm the diagnosis and even with the use of other imaging techniques, a definitive diagnosis often cannot be established. Thus, our recommendation based on the current situation is that operation with intraoperative diagnosis using frozen section should be conducted if hypercalcemia and high I-PTH are observed and when localization sites in MIBI and US coincide.

Keywords: Intrathyroid parathyroid adenoma, Ultrasonography, ^{99m}Tc-MIBI, Difficult-to-diagnose

Introduction

The basis of treatment of primary hyperparathyroidism (pHPT) is parathyroidectomy of the responsible lesion, and thus, preoperative localization is crucial. With advances in diagnostic imaging such as ultrasonography (US), computed tomography (CT), and ^{99m}Tc-MIBI-sestamibi (MIBI) scintigraphy, localized diagnosis of pHPT has become possible with considerable accuracy [1]. However, even with the use of these imaging techniques, since intrathyroid parathyroid tumors exist as a mass within the thyroid, it is often difficult to distinguish from thyroid masses. Although there have been various reports [1–3] on US images of intraparathyroid tumors,

*Correspondence: monochrome-rainbow@iijmio.mail.jp
[1] Department of Breast & Endocrine Surgery, Japan Medical Alliance East Saitama General Hospital, 5-517, Yoshino, Saitama-Pref, Satte 340-0153, Japan
Full list of author information is available at the end of the article

we experienced a case with US images that were distinct from previous reports. Herein we present a case of an intrathyroid parathyroid adenoma (IPA) that was difficult to diagnose, with a main focus on US images.

Case presentation

A 53-year-old man with a diagnosis of hyperparathyroidism was referred to our department in December 2018. The results of laboratory examinations were compatible with hyperparathyroidism: intact-PTH 94 pg/ml (normal range 10–65 pg/ml), serum Ca 11.9 mg/dl (normal range 8.2–10.4 mg/dl), and serum P 2.4 mg/dl (normal range 2.5–4.6 mg/dl). Thyroid function tests (TSH, Free-T3, Free-T4) were all within normal limits. Cervical tumors and lymphadenopathy were not identified on palpation. The patient showed no signs of hoarseness, dysphagia and dysphonia. His past medical history included ureter stones and type 2 diabetes, and he had no kidney diseases that can cause secondary hyperparathyroidism. There were no notable family medical histories. US was performed with a 7.5-MHz linear transducer (TOSHIBA MEDICAL SYSTEMS; SSA-790A, TOCHIGI, JAPAN). A tumor was found in the inferior pole of the right lobe of the thyroid gland and no parathyroid mass was observed. The tumor had an irregular round shape and showed heterogeneous hyperechogenicity with a defined margin, but within it, there were a few unclear margins, irregular and hypoechogenic area, and the tumor had a mosaic appearance at first glance (Fig. 1a, b). The size of the tumor was 18 × 13 × 11 mm (anteroposterior × transverse × craniocaudal dimension). Color Doppler sonography showed that the blood vessels flowing into the tumor were thick and marked blood flow was observed within the tumor (Fig. 1c). No lymph node swelling was observed in the cervical regions.

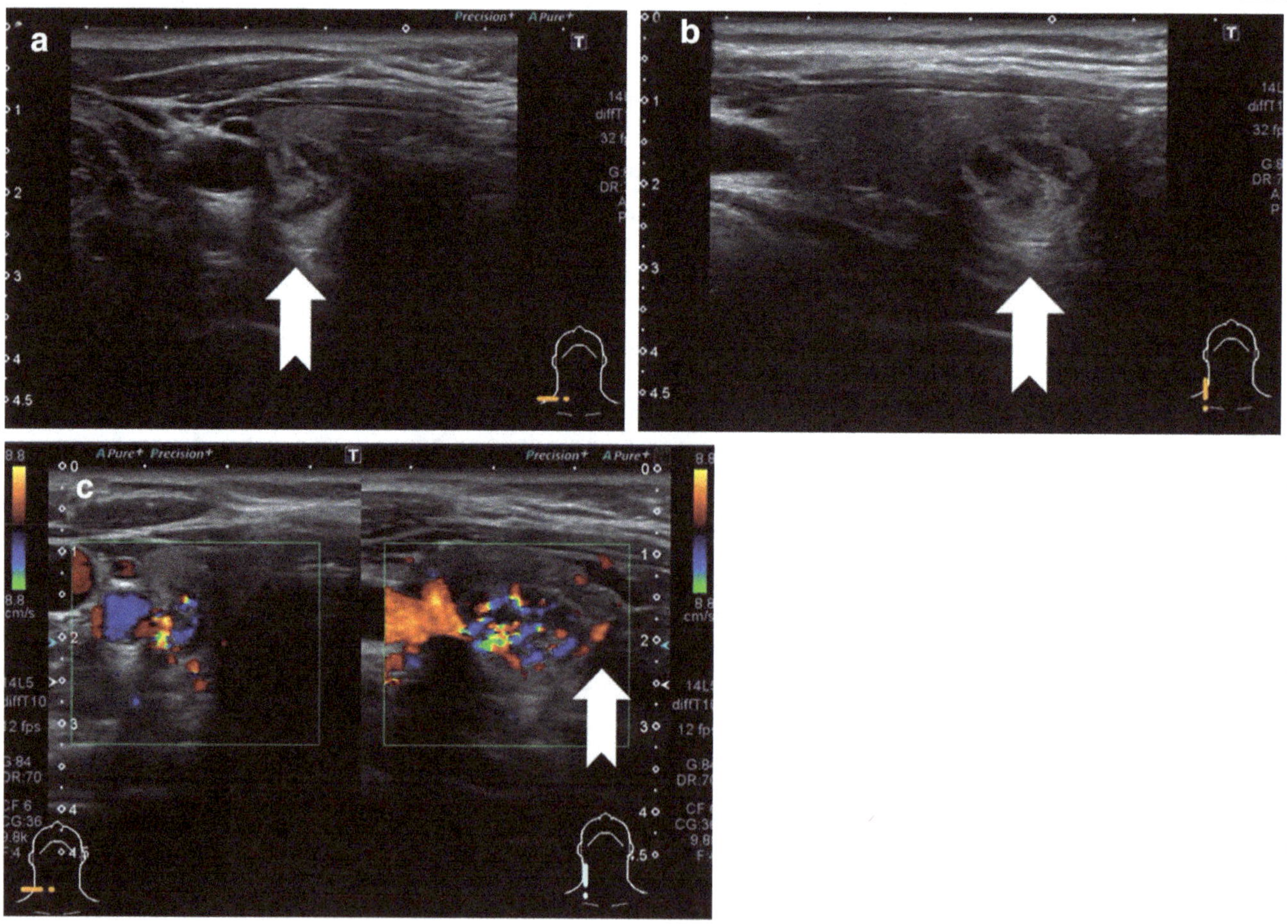

Fig. 1 Ultrasonographic imaging. **a** Transverse image. **b** Longitudinal image. **c** Color Doppler imaging. The tumor ((**a, b**) arrow) was located in the inferior pole of the right lobe of the thyroid gland and no parathyroid mass was observed. The size of the tumor was 18 × 13 × 11 mm (anteroposterior × transverse × craniocaudal dimension). The tumor had an irregular round shape and showed heterogeneous hyperechogenicity with a defined margin, but within it, there were a few unclear margins, irregular and hypoechogenic area, and the tumor had a mosaic appearance at first glance. Color Doppler sonography showed that the blood vessels ((**c**) arrow) flowing into the tumor were thick and marked blood flow was also observed within the tumor

Images obtained by CT revealed a low density mass which was slightly enhanced by contrast injection in the right thyroid lobe (Fig. 2a, b). No other abnormality was identified on thoraco-abdominal CT. The MIBI scintigraphy showed accumulation near the lower right pole and strong accumulation even in the delayed phase, suggesting parathyroid adenoma (Fig. 3). The image was very atypical for a parathyroid adenoma, and the possibility of hyperplasia and cancer was also considered. Considering the risk of dissemination, we decided not to carry out fine needle aspiration cytology (FNAC) but to attempt intraoperative diagnosis using frozen section and to treat at the same time.

The patient underwent resection of the tumor under collar incision on April 2019. As the tumor could not be identified on both naked eye and palpation, we used US intraoperatively and confirmed that the tumor was located in the inferior pole of the right lobe of the thyroid gland. The cranial side of the tumor was identified, from which the thyroid was incised and a right partial lobectomy was performed. Pathological examination revealed a parathyroid adenoma that was surrounded by a thin capsule and showed no variant type (Fig. 4b, d). However, there were some nodular areas composed of cells with clear cytoplasm (Fig. 4c), and there was scattered fatty infiltration. There was no evidence of malignancy. The final diagnosis was IPA. The patient recovered well after surgery and was discharged on the 5th day. Postoperatively, serum calcium and I-PTH were rapidly normalized, and no increase has been observed as of July 2019.

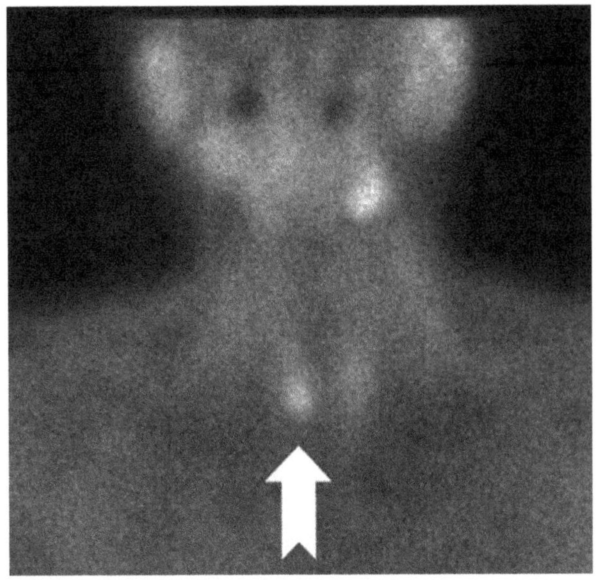

Fig. 3 MIBI scintigraphy The MIBI scintigraphy showed accumulation near the lower right pole and strong accumulation even in the delayed phase, suggestive of a parathyroid adenoma

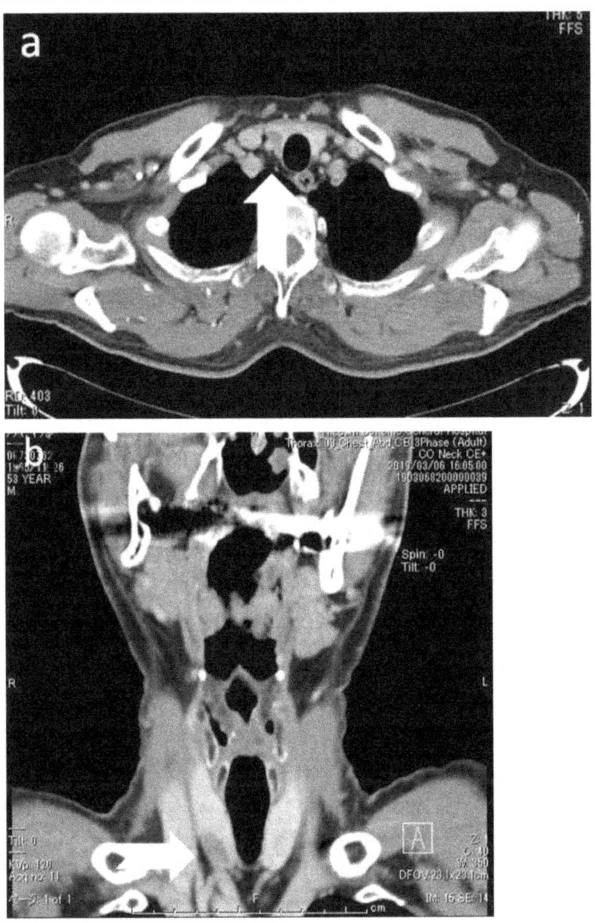

Fig. 2 Enhanced computed tomography. **a** Transverse image. **b** Sagittal image. Images obtained by CT revealed a low density mass which was slightly enhanced by contrast injection in the right thyroid lobe

Discussion

The parathyroid glands can become misaligned during development [2]. The vast majority of these displaced parathyroid glands are found in the inferior gland (90%) and those in the superior gland are rare [2, 4, 5]. This is because the developmental origin of parathyroid glands differs between the superior and inferior glands [2]. The superior parathyroid glands are derived from the fourth pharyngeal pouch and lie on the dorsal surface of the thyroid gland, while the inferior parathyroid glands originate from the third pharyngeal pouch accompanying the thymus, and are in a more inferior position than the superior parathyroid glands derived from the fourth pharyngeal pouch [6]. Therefore, the inferior glands are more likely to become misaligned due to more migration of embryological tissue.

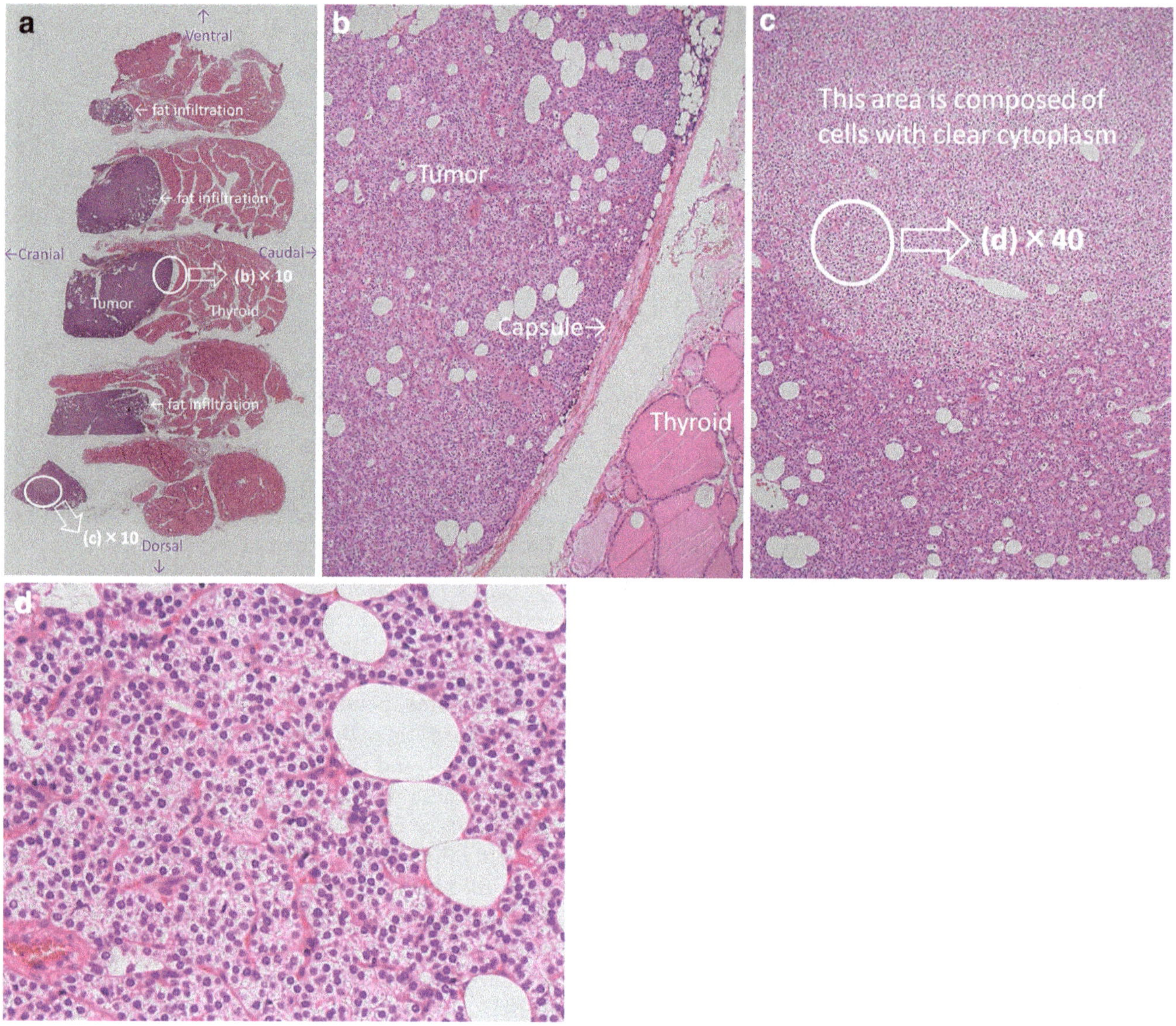

Fig. 4 Pathological findings (Hematoxylin and Eosin stain) **a** Semi-macroscopic view (loupe image). The longitudinal images of the tumor are arranged in order. **b** × 10. The parathyroid adenoma was surrounded by a thin fibrotic capsule. **c** × 10. There were some nodular areas, which are composed of cells with clear cytoplasm, and there was scattered fatty infiltration. **d** × 40. The parathyroid adenoma showed no variant type and was almost uniform throughout. There was no evidence of malignancy

Ectopic parathyroid gland is understood to be caused by the development of adenoma or hyperplasia from parathyroid glands that have been displaced, such as in the thyroid or in the thymus [2, 7]. Among pHPT, IPA is rare with its prevalence reported to be between 1.4 and 2.1% [3, 8]. IPA is more frequent on the right lobe [2–4], and is divided into complete and partial types in encircled form, but the frequency of these types are reported to be the same [2, 5, 9].

Cervical US, contrast-enhanced CT, and MIBI scintigram are useful for the localization of parathyroid tumors. The rate of correct diagnosis is very high especially when the localization in cervical US and MIBI scintigram coincide, and at present, the combination of US and 99mTc-MIBI SPECT/CT is most recommended [1]. However, in the case of IPA, the interpretation of imaging findings is difficult compared to pHPT cases that exist in the normal position [2].

When normal parathyroid tumor is observed in US, it is shown as a mass showing flat, elliptical, clear borderline, internal homogeneous hypoechoic mass on the dorsal side of the thyroid capsule depicted in high echo level, and in the color Doppler method, blood flow inside the mass is abundantly observed [1]. The previously reported US findings in IPA include the following: (a) the tumor is not flat but has an oval to near-spherical shape because the compression from the cervical spine and thyroid is weak [2]; (b) it often has the same properties as parathyroid tumor [2]; (c) it may be confused with cysts, but identification is possible by recognizing blood flow signals inside [1]; (d) Yubata [3] reported that the typical sonographic appearance of IPA consists of a regular shape, smooth border, hypoechoic level of internal echo, solid content, a hyperechoic line on the ventral surface of the parathyroid gland, and the presence of feeding vessels. In particular, a hyperechoic line on the ventral surface of the parathyroid gland has been reported as a finding characteristic of IPA. However, only 20% of reported cases had this hyperechoic line [2], and its diagnostic utility has not been determined.

In the US image of our case, the border of the mass was relatively clear, and the internal echo was homogeneous and hyperechoic, but within the mass, there were several irregularly shaped, unclear borders and hypoechoic areas, which resembled a mosaic at first glance. In the US transverse image, the hyperechoic line reported by Yubata et al. [3] appeared to be present on the ventral side of the adenoma, but the longitudinal image showed that the line was present almost all around the mass. The line was not ventrally specific, and is likely to have been the capsule of the mass. These findings were not specific enough to provide a definitive diagnosis of IPA based on US only.

There are several possible reasons for the atypical US image found in our case. First, Fig. 4a is a pathological picture in which the longitudinal images of the mass are arranged in order, but notice that the shape of the mass is different from the US image (Fig. 1b). However, when the US Probe was placed on the mass and compression was applied, the mass fell to the cranial side, and the image in Fig. 1b was obtained. The fat concentrated on the thyroid side (= caudal side) of the mass moved to the ventral side, so this may have been depicted as irregular hypoechoic (i.e., mosaic-like findings).

Also, when the pathological picture is reviewed, there is a nodular area in one part of the mass, and the area consists of clear cytoplasm in the surrounding area. Although speculative, since the US visualizes a mass as a shadow, factors such as density of cells, water content of each cell, and inherent properties of US such as scattering, absorption, attenuation, refraction, reflection, etc. may have interacted to create this image.

Next, MIBI is an essential modality for diagnosis of pHPT due to its high specificity, but may give rise to false-negatives for small parathyroid glands smaller than 300 mg [1]. In addition, pHPT is likely to be associated with various nodular thyroid lesions [10, 11], and MIBI is known to be frequently accumulated in thyroid-derived nodules and to give rise to false-positives [1, 3]. However, thyroid tumors tend to be excreted in the delayed phase because they wash out faster than the parathyroid gland, and there is also a report that differentiation is possible to some extent [12]. In this case, strong accumulation was observed even in the delayed phase, and retrospective observation suggests that it was more likely to be IPA rather than a goiter.

In addition, CT has recently been used to provide diagnosis for enlarged parathyroid glands by contrast pattern [13], but in the case of IPA, it is strongly affected by contrast enhancement of the background thyroid, so it is very difficult to confirm the tumor contrast pattern. Although the existence of a tumor can be confirmed by CT, currently, definitive diagnosis is difficult to establish.

Recently, it has been reported that a single-photon emission computed tomography/computed tomography (SPECT/CT) imaging is useful for localization of parathyroid lesions and identification of the size of adenomas or hyperplastic glands [14, 15]. SPECT/CT has been reported to be capable of detecting parathyroid adenomas even with a greatest axial diameter of 0.6 cm [14]. In Japan, this equipment is still not widely available; however, workstations to create a fusion image of MIBI SPECT and CT are being used in some facilities without an exclusive SPECT/CT device [16]. There is a growing expectation for wider availability of this method.

Some authors have suggested that it may be possible to determine whether a tumor is of parathyroid origin or not by measuring intact-PTH of the lavage fluid from fine needle aspiration of the lesion [17]. However, in facilities where the number of cases is limited, this may not be feasible in terms of cost. Furthermore, given that the parathyroid tissue is a tissue that can easily engraft [18] and disseminate [2], while puncture can cause bleeding, this method may not be practical especially for cases where parathyroid cancer is suspected. Indeed, FNAC is contraindicated for parathyroid cancer [19], and even if IPA is suspected clinically, performing FNAC carries a risk as preoperative diagnosis of parathyroid cancer is difficult.

At present, it is difficult to make a definitive diagnosis of IPA before operation, although the accuracy of diagnosis of IPA can be increased by combining various imaging techniques. In particular, there are no typical images that are specific enough to establish a definitive diagnosis with US. In the case of suspected IPA, currently, the optimal measure may be to perform resection together with intraoperative US and to confirm parathyroid tissue with frozen section. Development of new diagnostic imaging techniques is warranted for preoperative diagnosis of IPA.

Conclusion

We experienced an IPA presenting an US image that was atypical and has previously not been reported. IPA has no established US image to confirm the diagnosis and even with the use of other imaging techniques, a definitive diagnosis often cannot be established. Thus, our recommendation based on the current situation is that operation with intraoperative diagnosis using frozen section should be conducted if hypercalcemia and high I-PTH are observed and when localization sites in MIBI and US coincide.

Abbreviations

US: Ultrasonography; CT: Computed tomography; MIBI: ^{99m}Tc-MIBI-sestamibi; pHPT: Hyperparathyroidism; IPA: Intrathyroid parathyroid adenoma; FNAC: Fine needle aspiration cytology.

Acknowledgements

Not applicable.

Authors' contributions

NT performed both ultrasound imaging and operation, conducted the literature review, and wrote the manuscript. AK reviewed and edited the manuscript. MY performed the histological examination of the parathyroid. YY provided advice on diagnosis. HY assisted in the operation. All authors read and approved the final manuscript.

Author details

[1] Department of Breast & Endocrine Surgery, Japan Medical Alliance East Saitama General Hospital, 5-517, Yoshino, Saitama-Pref, Satte 340-0153, Japan. [2] Research and Development Unit, Parc Sanitari Sant Joan de Déu, Fundació Sant Joan de Déu, CIBERSAM, Sant Boi de Llobregat, Barcelona, Spain. [3] ICREA, Pg. Lluis Companys 23, Barcelona, Spain. [4] Department of Pathology, Saitama Medical University International Medical Center, 1397-1, Yamane, Hidaka, Saitama-Pref, Japan. [5] Department of Endocrine Internal Medicine, Japan Medical Alliance East Saitama General Hospital, 5-517, Yoshino, Satte, Saitama-Pref, Japan. [6] Geriatric Health Service Facility (COSMOS), Japan Medical Alliance Yokohama Stroke and Brain Center, 1-2-1 Takigashira, Isogoku, Yokohama, Kanagawa-Pref, Japan.

References

1. JABTS (2017) Thyroid ultrasound—a guidebook for diagnosis and management, 3rd edn. Nankodo, Tokyo, pp 135–143 **[Japanese]**
2. Satoh S, Mori Y, Tachibana T et al (2014) Ten cases of intrathyroid parathyroid adenoma. J Jpn Soc Head Neck Surg 24(2):207–216 **[Japanese]**
3. Yubta T, Tsushima Y, Masuoka H et al (2011) Ultrasonographic features of intrathyroidal parathyroid adenoma causing primary hyperparathyroidism. J Endocr 58:989–994
4. Proye C, Bizard JP, Quiévreux JL et al (1994) Hyperparathyroidism and intrathyroid parathyroid gland. Ann Chir 48:501–506
5. Goodman A, Politz D, Normal J et al (2011) Intrathyroid parathyroid adenoma: incidence and location—the case against thyroid lobectomy. Octolaryngol Head Neck Surg 14:867–871
6. Moore Keith L, Persaud TVN (2008) The Developing Human, 8th edn. Elsevier/Saunders, Philadelphia, pp 237–240
7. Fujita Y, Suzuki K, Mori Y et al (2012) A case of intrathyroidal parathyroid adenoma with primary hyperparathyroidism. Otologia Fukuoka 58:278–284 **[Japanese]**
8. Bahar G, Feinmesser R, Joshua BZ et al (2006) Hyperfunctioning intrathyroid parathyroid gland: a potential cause of failure in parathyroidectomy. Surgery 139:821–826
9. Abbound B, Sleitaly G, Abadjian G et al (2007) Intrathyroid parathyroid adenoma in primary hyperparathyroidism: can it be predicted preoperatively? World J Surg 31:817–823
10. dell'Erba L, Baldari S, Borsato N et al (2001) Retrospective analysis of the association of nodular goiter with primary and secondary hyperparathyroidism. Eur J Endocrinol 145(4):429–434
11. Feliciano DV (1992) Parathyroid pathology in an intrathyroidal position. Am J Surg 164:496–500
12. Takami H, Ooshima M, Harasawa Y et al (1997) Localization of thyroid and parathyroid masses by 99mTc-MIBI scintigraphy. J Clin Surg 52(9):1125–1129
13. Rodgers SE, Hunter GJ, Hamberg LM et al (2006) Improved preoperative planning for directed parathyroidectomy with 4-dimensional computed tomography. Surgery 140(6):932–940
14. Shafiei B, Hoseinzadeh S, Fotouhi F et al (2012) Preoperative 99mTc-sestamibi scintigraphy in patients with primary hyperparathyroidism and concomitant nodular goiter: comparison of SPECT-CT, SPECT, and planar imaging. Nucl Med commun 33(1070):1076
15. Monzen Y, Tamura A, Okazaki H et al (2015) SPECT/CT fusion in the diagnosis of hyperparathyroidism. Asia Ocean J Nucl Med Biol 3(1):61–65
16. Nakada K, Takahashi H, Sakuma I et al (2010) Clinical value of fusion images of MIBI SPECT and enhanced MDCT registered by workstation in primary hyperparathyroidism. J Nucl Med 51(Suppl2):p56
17. Ishimori N, Kawamata A, Horiuchi K et al (2011) A case of hyperparathyroidism due to intrathyroidal parathyroid adenoma. J Tokyo Women's Med Univ 81(4):272–275 **[Japanese]**
18. Wells SA, Gunnells JC, Sherwood LM et al (1975) Transplantation of the parathyroid glands in man: clinical indications and results. Surgery 78:34–44
19. Wei CH, Harari A (2012) Parathyroid carcinoma Update and guidelines for management. Curr Treat Options Oncol 13:11–23

17

Sonographic presentation of rice bodies in subacromial-subdeltoid chronic bursitis

Raham Bacha[1], Iqra Manzoor[2*] and Syed Amir Gilani[3]

Abstract

Background: subacromial-subdeltoid chronic bursitis is one of the main causes of shoulder pain syndrome. There are various causes of shoulder pain syndrome including chronic bursitis. The sonographic appearances of chronic bursitis vary from patient to patient, depending upon the underlying cause. However, rice bodies are the rare sonographic presentation among them. Rice bodies can be associated with atypical mycobacterial tenosynovitis, bursitis, mycobacterium tuberculosis and infections, but very rarely occur in the chronic subacromial-subdeltoid bursitis. Its unique sonographic presentation makes it easy to be diagnosed confidently, but it is difficult to be recognized, interpret and distinguish from other pathologies due to its rare occurrence. It is therefore intended to present this rare and interesting sonographic presentation of chronic subacromial-subdeltoid bursitis as a case report.

Case-presentation: A 36-year-old male suffering from swelling and pain on his left shoulder for 6 months came to the clinic with Grade-3 impingement syndrome. Free-floating echogenic rice bodies were identified in the subacromial-subdeltoid bursa during ultrasound examination, which was also confirmed with Magnetic resonance imaging (MRI) and serological tests of the specimen after surgery.

Conclusion: The unique sonographic presentation of rice bodies in the chronic subacromial-subdeltoid bursitis makes it easy to be diagnosed confidently, but it is difficult to be recognized, due to its rare occurrence.

Keywords: Rice bodies, Shoulder joint, Bursitis, Ultrasound, subacromial-subdeltoid bursa

Introduction

Shoulder pain is a disabling clinical entity contributing to a great extent to the individual dependency. It is the third most common musculoskeletal complaint in orthopedic practice [1]. There are various causes of shoulder pain syndrome ranging from capsulitis to tendon tear and joint dislocation. Chronic bursitis is one of the main causes of shoulder pain; however, the sonographic presentation of the shoulder pain varies from individual to individual due to underlying causes [2]. Rice bodies are a rare and unique sonographic presentation of chronic bursitis. In chronic bursitis, whitish rice resembling biconcave grains are formed; hence, named as rice bodies [3]. It can also be formed during chronic rheumatoid arthritis and also seen in patients without any underlying causes [4]. They can be formed in different joints of the body including shoulder, knee, wrist, elbow and ankle, but the joint which is affected mostly is shoulder and knee joint. Rheumatoid arthritis is a common complication during which rice bodies can be formed and they are also present in patients without any underlying causes [5]. Under the microscope, the rice bodies are seen as white and shiny grains of rice while on histological examination they are seen as inner amorphous core of acidophilic material which is surrounded by fibrin and collagen. It is often debated, that rice bodies are a nonspecific response to synovial inflammation [6]. The exact pathophysiology of the rice bodies is still unknown. According to some researchers, the rice bodies arise from the microinfarcts of the synovial membrane which leads to the shedding of the synovium [7]. Contrary to this, some researchers say that these bodies are produced impulsively in the synovial fluid and enlarge progressively with the accumulation of the fibrin [8]. Rice bodies are the products of the

*Correspondence: iqramanzoor36@gmail.com
[2] University Institute of Radiological Sciences and Medical Imaging Technologies (UIRSMIT), The University of Lahore, G 10\2 Canal Berg, Lahore 54000, Pakistan
Full list of author information is available at the end of the article

acute and chronic inflammation of the synovium, but they are not the part of chondroid tissues. Infection can also be ruled out when the count of WBC is in normal physiological range [9]. Rice bodies can be detected with the help of different imaging modalities including plain X-ray, Computed tomography (CT) scan, MRI and Ultrasound. Sonoelastography is also useful in the detection of various musculoskeletal pathologies with sensitivity and specificity of 100% and 89%, respectively [10]. However, the advent of state-of-the-art modality and technological development in ultrasound makes it more helpful in the evaluation of superficial structures and their pathologies [11]. As diagnostic ultrasound has no bioeffects and is free of radiation hazards, it is justified to conduct more and more studies on the application of ultrasound in the diagnosis of various diseases.

Case-presentation

A 36-year-old married male came to the Gilani ultrasound center, Lahore, Pakistan. He was a medical lab assistant by profession. On physical examination, he was suffering from shoulder pain for last 6 months but his pain was aggravated from last 1 month and his pain was so severe that he was not able to lie on the affected shoulder. No fever, warmth, and change in color were noted on the affected shoulder. Prominent difference between two shoulders and compressible swelling on the affected shoulder was seen during the scan. On laboratory examination, erythrocyte sedimentation rate (ESR) of the patient was not significantly raised (21 mm/h). The white blood cells (WBC's) were in normal range, Rheumatoid factor (RF) was negative, and C-reactive protein (CRP) concentration level and urine analysis were normal. The patient was scanned in sitting position with the real-time ultrasound examination technique with Toshiba (Xario 200) with linear transducer frequency ranging from 7 to 14 MHz. Left bursa was massively enlarged while measuring from 18 to 24 mm in vertical dimension (Figs. 1, 3). There were multiple biconcave bodies like RBCs with moderate echogenicity in the subacromial-subdeltoid bursa (Fig. 1). These bodies were freely moving and compressible with the transducer compression and joint movement (Additional file 1: Video S1). The size of the rice bodies was measured as 4.6 to 7.1 mm (Fig. 2). Mid-range movement was impaired but movement became normal while abducted with the help of contralateral hand. The cracking sound was also heard with active shoulder movement. The moment of

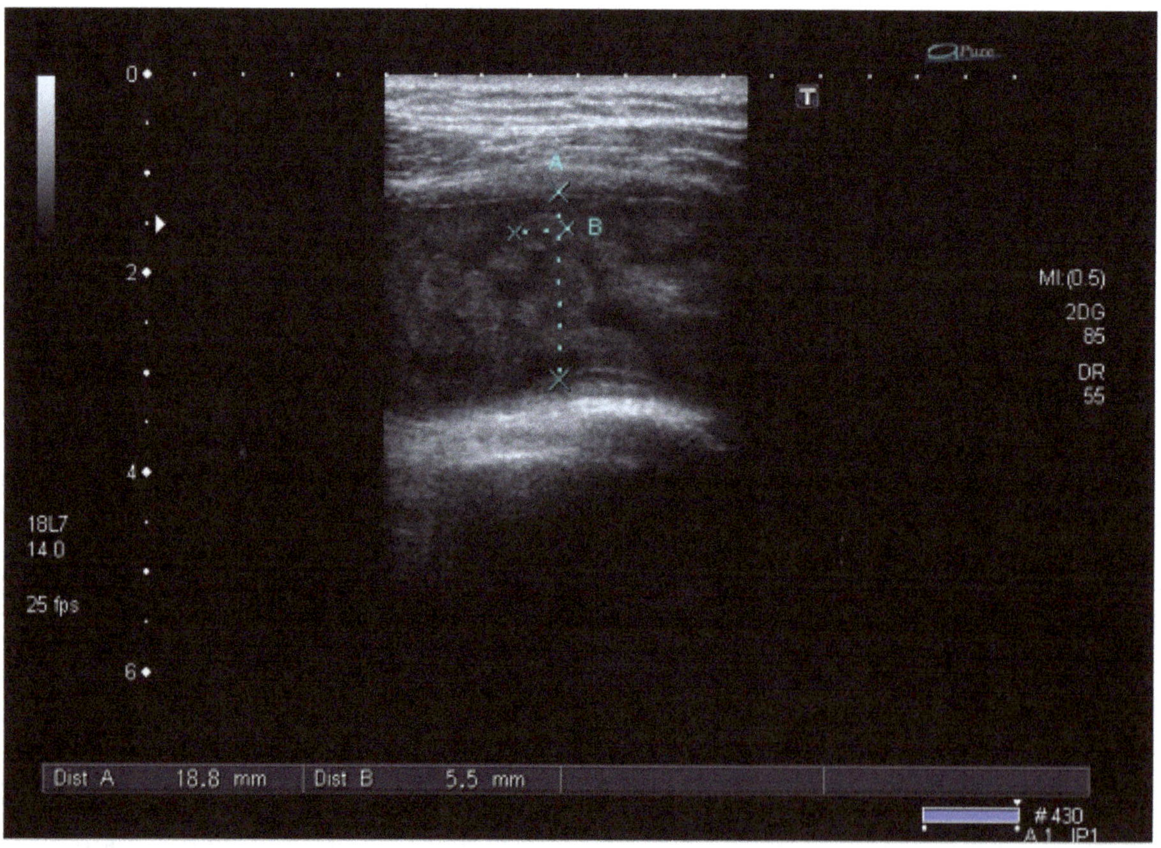

Fig. 1 Rice bodies in the subacromial-subdeltoid bursa

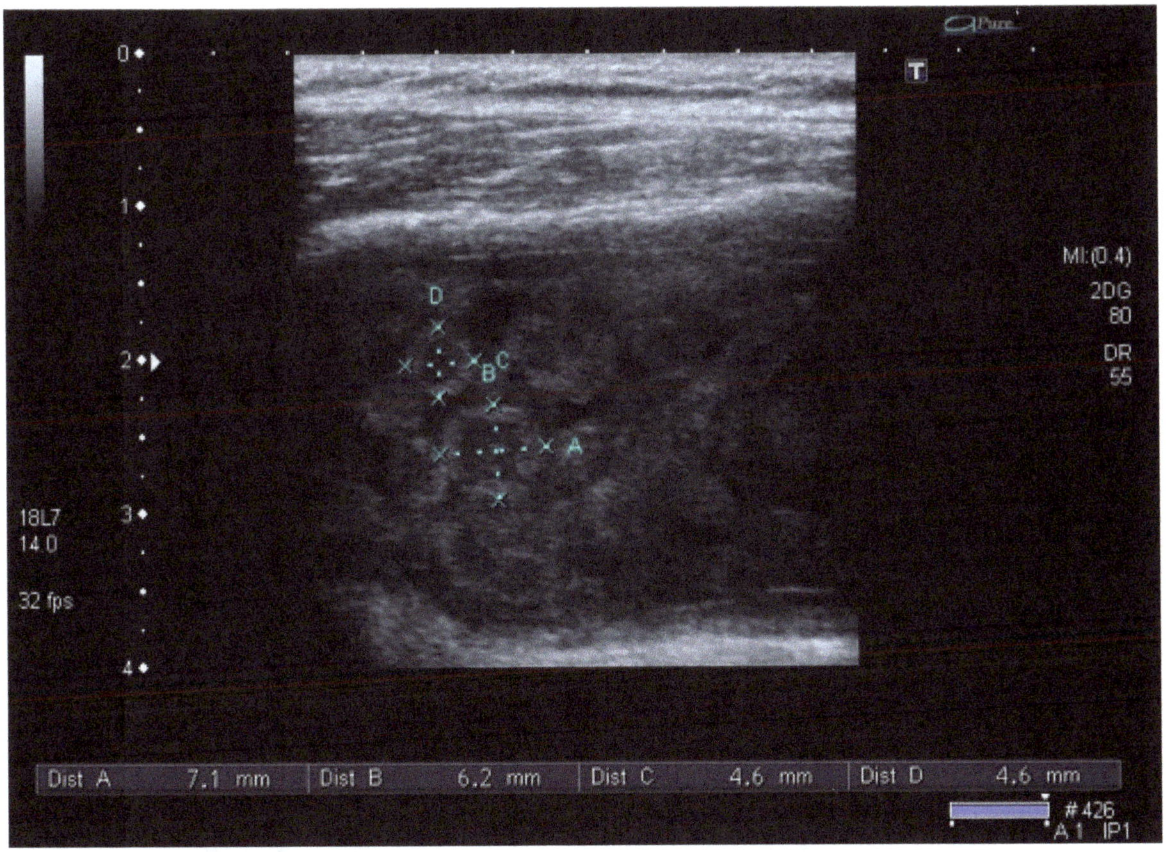

Fig. 2 Measurement of the rice bodies

the glenohumeral joint was restricted having grade-3 impingement. Panoramic view of the subacromial-subdeltoid bursa showing numerous round lentil-like bodies which are named as rice bodies was also taken (Fig. 3). No tear was found in the rotator cuff tendon. Posterior glenoid labrum was normal. Long head of biceps tendon was found in the bicipital groove and was normal. Deltoid muscle and pectoralis muscles were normal (Additional file 1: Video S1). X-ray was also performed after the ultrasound examination which revealed no abnormalities except soft tissue swelling. Next day, MRI was performed which confirms the presence of rice bodies in the subacromial-subdeltoid bursa.

Discussion

The rice bodies were first described by Riese in association with tuberculosis arthritis about a century ago [12]. They are termed as rice bodies because of their close resemblance with the shape and size of the polished rice grains. A great variation is seen in the prevalence of the rice bodies in patients of rheumatoid arthritis, but in one study reported that they are found microscopically as high as 72% [13]. Significant improvement in the complaints of the patients was evident with surgical removal of rice bodies from the affected bursa [3]. The differential diagnosis made for these tiny echogenic materials revealed pigmented villonodular synovitis and synovial chondromatosis especially in the latter stages. In primary synovial chondromatosis, normal joints can be affected but the rice bodies can be associated with tuberculous arthritis, rheumatoid arthritis, osteoarthritis and infective arthritis. This is because synovial chondromatosis results due to metaplasia of subsynovial connective tissue into cartilage nodules. If the rice bodies are mineralized, they can easily be visualized on plain radiographs. Otherwise, MR T-2-weighted scans are very helpful for its diagnosis [14]. An article published in 1996 by Griffith et al. presented 2 cases of the subacromial-subdeltoid bursitis with rice bodies in the size of the rice bodies ranging from 3 to 10 mm, while in our study, the size was ranging from 4.6 to 7.1 mm [15]. Another study reported a similar case of subacromial bursitis with multiple small rice bodies. The findings of X-ray, MRI and Ultrasound were compared for the diagnosis of rice bodies [16]. Similarly, a case was reported by Adriana and colleagues in 2012, while observing a massive subacromial-subdeltoid bursitis with rice bodies secondary

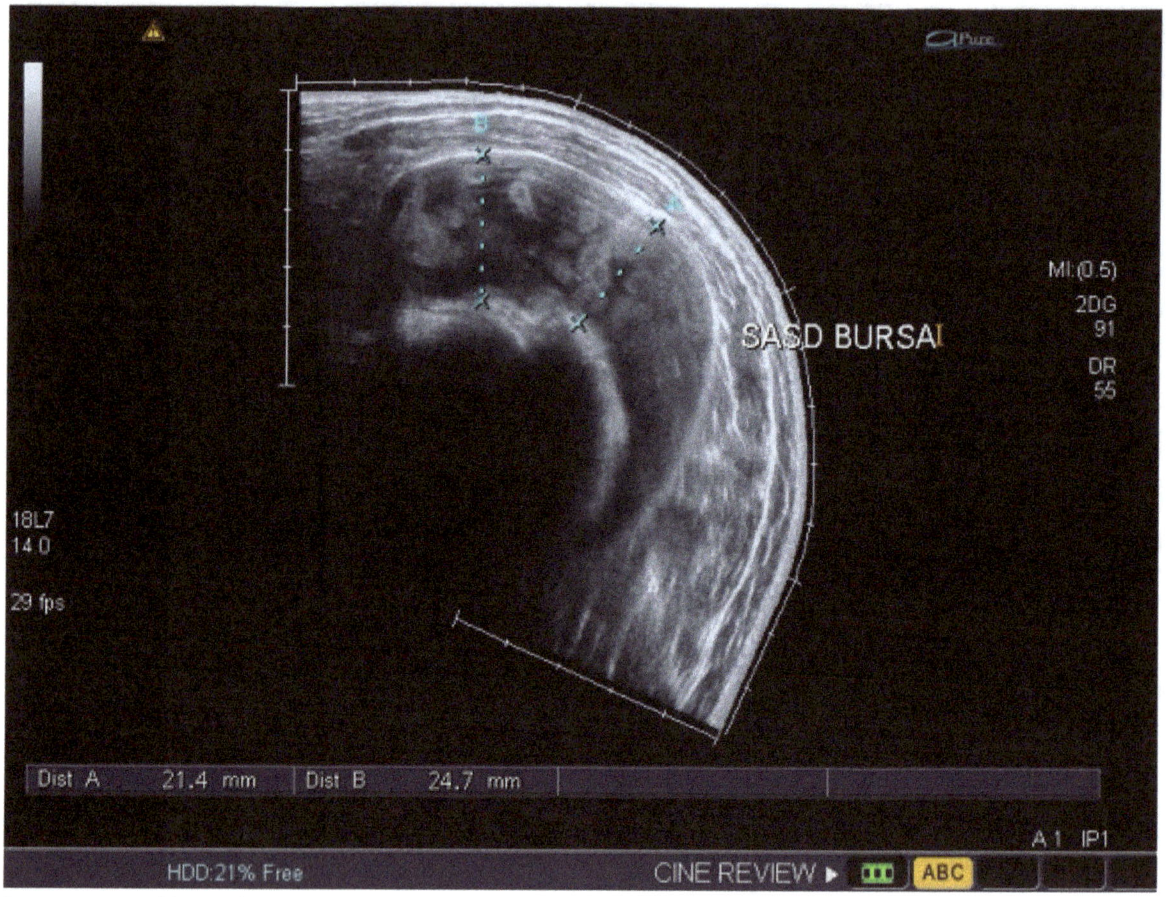

Fig. 3 Panoramic view of the rice bodies

to an orthopedic implant. A large encapsulated fluid was found in the subacromial-subdeltoid bursa, which contained several hundred small 5-mm rice bodies [17]. Various protocols and indications are applicable in different countries of the world. With the prudent use of ultrasound, various diseases could be diagnosed easily which were previously not included in the spectra of its diagnosis [18].Our case report demonstrated a rare case of isolated subacromial-subdeltoid bursitis with rice bodies; the size and appearance were similar to the international studies. But the name rice bodies are suitable for these particles in the subacromial-subdeltoid bursa due to its white color but the sonographic appearance of these bodies was more round-like lentils (Figs. 1, 2, 3).

Conclusion

The unique sonographic presentation of rice bodies in the chronic subacromial-subdeltoid bursitis makes it easy to be diagnosed confidently, but it is difficult to be recognized, due to its rare occurrence.

Additional file

Additional file 1: Video S1. Additional videos.

Abbreviations

MRI: magnetic resonance imaging; CT: computed tomography; WBCs: white blood cells; ESR: erythrocyte sedimentation rate; RF: rheumatoid factor; CRP: c-reactive protein; SASD bursa: subacromial-subdeltoid bursa.

Acknowledgements

I would like to thank our clinical staff members; Komal, Ayesha and Kiran; for their continuous support, and also want to say thank to my family because without their prayers and continuous support nothing will be possible.

Authors' contributions

RB (Scanned the patient, article preparation). IM (Corresponding author, article preparation). SAG (Reviewer). All authors read and approved the final manuscript.

Author details

[1] University Institute of Radiological Sciences and Medical Imaging Technologies (UIRSMIT), Faculty of Allied Health Sciences (FAHS), The University of Lahore, Lahore, Pakistan. [2] University Institute of Radiological Sciences and Medical Imaging Technologies (UIRSMIT), The University of Lahore, G 10\2 Canal Berg, Lahore 54000, Pakistan. [3] Dean Faculty of Allied Health Sciences (FAHS), The University of Lahore, Lahore, Pakistan.

References

1. Garving C, Jakob S, Bauer I, Nadjar R, Brunner UH (2017) Impingement syndrome of the shoulder. Deutsches Ärzteblatt Int 114(45):765
2. Manzoor I, Bacha R, Gilani SA, Liaqat M (2019) The role of ultrasound in shoulder impingement syndrome and rotator cuff tear. Ann Orthop Trauma Rehabil 2(1):126
3. Joshi P (2018) severe sub-acromial bursitis with rice bodies in a patient with rheumatoid arthritis: a case report and review of literature. Malays Orthop J 12(2):52
4. Bayram S, Erşen A, Altan M, Durmaz H (2016) Tuberculosis tenosynovitis with multiple rice bodies of the flexor tendons in the wrist: a case report. Int J Surg Case Rep 27:129–132
5. Chalasani P, Koduru S, Mikkineni K (2016) A rare case of multiple rice bodies in glenohumeral joint, subscapular recess and along long head of biceps. J Orthop Case Rep 6(3):53
6. Dharmshaktu GS, Singh B, Pangtey T (2017) Rice bodies: an uncommon incidental finding inside a bursa over a hip implant. J Musculosk Surg Res 1(1):19
7. Edison MN, Caram A, Flores M, Scherer K (2016) Rice body formation within a peri-articular shoulder mass. Cureus. 8:8
8. Druschel C, Funk JF, Kallinich T, Lieb A, Placzek RP (2013) Development of rice bodies in 2 children younger than 3 years. JCR. 19(1):35–37
9. Hong SE, Pak J-H, Suh HS, Kang S-R, Park BY (2015) Rice body tenosynovitis without tuberculosis infection after multiple acupuncture procedures in a hand. Archiv Plastic Surg 42(4):502
10. Manzoor I, Bacha R, Gilani SA (2018) Diagnostic accuracy of sonoelastography in different diseases. J Ultrasonogr 18(72):29
11. Gilani SA (2012) An overview of musculoskeletal ultrasound—a thirteen years experience in Pakistan. Persp Med 1(1–12):427–430
12. Ali N, Bhat A, Bangroo FA, Wani AH, Kalhan S, Dhanda MS (2016) Rice bodies: a rare presentation of tubercular arthritis of the knee joint. Prog Orthop Sci. 2(2):17–19
13. Pimprikar MV, Kekatpure AL (2014) Subdeltoid bursa tuberculosis with rice bodies formation: case report and review of literature. J Orthop Case Rep 4(2):57
14. Turan A, Çeltikçi P, Tufan A, Öztürk MA (2017) Basic radiological assessment of synovial diseases: a pictorial essay. Eur J Rheumatol 4(2):166
15. Sivaloganathan S, Amr R, Shrivastava R, Relwani J (2015) The Risotto sign—a severe inflammatory bursitis with rice body formation, complicating a rotator cuff repair with a bioabsorbable suture anchor. JRSM Open. 6(1):2054270414562986
16. Mishra BN, Poudel RR, Jha A, Mainali N, Bhattarai M (2018) Rheumatoid subacromial-subdeltoid bursitis with rice bodies: a case report. J Clin Orthop Trauma 10(3):514–517
17. Urruela AM, Rapp TB, Egol KA (2012) Massive subacromial-subdeltoid bursitis with rice bodies secondary to an orthopedic implant. Am J Orthop 41(9):418
18. Gilani SA. Ultrasound Education & Research in Developing Countries. 2011

18

Ultrasound at the patient's bedside for the diagnosis and prognostication of a renal colic

Jean-Eudes Bourcier[1,2*], Emeric Gallard[1], Jean-Philippe Redonnet[1], Morgan Abillard[1], Quentin Billaut[1], Laura Fauque[1], Anna Jouanolou[1] and Didier Garnier[1]

Abstract

Background: Diagnosing a ureteral colic is sometimes difficult; however, clinicians should not fail to detect a surgical emergency. This is why diagnostic strategies depend on the imaging examinations, especially ultrasound. Prior studies have investigated the accuracy of Point of Care Ultrasound (PoCUS), but there are relatively few. This study aimed to evaluate the performance of the PoCUS in the diagnosis of renal colic. The secondary objective was to evaluate the relationship between the imaging results and the treatment performed.

Methods: After the clinical evaluation of patients aged > 18 years with suspected ureteral colic, the Emergency Physician (EP) trained in ultrasound performed PoCUS to conclude whether a diagnosis of "renal colic" should be made. A computed tomography (CT) examination was subsequently performed, to determine whether ureteral or bladder lithiasis was present to diagnose a ureteral colic. The patient's management was decided according to the to degree of urinary tract dilatation, presence of perinephric fluid, size, and localization of stones.

Results: Of the 12 Eps in our units, seven met the training criteria for the inclusion of patients. A total of 103 patients were analyzed, and the renal colic diagnosis was retained in 85 cases after the CT examination. The accuracy of PoCUS was 91% (86; 95%) for detecting urinary tract dilatation, 83% (76; 90%) for detecting perinephric fluid, and 54% (44; 64%) for detecting lithiasis. Only high urinary tract stones with ≥ 6 mm diameter were surgically managed ($p < 0.01$). Conversely, distal ureteral stones with a diameter of < 6 mm were managed with medical ambulatory treatment ($p < 0.05$).

Conclusion: PoCUS is a good diagnostic tool, for renal colic, and could help reduce the requirement for the CT examinations and, hence, reduce induced radiation exposure.

Introduction

Ureteral colic, which is usually revealed by the occurrence of acute lumbar or abdominal pain accounts for 1–5% of the admissions in emergency Unit [1]. Some of its clinical symptoms are similar to those of other pathologies, such as appendicitis, renal infarction, or aortic aneurysm fissuration. Furthermore, in 5% of the cases, ureteral colic is complicated by condition, such as obstructive acute renal failure, suppurated urinary retention, and rupture of the urinary tract, and may require emergency drainage [2, 3]. This is why imaging is often necessary from the initial stage of the patient's management. Computed tomography (CT) without the injection of a contrast agent is the gold standard imaging modality; however, its reasonable use is necessary owing to the involved radiation exposure [4]. Moreover, CT equipment or a radiologist is not always immediately available [5]. Point of Care Ultrasound (PoCUS), performed by the

*Correspondence: je.bourcier@gmail.com
[2] Pôle Anesthésie-Réanimation-Urgences, Hôpital de Lourdes, 2 Avenue Alexandre Marqui, 65100 Lourdes, France
Full list of author information is available at the end of the article

emergency physician (EP), eliminates these drawbacks; however, its reliability remains to be demonstrated [6, 7].

In addition, although imaging is recommended, the impact on patient management is unclear [8–10].

Therefore, the aim of this study was to compare the performance of PoCUS performed by the emergency physician relative to a CT scan interpreted by a radiologist.

The secondary goal was to evaluate the impact of the imaging findings on the patients management.

Patients and methods

Study design

This was a 1-year, single-center, prospective observational study in an emergency unit recording 19,000 visits per year.

Ethic approval statement

The study protocol was approved by ethics Committee of our institution (PV 170216), according to the Jardé law (France). The IRB (Institutional Review Board) considered that the standard of care was not modified. Indeed, in our institution, we did not have access to ultrasound performed by a radiologist. That is why CT scan was the first line examination in case of suspected nephritic colic.

Patients

Any patient aged ≥ 18 years old presenting at the emergency department with a nontraumatic pain suggesting a ureteral colic (i.e., lumbar and/or pelvic pain that suddenly appeared, with or without pollakiuria and hematuria) was considered eligible, by EP. Patients were included if their attending physician was trained in clinical ultrasound.

Physician qualification was based on the completing a 5-day theoretical and practical training session at a certified center, followed by 18 months of e-learning. This course was in accordance with the recommendations of the American College of Emergency Physicians [11].

Pregnant women and patients with the previous imaging examinations were excluded. Patients who did not have an imaging session or without imaging report were also excluded.

Clinical–biological data

After the patient interview and clinical examination, the patients received an analgesia and underwent routine blood and urinary examinations.

Ultrasound data

The EP in charge of the patient performed the ultrasound examination using an Xporte© SonoSite device (SonoSite, Bothell, WA, USA). A convex abdominal probe (3.5–5 MHz) was used, according to a longitudinal grid technique (with the probe parallel to the plane of the bed). The EP followed the two axillary lines, to analyze the epigastric region, and the under-umbilical area. This permitted analyzing both the kidneys and ureters using low longitudinal and transverse intercostal slices, to measure and compare the pyelic and caliceal cavities.

The EP searched for dilatation of the pyelocalyceal cavities,which was graded according to severity, as follow: grade 1, pyelic dilatation alone; grade 2 with confluent calyceal dilatation of >1 cm; grade 3 same as grade 2, but with a confluent dilatation of 1.5 cm diameter; grade 4 same as grade 3, but with additional cortical thinning. Grade 3 or 4 dilatation was considered severe [12]. An equal focus was given to detect perirenal effusion, which indicates a rupture of the excretory tract.

The proximal ureter was evaluated to detect lithiasis in the pyelo-ureteral junction. The EP also ultrasonologically examine the area next to the iliac vessels and the supra pubic region, to detect lithiasis in the iliac or pelvic ureter, or in uretero-vesical meatus (Figs. 1 and 2).

The ultrasound examination also included the detection of peritoneal effusion and measurement of the abdominal aortic caliber to exclude an aneurysm.

Once PoCUS was completed, the EP wrote a report of the examination findings, including: the degree of

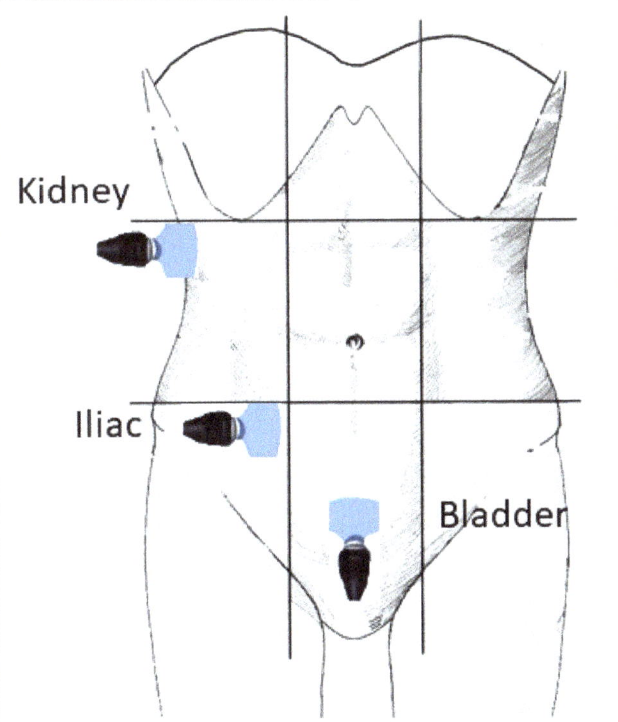

Fig. 1 Successive probe positions to explore urinary tract

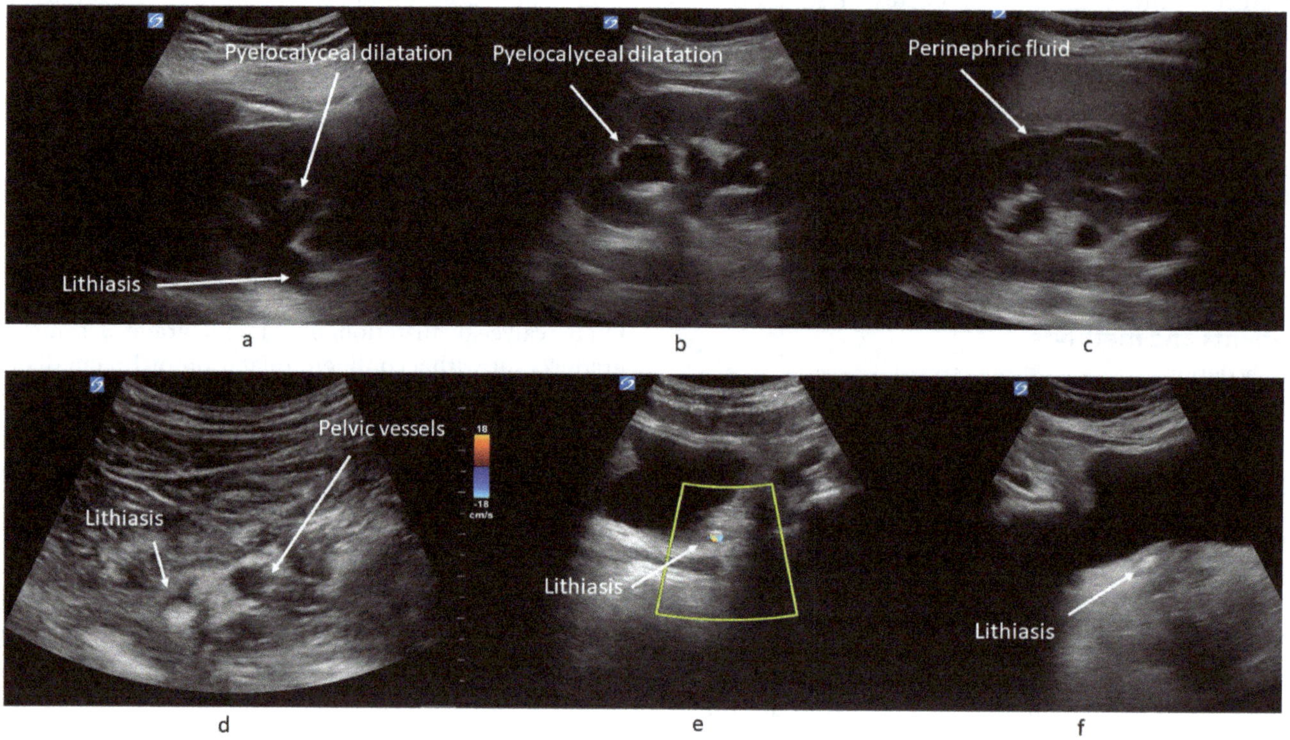

Fig. 2 Ultrasound images: **a** pyelocalyceal dilatation and proximal lithiasis, **b** pyelocalyceal dilatation, **c** perinephric fluid, **d** pelvic lithiasis, **e** bladder lithiasis and twinkle artifact in color doppler; and **f** bladder lithiasis

dilatation, presence, or absence of lithiasis including the size and location of stone, if present; and the presence or absence of perinephric fluid. Finally, the EP concluded whether the patient had "ureteral colic or not".

CT scan data

After PoCUS performed, all patients underwent an abdominopelvic CT without contrast examination with TOSHIBA© Aquilion Prime (Canon Medical System Coroporation, Otowara, Japan), the induced dose was 213 milligray. A radiologist who was blinded to the ultrasound examination result checked for the presence or absence of pyelocaliceal dilatation, perirenal effusion, or ureteral lithiasis, reporting the location and size of the stones, if present. Finally, the radiologist concluded whether or not "the patient had renal colic".

Ureteral colic diagnosis

The diagnosis of ureteral colic was retained when ureteral lithiasis with or without an upstream dilatation or bladder lithiasis was detected on CT. It was also retained if the expulsion of the stones had been clinically confirmed.

Judgment criteria

The primary end point of the study was the diagnostic agreement rate between PoCUS and CT.

The secondary objective was to evaluate the relationship between the result of the ultrasound examination and the treatment performed.

Statistical analysis

A physician not involved in the study, but collected the results of the examinations (PoCUS and CT scan) for analysis and comparison.

The data were analyzed using Excel © software. Quantitative variables are expressed as mean ± standard deviation. Qualitative variables are expressed as number and percentage. The performance of PoCUS in detecting of pyelocalyceal dilatation, perirenal fluid, and ureteral lithiasis was expressed as sensitivity, specificity, positive predictive value, negative predictive value, and accuracy. Accuracy was defined according to the proportion of confirmed cases, or the ratio of true positives and true negatives to the total population. Further 95% confidence intervals (95% CI) were calculated.

To assess the impact of imaging on treatment, a Fischer's exact test was performed for severe dilatation of the urinary tract, perinephric fluid, and size and location of stones, with a significance level set at 0.05.

Results

Patient characteristics

Of the 12 EPs on duty, seven met the training criteria for the inclusion of patients.

A total of 184 patients suspected to have renal colic from July 2017 to June 2018 were eligible, and 103 patients were finally analyzed (Fig. 3). The patients' demographic data are reported in Table 1.

Main results

Clinical and ultrasound examinations revealed that 18 patients were mistakenly suspected of having ureteral colic. Further, in 15 of these 18 patients, ultrasound examinations mainly found pyelocalyceal dilatation. The diagnoses after the CT were as follow: pyelonephritis ($n=4$), kidney neoplasia ($n=1$), adrenal hematoma ($n=1$), renal cyst ($n=1$), prostatism ($n=1$), uncomplicated diverticulitis ($n=2$), uncomplicated appendicitis ($n=1$), nonspecific inflammation of the digestive tract ($n=2$), uncomplicated ovarian cyst ($n=1$), nonspecific abdominal pain ($n=3$), and low back pain ($n=1$). PoCUS detected one case of ovarian cyst and one case of diverticulitis. Before CT, ultrasound examinations did not exclude any diagnosis of ureteral colic. The PoCUS finding compared to CT are reproted in Table 2.

Eight patients diagnosed with renal colic had no ureteral lithiasis on CT, but had pyelocalyceal cavity dilatation. Six of them had bladder lithiasis and two had spontaneous elimination of stones between the PoCUS and CT examinations.

The performance of PoCUS in detecting the abnormalities sought as compared to CT is reported in Table 3.

Among the 85 patients diagnosed with ureteral colic, 43 had lithiasis not detected on ultrasound (14 in the bladder–ureteral junction, six in the pelvic ureter, 21 in the lumbar ureter, and two in the proximal ureter) (Table 4).

Sixteen patients underwent surgical treatment in the emergency setting, three of whom had ureteral obstruction and urinary sepsis (Table 3).

Among the nine patients who presented with pelvic stones > 6 mm, two underwent urgent drainage. Among the seven remaining patients, four were secondarily treated with extracorporeal lithotripsy.

Among the 69 outpatients, 3 (4%) had a secondary readmission for a recurrent pain and four others underwent delayed lithotripsy.

Discussion

This study assesses the performance of PoCUS compared with CT in the simultaneous detection of urinary tract dilatation, lithiasis, and perirenal effusion. Our results suggest that ultrasound allows the reasonable use of CT a secondary intervention when the ultrasound findings are inconclusive.

In this work, the accuracy of PoCUS in detecting a pyelocalyceal dilatation was 91%. This is comparable to what is reported in the literature, regardless of whether the examination was performed by an EP or a radiologist [13–15]. Overestimations occur owing to the difficulty posed by structure, such as Malphigi pyramids, parapyelic cysts, or cortical cysts, which can be incorrectly interpreted as a dilatation of the urinary tract (not central confluents findings). Moreover, ultrasound examinations were performed ≤ 6 h after the beginning of symptoms

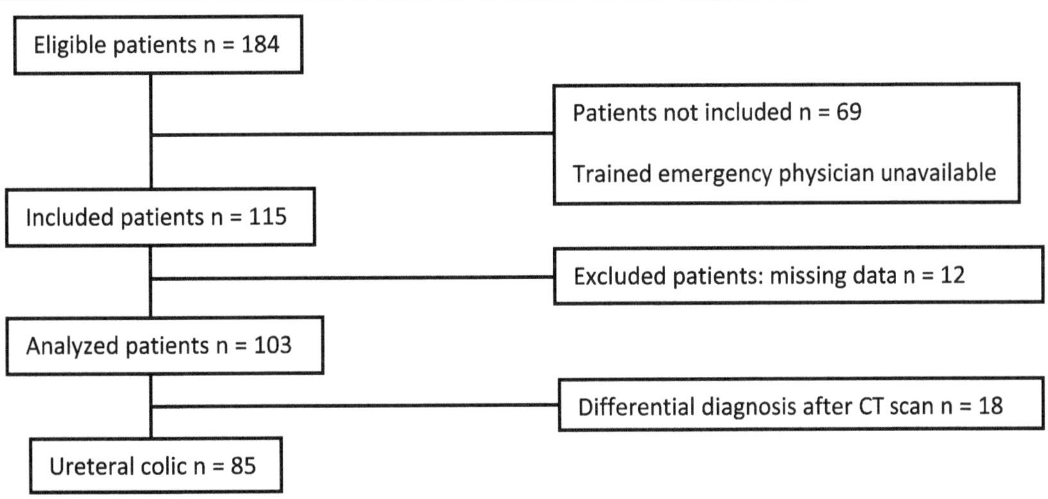

Fig. 3 Patient flowchart

Table 1 Characteristics of patients with confirmed ureteral colic

	Ureteral colic ($n=85$)	Differential diagnosis ($n=18$)
Age years (mean ± standard deviation)	52.1 ± 15.9	52 ± 12.3
Sex		
Female	28 (33%)	11 (61%)
Male	57 (67%)	7 (39%)
Antecedents		
Ureteral colic	38 (44%)	6 (33%)
Uropathy	6 (7%)	4 (22%)
Pain relief		
Level 1	44 (52%)	8 (44%)
Level 2	11 (13%)	5 (28%)
Level 3	28 (34%)	5 (28%)
NA	2 (2%)	0
Pain duration before admission		
<6 h	51 (60%)	4 (22%)
6–24 h	6 (7%)	5 (28%)
>24 h	20 (24%)	9 (50%)
NA	8 (9%)	0
Size of stone, mm		
<6	60 (70%)	0
>6	25 (30%)	0
Location of stone		
Pyelo-ureteral junction	7 (8%)	0
Lumbar ureter	21 (25%)	0
Lower third of the urinary tract	57 (67%)	0
Hospitalization	16 (18%)	2 (11%)

NA, not applicable

in 50% of the patients, explaining the false negative results due to delayed dilatation. Meanwhile, the dilatation found on ultrasound was sometimes due to other diseases such as appendicitis, colic inflammation, and kidney or pelvic mass. However, PoCUS did not exclude the diagnosis of renal colic. It would require widening the exploration of the digestive tract, with a high-frequency probe.

The accuracy of BUS in detecting a perinephric fluid was 83%, and we found no data in the literature about this topic.

The performance of PoCUS in detecting lithiasis, and therefore ureteral colic was as follow: accuracy, 54%; sensitivity, 43%; and specificity, 92%. These results are comparable to available data from examination performed by a radiologist [16–18]. Our study is the only study to involve an EP in this setting. Among the 43 lithiasis cases not detected by ultrasound, 14 were located in the pelvic ureter or at the junction between bladder, and ureter and their detection could have been improved. An explanation for the failed detection was that bladder was often empty at the time of PoCUS owing to prior completion of a urine dipstick test.

In our study, a urinary bypass was performed only for stones ≥6 mm in diameter located in the proximal or lumbar ureter. Patients with stones <6 mm were treated as outpatients.

Severe dilatation of the urinary tract (grade 3 or 4) was correlated with hospital stay in many studies [19], as in ours. However, in our study, there was a relationship between perinephric fluid and urgent surgical treatment. In the literature, this point is not clarified [10, 20].

In summary, our results suggests that findings on the ultrasound correlate well with the CT and ultimate surgical treatment such that the ED physician may be able to make an early decision regarding the referral pathway and possible discharge of patients with small distal stones [21, 22]. PoCUS could be sufficient to manage a subset of uncomplicated patients unlikely to require further surgical management. A "clinical-ultrasound" step can be

Table 2 PoCUS findings compared to CT

	CT		
	Pyelo-caliceal dilatation +	**Pyelo-caliceal dilatation –**	**Total**
PoCUS			
Pyelo-caliceal dilatation +	83	5	88
Pyelo-caliceal dilatation –	4	11	15
Total	87	16	103
	CT		
	Perinephric fluid +	**Perinpehric fluid –**	**Total**
PoCUS			
Perinephric fluid +	12	8	20
Perinephric fluid –	9	74	83
Total	21	82	103
	CT		
	Stone +	**Stone –**	**Total**
PoCUS			
Stone +	34	2	36
Stone –	45	22	67
Total	79	24	103

Table 3 Summary of diagnosis performance of PoCUS

	Pyelocalyceal dilatation	Lithiasis	Perinephric fluid
Se [95% CI]	95 [89–100]	43 [32–54]	57 [36–78]
Sp [95% CI]	68 [58–77]	92 [80–100]	90 [83–97]
PPV [95% CI]	94 [88–99]	94 [87–99]	60 [38–81]
NPV [95% CI]	73 [63–82]	33 [21–44]	89 [82–95]
A [95% CI]	91 [86–95]	54 [44–64]	83 [76–90]

Se, sensitivity; Sp, specificity; PPV, positive predictive value; NPV, negative predictive value; A, accuracy

recommended, as 40% of lithiasis cases were detected by PoCUS in our study. CT could be performed only as a secondary intervention in the other patients, to avoid radiation exposure and reduce the cost in this patient population [23, 24].

Moreover, PoCUS is immediately available after admission, thus allowing early evaluation, and is more comfortable and safer than CT. In addition, it does not require patients to be transferred from the emergency unit, which is beneficial for more severe cases.

Our study had some limitations. This was a single-center study involving a relatively small number of patients, in which 37% of eligible patients were not included because their EP did not meet the training criteria. Further, it would have been interesting to evaluate the

Table 4 Patients' management and imaging findings on CT

Pathological imaging findings	Surgical management < 24 h ($n=16$)	Ambulatory management ($n=69$)	Total ($n=85$)	p
Perinephric fluid	9	12	21 (24%)	< 0.05
Severe pyelocalyceal dilatation	6	9	15 (17%)	< 0.05
Location and size of stones				
Proximal > 6 mm	12[a]	4	16 (19%)	< 0.05
Proximal < 6 mm	2	10	12 (15%)	1
Distal > 6 mm	2	7	9 (10%)	0.67
Distal < 6 mm	0	48	48 (56%)	< 0.05

[a] Three patients who initially received ambulatory treatment were readmitted within 48 h and underwent surgical treatment

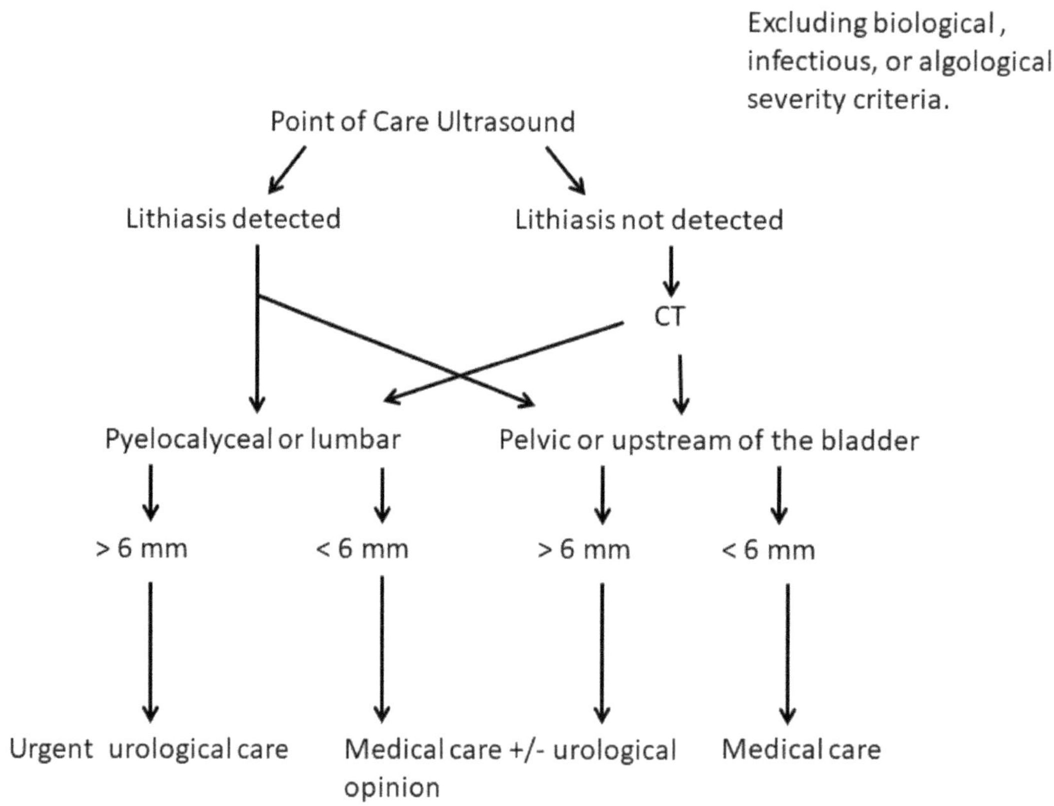

Fig. 4 Use of imaging (PoCUS and CT) for the management of patients presenting with ureteral colic

patients' length of stay in the emergency unit, as some studies demonstrated a clear decrease in this setting [25].

Our results suggest that patient management could follow the algorithm shown in Fig. 4 involving the complementary use of BUS and CT for detecting lithiasis.

Conclusion

PoCUS is a good tool for the diagnostic and therapeutic evaluation of patients for renal colic. Its availability at the bedside, in addition to allowing the reasonable use of CT could optimize patient care, particularly in the most acute cases.

Abbreviations

EP: Emergency physician; BUS: Bedside ultrasound; CT: Computerized tomography; PPV: Positive predictive value; NPV: Negative predictive value; Se: Sensitivity; Sp: Specificity.

Authors' contributions

JEB planned the study; JEB, EG, JPR and LF performed patients inclusion; MA and QB reviewed the data; AJ and DG reviewed the manuscript. All authors read and approved the final manuscript.

Author details

[1]Emergency, Anesthesiology and Critical Care Department, Lourdes Hospital, Lourdes, France. [2]Pôle Anesthésie-Réanimation-Urgences, Hôpital de Lourdes, 2 Avenue Alexandre Marqui, 65100 Lourdes, France.

References

1. Johnson CM et al (1979) Renal stone epidemiology: a 25-year study in Rochester. Minnesota Kidney Int 16(5):624–631
2. Cupisti A et al (2008) Renal colic in Pisa emergency department: epidemiology, diagnostics and treatment patterns. Intern Emerg Med 3(3):241–244
3. Schoenfeld EM et al (2019) Association of patient and visit characteristics with rate and timing of urologic procedures for patients discharged from the emergency department with renal colic. JAMA Netw Open 2(12):e1916454
4. Rodger F, Roditi G, Aboumarzouk OM (2018) Diagnostic accuracy of low and ultra-low dose CT for identification of urinary tract stones: a systematic review. Urol Int 100(4):375–385
5. Xiang H et al (2017) Systematic review and meta-analysis of the diagnostic accuracy of low-dose computed tomography of the kidneys, ureters and bladder for urolithiasis. J Med Imaging Radiat Oncol 61(5):582–590
6. Dalziel PJ, Noble VE (2013) Bedside ultrasound and the assessment of renal colic: a review. Emerg Med J EMJ 30(1):3–8
7. Smith-Bindman R et al (2014) Ultrasonography versus computed tomography for suspected nephrolithiasis. N Engl J Med 371(12):1100–1110
8. Pradère B et al (2018) Evaluation of guidelines for surgical management of urolithiasis. J Urol 199(5):1267–1271
9. Hiller N et al (2012) The relationship between ureteral stone characteristics and secondary signs in renal colic. Clin Imaging 36(6):768–772

10. Nadav G et al (2018) Evaluation of the clinical significance of sonographic perinephric fluid in patients with renal colic. Am J Emerg Med 37(10):1823–1828
11. Ultrasound guidelines: emergency, point-of-care and clinical ultrasound guidelines in medicine. Ann Emerg Med 69(5):e27–54; 2017
12. Green WM, King DL (1976) Diagnostic ultrasound of the urinary tract. J Clin Ultrasound JCU 4(1):55–64
13. Herbst MK et al (2014) Effect of provider experience on clinician-performed ultrasonography for hydronephrosis in patients with suspected renal colic. Ann Emerg Med 64(3):269–276
14. Rosen CL et al (1998) Ultrasonography by emergency physicians in patients with suspected ureteral colic. J Emerg Med 16(6):865–870
15. Watkins S et al (2007) Validation of emergency physician ultrasound in diagnosing hydronephrosis in ureteric colic. Emerg Med Australas EMA 19(3):188–195
16. Fowler KAB et al (2002) US for detecting renal calculi with nonenhanced CT as a reference standard. Radiology 222(1):109–113
17. Kanno T et al (2014) Determining the efficacy of ultrasonography for the detection of ureteral stone. Urology 84(3):533–537
18. Vijayakumar M et al (2018) Review of techniques for ultrasonic determination of kidney stone size. Res Rep Urol 10:57–61
19. Gaspari RJ, Horst K (2005) Emergency ultrasound and urinalysis in the evaluation of flank pain. Acad Emerg Med Off J Soc Acad Emerg Med 12(12):1180–1184
20. Farrell MR et al (2018) Perinephric fat stranding is associated with elevated creatinine among patients with acutely obstructing ureterolithiasis. J Endourol 32(9):891–895
21. Sasmaz Mİ, Kirpat V (2019) The relationship between the severity of pain and stone size, hydronephrosis and laboratory parameters in renal colic attack. Am J Emerg Med 37(11):2107–2110
22. Moesbergen TC et al (2011) Distal ureteral calculi: US follow-up. Radiology 260(2):575–580
23. Brenner DJ, Hall EJ (2007) Computed tomography—an increasing source of radiation exposure. N Engl J Med 357(22):2277–2284
24. Brisbane W, Bailey MR, Sorensen MD (2016) An overview of kidney stone imaging techniques. Nat Rev Urol 13(11):654–662
25. Park YH et al (2016) Does the use of bedside ultrasonography reduce emergency department length of stay for patients with renal colic?: a pilot study. Clin Exp Emerg Med 3(4):197–203

Mechanical ventilation weaning issues can be counted on the fingers of just one hand: part 1

Luigi Vetrugno[1*†], Giovanni Maria Guadagnin[1*†], Alessandro Brussa[1], Daniele Orso[1], Eugenio Garofalo[2], Andrea Bruni[2], Federico Longhini[2] and Tiziana Bove[1]

Abstract

Although mechanical ventilation may be a patient's vital ally during acute illness, it can quickly transform into an enemy during chronic conditions. The weaning process is the fundamental phase that enables the resumption of physiological respiratory function; however, it is also associated with a number of life-threatening complications, and a large percentage of critically ill patients never achieve airway device removal or require the resumption of mechanical ventilation just a few days post-weaning. Indeed, the weaning process is, at present, more of an art than a science. As such, there is urgent need for novel contributions from the scientific literature to abate the growing rates of morbidity and mortality associated with weaning failure. The physician attempting to wean a patient must integrate clinical parameters and common-sense criteria. Numerous studies have striven to identify single predictive factors of weaning failure and sought to standardize the weaning process, but the results are characterized by remarkable heterogeneity. Despite the lack of benchmarks, it is clear that the analysis of respiratory function must include a detailed overview of the five situations described below rather than a single aspect. The purpose of this two-part review is to provide a comprehensive description of these situations to clarify the "arena" physicians are entering when weaning critically ill patients from mechanical ventilation.

Keywords: Weaning, Mechanical ventilation, Ultrasound, Echocardiography, Diaphragm, Diaphragm dysfunction

Introduction

Up to 25% of critically ill patients experience difficulties in weaning from invasive mechanical ventilation (IMV), burdening the intensive care unit (ICU) with long lengths-of-stay, prolonged mechanical ventilation (IMV), and increased morbidity and mortality [1]. Weaning failure is commonly described as a failed spontaneous breathing trial (SBT) or the reinstitution of mechanical ventilation within 2 to 7 days after extubation [2]. Failed extubation complicates up to 30% of successful spontaneous breathing trials [3] and correlates with higher morbidity and mortality rates [4, 5].

Determining the optimal time to extubate a patient continues to be a challenge. Prolonged mechanical ventilation is associated with a series of adverse effects (e.g., tracheal lesions, ventilator-associated pneumonia, ventilator-induced lung injury, and ventilator-induced diaphragm injury) [6, 7], whereas premature extubation exposes the patient to cardiovascular stress due to spontaneous breathing, often requiring the reinstitution of ventilatory support [8]. Although international guidelines recommend the implementation of spontaneous breathing trials [9], used alone this practice is ineffective in predicting weaning failure and reintubation [10–13]. A number of studies have investigated and proposed

*Correspondence: luigi.vetrugno@uniud.it; giovannimaria.guadagnin@gmail.com

†Luigi Vetrugno and Giovanni Maria Guadagnin contributed equally to this work.

[1] Anesthesiology and Intensive Care Clinic, Department of Medicine, University of Udine, Via Colugna 50, 33100 Udine, Italy

Full list of author information is available at the end of the article

different parameters as outcome predictors of weaning from mechanical ventilation; however, a clear understanding of the ideal time to proceed with extubation for a successful outcome continues to elude us [14, 15]. Cardiac failure, diaphragmatic dysfunction and acute respiratory illness (lung parenchyma disease, or upper or lower airway obstructions), neurological status, and intra-abdominal issues are among the known leading causes of failed weaning [3, 16].

Significant advancements have been achieved in ultrasound technology over the last 20 years, most notably in bringing these techniques to the bedside, with all the advantages that this conveys. In fact, our capacity to study the individual organs ultrasonographically has become so finely tuned and specialized that physicians risk overlooking a more integrated examination of the patient. A comprehensive approach to invasive mechanical ventilation should include an extensive ultrasonographic assessment of cardiac function, diaphragmatic activity, and lung parenchyma. In particular, much light has been shone on the use of ultrasonographic assessment of diaphragmatic dysfunction as a predictor of weaning failure. That said, it is fundamental that the diaphragm does not receive excessive attention at the expense of other predictive factors. A simultaneous and comprehensive ultrasound examination of the cardio-pulmonary-diaphragmatic district may confer valuable predictive information regarding successful weaning from mechanical ventilation, although literature in this regard is still limited [17]. It is also important to bear in mind that other factors able to negatively influence the weaning outcome exist outside the cardio-pulmonary-diaphragmatic area (i.e., the neurological status and intra-abdominal hypertension) that cannot be evaluated with ultrasound [18, 19].

Mechanical ventilation can negatively affect the actors involved in respiratory function; for example, ventilator-induced lung injury, impaired cardiac performance, and ventilator-induced diaphragmatic dysfunction are all possible consequences. Although the concept of 'lung protection' during mechanical ventilation is well established, a more precise definition of a 'protective modality' to help preserve all the elements involved in the respiratory function is also desirable.

The purpose of this two-part review is to illustrate the main causes of unsuccessful weaning and recent advancements on the application of bedside ultrasound evaluation in these topics.

The weaning path

Weaning from mechanical ventilation starts with the institution of mechanical ventilation; from the outset, the physician assesses the patient on a daily basis to determine when they might be ready to wean. Invasive mechanical ventilation is a risky journey for a critically ill patient admitted to the intensive care unit because of acute illness, IMV itself, or a failed weaning attempt. Weaning is the process in which the breathing effort is progressively returned from the machine to the patient. This process consists of 3 key steps, Fig. 1: first, when the patient's clinical conditions permit it, ventilation supports are progressively decreased (*Ready, weaning!*); second, a spontaneous breathing trial (SBT) assesses the patient's capability to breathe autonomously (*Ready, breathing!*); and third, the patient is liberated from mechanical ventilation (*Ready, extubation!*) [20, 21]. Three main SBT strategies are described in the literature: the T-piece trial; the continuous positive airway pressure (CPAP) trial—in which the CPAP applied is equal to the previously applied positive end-expiratory pressure (PEEP); and positive support ventilation, which uses a low level of pressure support (5–8 cmH_2O).

No standardized SBT method has been identified to date in terms of type or duration (30–120 min) that can ensure a higher rate of successful weaning. However, strong evidence does exist supporting the employment of a short-term (30 min) breathing trail and low-level pressure support (8 cmH_2O) [22]. If the SBT is accompanied by patient discomfort (i.e., anxiety or fatigue) and/or cardio-respiratory distress (i.e., $RR \geq 35$ bpm, $SpO_2 < 90\%$, HR variability $> 20\%$, hemodynamic instability) [23], then it is considered to have failed. In the absence of such responses, the SBT is deemed successful and the patient can be considered for airway removal (*Ready, extubing!*). Although heterogeneity exists in the definition of successful weaning, it is generally taken as the patient's capacity to maintain spontaneous breathing for at least 48 h following extubation [3]. As mentioned above, despite international guidelines recommending the implementation of spontaneous breathing trials [3, 9], used alone SBTs are ineffective in predicting weaning failure and reintubation [10–13]. One possible solution to this may be the implementation of integrated cardio-pulmonary-diaphragmatic assessments for the detection of predictive indicators of weaning failure.

The (he)art of weaning from mechanical ventilation

In the case of shock patients admitted to intensive care, most are resuscitated with the use of mechanical ventilation and intravenous fluid for respiratory and circulatory support. Regarding fluid management procedures in shock patients, recent literature has schematized its practice into four different phases, adopting the acronym ROSE: resuscitation (R), optimization (O), stabilization (S), and evacuation (E) [24]. Resuscitation, in some cases, could be too aggressive with the risk of fluid-overload,

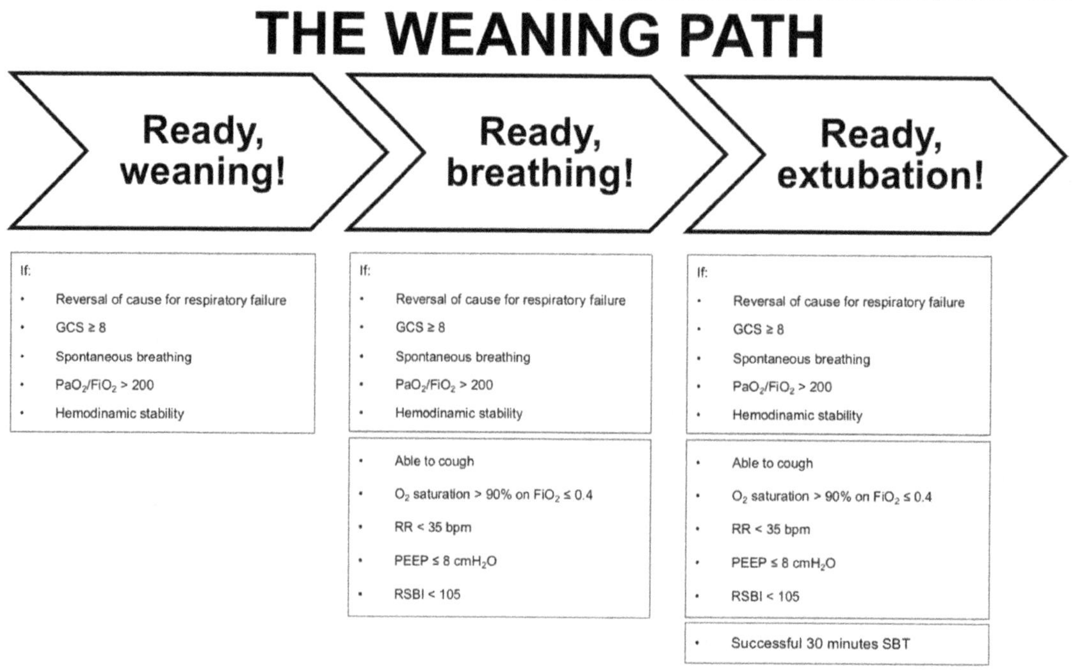

Fig. 1 The weaning path. *GCS* Glasgow Coma Scale, *RR* respiratory rate, *PEEP* positive end-expiratory pressure, *RSBI* rapid shallow breathing index, *SBT* spontaneous breathing trial

whereas evacuation could be too fast with the risk of hypovolemia and low cardiac output state (see below). In the first case, previous over-hydration with a positive fluid balance has been associated with death and an increased risk of failed weaning from mechanical ventilation in surviving patients [25, 26]. This could be explained by the fact that shifting the patient from mechanical ventilation (positive airway pressure) to a T-piece trial (negative airway pressure) can increase cardiac preload and unmask an underlying cardiac problem. Lemaire and colleagues were the first to demonstrate this vicious circle [8]. Potential cardiac complications can be monitored in 3 main ways: one is direct but invasive—measurement of the cardiac filing pressure by pulmonary arterial catheter (PAC); the remaining two are indirect and un-invasive—one entails the use of heart or lung ultrasound, and the other the rapid measurement of natriuretic peptide for the diagnosis of acute heart failure [27, 28].

Monitoring for cardiac complications is necessary because the sensitivity and specificity of clinical signs of acute heart failure in intensive care patients are poor [29]. PAC is reserved for specific severe cases. It is used for the diagnosis and treatment of pulmonary arterial hypertension and to guide fluid and catecholamine management; however, its routine use has been abandoned globally due to the lack of any outcome benefits [30, 31]. Ultrasound, on the other hand, has become an invaluable tool in the ICU thanks to its widespread availability at the patient's bedside and the absence of any known side effects [28]. Moreover, the role of echocardiography in the detection of cardiac origins of weaning failure has grown significantly over the last 15 years. In particular, we now know that impaired systolic function (i.e., a small left ventricular ejection fraction [LVEF]) is less frequently associated with weaning failure in patients who failed the SBT (33% of cases) than left ventricular diastolic dysfunction (67% of cases) [28, 32, 33]. To investigate this latter condition, trans-mitral flow is interrogated using a pulse wave Doppler placed over the mitral valve in an apical four-chamber view. An early wave (E wave) is displayed on the monitor, Fig. 2a, that represents the first phase of the diastole as a passive phenomenon, limited only by the stiffness of the left ventricle or by interventricular interdependence—right ventricular push over the left ventricle via the septum. A stiff ventricle generates an elevated filling pressure, leading to pulmonary edema. In addition to trans-mitral Doppler, an E wave inpatient with sinus rhythm is followed by atrial contraction (A wave, Fig. 2a). The left ventricular preload is the sum of the E and A waves at a price of low or average left ventricular end-diastolic pressure (LVEDP) less than 12–14 mmHg. However, to estimate the LVEDP non-invasively, the E/A ratio has shown to be preload dependent and insufficient [34]. On the other hand, tissue Doppler directly measures myocardial velocities by means of the E′ wave in a load-independent way, Fig. 2b. The combination of the trans-mitral Doppler E wave, the tissue Doppler E′ wave, and the *E*/*E*′ ratio at the end of an SBT also seems to be

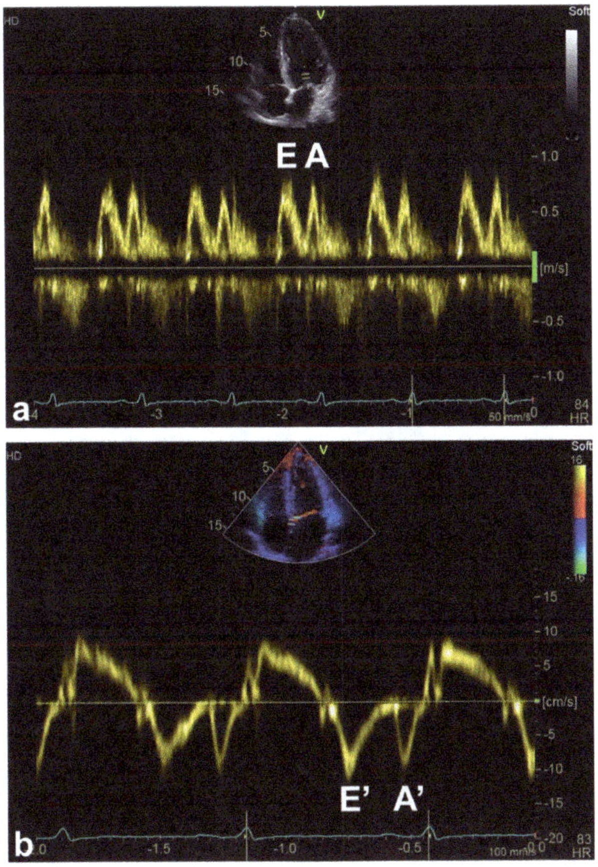

Fig. 2 Pulse wave Doppler and tissue Doppler. **a** Trans-mitralic Doppler; an early wave (E wave) is displayed on the monitor that represents the first phase of the diastole as a passive phenomenon, limited only by the stiffness of the left ventricle or by interventricular interdependence—right ventricular push over the left ventricle via the septum. The E wave in patient with sinus rhythm is followed by atrial contraction (A wave). **b** Septal tissue Doppler; tissue Doppler directly measures myocardial velocities by means of the E′ wave in a load-independent way. The combination of the trans-mitral Doppler E wave, the tissue Doppler E′ wave, and the *E/E′* ratio at the end of an SBT also seems to be capable of predicting weaning failure from diastolic dysfunction

capable of predicting weaning failure from diastolic dysfunction in patients with arrhythmia, immediately after and 10 min after extubation, with an area under the curve (AUC) of 0.75 and 0.86, respectively [33]. However, two main limitations of these methods need to be recognized. First, although an E/E' value < 8 can accurately identify patients with a normal LVEDP, and an E/E' value > 15 can identify those with an elevated LVEDP, a gray zone exists between the values of 8 and 15 [33–35]; second, not all intensive care clinicians possess advanced echocardiography skills; and third, LVEDP may also be elevated in cases of increased intra-abdominal pressure (see below).

In a very recent study, lung ultrasound evaluating the delta-B-lines before and after SBT in the four anterior chest wall regions was shown to provide excellent correlation with successful weaning [36]. However, the shift from mechanical to spontaneous ventilation may alone justify the appearance of such artifacts. Furthermore, distinguishing between cardiogenic and inflammatory causes of delta-B-lines may be a challenge.

Lastly, natriuretic peptides, and in particular brain natriuretic peptide (BNP), have been studied for their potential to predict weaning failure. In their study, Mekontso-Dessap et al. reported the outcome of two weaning strategies, one of which was driven by BNP level, whereas the other followed no explicit protocol [37]. They found that the BNP-guided fluid strategy was associated with increased use of diuretics, more negative fluid balance leading to a shorter mechanical ventilation time, and more ventilator-free days, but no change in ICU length-of-stay, morbidity, or mortality. The authors suggest that the changes in BNP that occur in the ICU are relatively slow and may be influenced by renal insufficiency or by the use of extracorporeal renal replacement therapy.

As previously mentioned, one-third of weaning failures with a cardiac origin depend on systolic dysfunction. In the case of cardiogenic shock, the diaphragmatic blood flow decreases and diaphragm muscular function can become compromised. In normal conditions, the diaphragmatic blood flow significantly increases with a high level of muscle contraction [38]. Indeed, the diaphragmatic blood flow is strictly dependent on cardiac output in both individuals at rest and with increased muscular activity [39]. Thus, since the diaphragm requires a high blood flow—in fact it is the skeletal muscle receiving the largest volume of blood per gram of tissue—diaphragm function may be impaired by a reduction in blood flow [40].

In patients with cardiogenic shock, respiratory muscles, which are the only muscles working during low cardiac output, shift to anaerobic metabolism resulting in lactate production even though they may be receiving a large fraction of the cardiac output [41]. As a consequence, skeletal muscles and vital organs receive less blood flow, contributing to an increased production and impaired removal of lactate [41]. The onset of acidemia and hypoxemia then leads to an increase in the work of breathing due to induced compensatory hyperventilation. Of note, whenever the muscle oxygen and nutrient demands exceed the supply, the diaphragm's ability to generate and sustain force decreases and muscle failure ensues [42]. During cardiogenic shock, the imbalance between demand and supply is facilitated by the reduced cardiac output and diaphragmatic blood flow (see Fig. 3).

In 1982, Aubier and colleagues investigated the influence of respiratory muscle activity on lactic acidosis and survival time in a cardiogenic shock canine model [41].

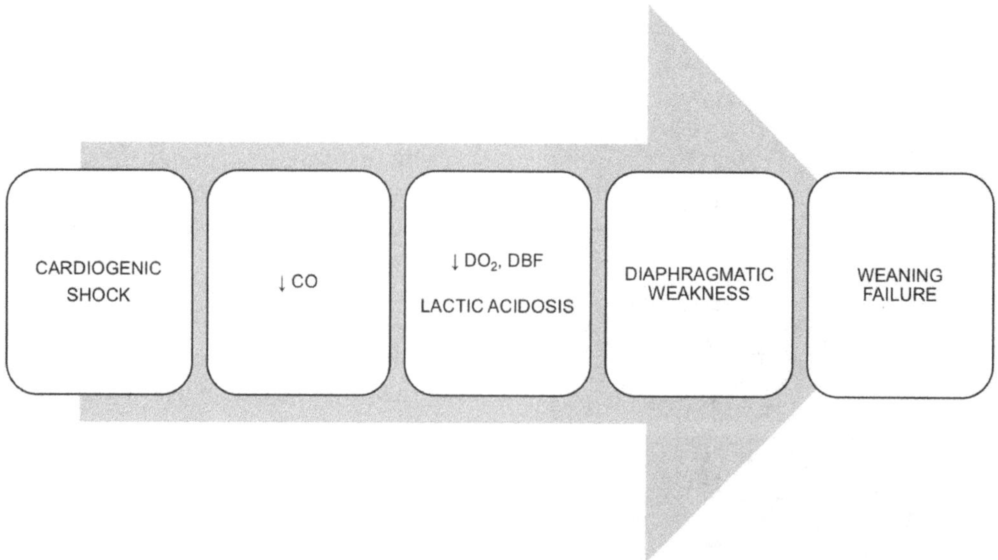

Fig. 3 Cardiogenic shock impairing diaphragm activity. *CO* cardiac output, *DO_2* oxygen delivery, *DBF* diaphragm blood flow

As opposed to mechanically ventilated dogs, the spontaneously breathing ones showed higher lactate levels and lower glycogen concentration due to the increased minute ventilation and respiratory workload occurring in the first hour after the onset of cardiogenic shock; afterward, minute ventilation rapidly decreased, due to diaphragmatic fatigue, till the death of the animal [41]. Furthermore, the use of neuromuscular blocking agents in mechanically ventilated dogs may have reduced lactate production due to the absence of diaphragmatic activity [41]. Impairment of the diaphragmatic contraction process during cardiogenic shock may be the

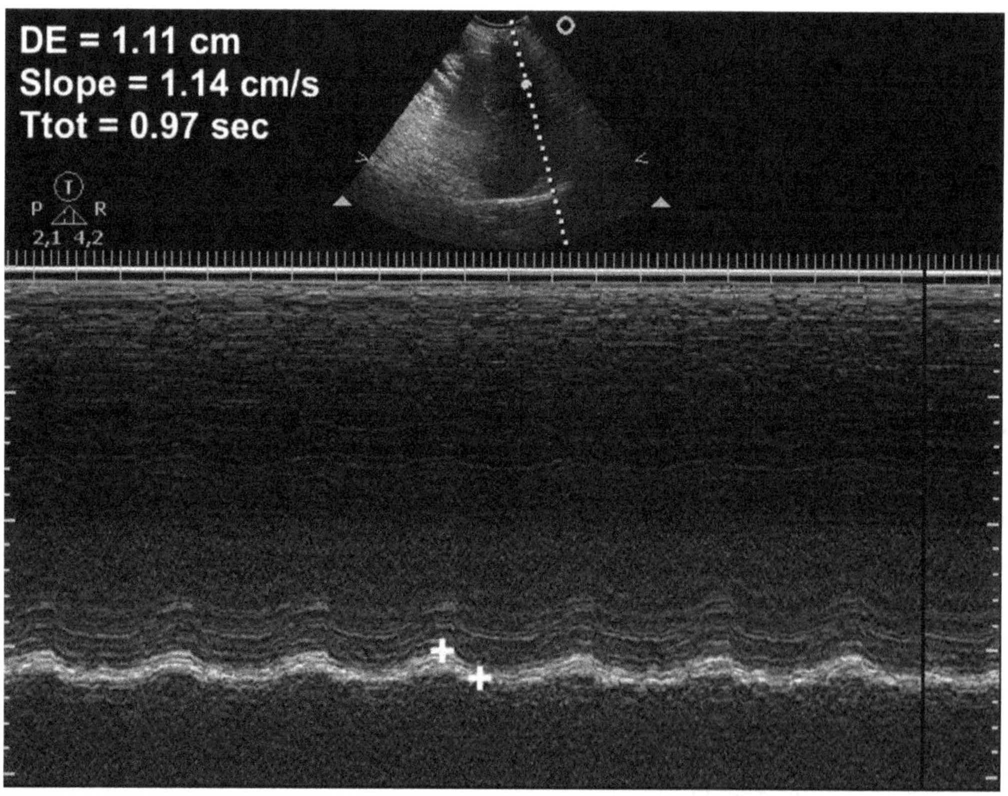

Fig. 4 Diaphragm excursion. *DE* diaphragmatic excursion, *Slope* diaphragmatic contraction speed, *Ttot* inspiration + expiration time

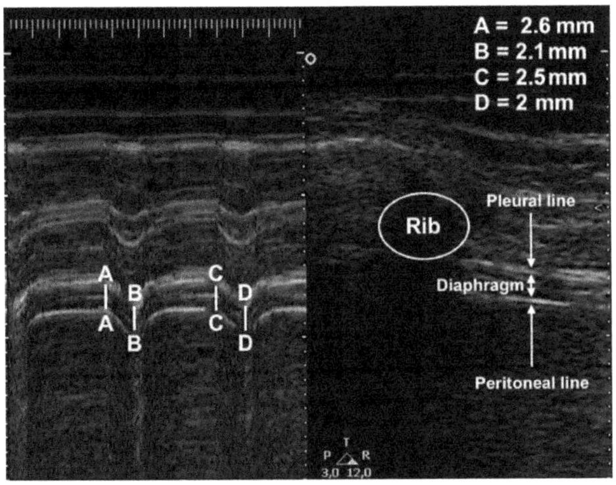

Fig. 5 Diaphragm thickening fraction assessment. **a**, **c** End of inspiration thickness; **b**, **d** End of expiration thickness

underlying mechanism responsible for ventilatory failure (see below) [43]. No studies have so far evaluated the ultrasonographic modifications of the diaphragm during the course of or after cardiogenic shock, or their impact on short- and long-term outcomes.

Table 1 Most common bias to consider before an ultrasound assessment of diaphragmatic function

	Affected parameters	
	DE	DTF
Poor echographic transthoracic window		
Obesity	Ø	Ø
Splenectomy (left hemidiaphragm)	Ø	Ø
Altered starting position of hemidiaphragm		
Downward: COPD, asthma, PLEFF	Ø	
Upward: abdominal hypertension, ascites, supine position	Ø	
Iatrogenic impaired function		
Drugs (sedative, myorelaxants, etc.)	Ø	Ø
Mechanical ventilation		
Inspiratory positive pressure	Ø	
PEEP	Ø	
Operator-dependent factors		
a angle other than 90°	Ø	
ZOA identification[a]		Ø

DE diaphragmatic excursion, *DTF* diaphragm thickening fraction, *COPD* chronic obstructive pulmonary disease, *PLEFF* pleural effusion, *PEEP* positive end-expiratory pressure, *a angle* angle between M-Mode and hemidiaphragm examined, *ZOA* zone of apposition

[a] The further away from the ribs, the smaller the DTF will be

Diaphragm ultrasound (DUS)

The diaphragm, being the primary respiratory muscle, performs the majority of the work entailed in breathing. Diaphragm dysfunction, defined as the inability of the diaphragm to generate reasonable levels of maximal force, is an under-recognized pathological condition in critically ill patients and can render weaning from mechanical ventilation extremely difficult, resulting in protracted mechanical ventilation and prolonged intensive care unit length-of-stay [44]. The prevalence of diaphragm dysfunction in critically ill patients admitted to the intensive care unit and requiring IMV is over 60%, reaching 80% in patients requiring prolonged IMV and experiencing difficult weaning [45].

Considerable research attention has been focused on diagnosing diaphragm dysfunction over recent years, and there is strong evidence to sustain an association/correlation between diaphragm dysfunction and weaning failure [45–47]. The gold standard for evaluating diaphragm force is the measurement of trans-diaphragmatic pressure (Pdi) [48]. This test entails the insertion of a dedicated catheter with two balloons that measure the esophageal and gastric pressures, respectively. Diaphragm dysfunction occurs when Pdi < 11 cmH_2O [48].

Another adjunctive test to assess diaphragm activity is the electrical activity of the diaphragm (EAdi) test. EAdi is performed using a dedicated esophageal catheter that has four couples of electrodes at its distal end. Besides monitoring the diaphragm, EAdi is also used to drive the ventilator with a proportional mode of ventilation, the so-called neutrally adjusted ventilator assist (NAVA). Thus, EAdi can be used to monitor the diaphragm at the bedside, whereas NAVA can exert a rehabilitative role in the case of diaphragm dysfunction.

Bedside ultrasound assessment of the diaphragm in critically ill patients can also be used to detect diaphragm dysfunction (diaphragm activity is classified as: usual, reduced, or loss of function) [49]. Although it may help the clinician make therapeutic decisions, a possible role in ventilation and weaning from mechanical ventilation has yet to be fully determined [49–52].

Two diaphragm sonographic predictors of successful weaning have been proposed [45, 49–56]:

- Diaphragmatic excursion (DE, cm)—defined as the maximum displacement of the hemidiaphragm during breathing (Fig. 4);
- Diaphragmatic thickening fraction (DTF, %)—defined as the difference between the end-inspiration thickness (Te-Insp) and end-expiration thickness (Te-exp) divided by the end-expiration thickness (Fig. 5).

Table 2 Recent literature on predictive value of DUS

Variables	Study	Major findings
Diaphragm excursion (DE)	Jiang et al. [61]	Mean values of liver and spleen displacement during SBTs were higher in the successfully weaned group. Sensitivity and specificity for predicting successful extubation were 84.4% and 82.6%, respectively
	Spadaro et al. [62]	By replacing tidal volume (VTe) with DE in the formula for the Rapid Shallow Breathing Index (RSBI = RR/VTe), the authors created a new index called the diaphragmatic-RSBI (D-RSBI) The use of diaphragmatic excursion makes this index more accurate than the traditional rapid shallow breathing index in predicting outcome from weaning
	Kim et al. [43]	The authors describe an association between diaphragmatic dysfunction (DE < 10 mm obtained by M-Mode ultrasonography), a prolonged weaning period, and early or delayed weaning failures
	Luo et al. [63]	The authors find that a DE cut-off value < 12.6 mm was the most reliable predictor of reintubation within 1 week (sensitivity 80%, negative specificity 68.4%)
	Garrido-Aguirre et al. [64]	The authors propose a new weaning index (ULDIMex) that takes into consideration inspiration time (*a*), expiration time (*b*), and DE (*c*). With the conceived formula $(a + b)c/2$, the authors identified a cut-off slope value of 4.06 cm/s for ULDIMex in successfully weaned patients, with a negative predictive value of 96.5%
	Palkar et al. [65]	Greater diaphragm excursion, a longer inspiratory time, and a smaller decrease in the diaphragmatic excursion-time (E-T) index during SBT may help to predict successful extubation
	Carrie et al. [66]	According to the authors, DE was unable by itself to predict weaning failure with low sensitivity and specificity 59% and 71%, respectively
Diaphragm thickening fraction (DTF)	Jung et al. [67]	The authors reveal a significantly lower mean DTF in patients requiring reintubation versus patients who did not (12% vs. 20%, $p = 0.008$)
	Samanta et al. [68]	DTF assessment of the right diaphragm during pressure support ventilation (PSV) may be employed to predict successful weaning prior to a T-piece SBT
	Blumhof et al. [69]	A DTF > 20% is a robust predictor of extubation success during pressure support ventilation tests with 5/5 and 10/5 cmH_2O with sensitivity and specificity values of 84.6% and 79.0%, 88.9% and 75.0%, respectively
	DiNino et al. [70]	The authors find that a DTF threshold ≥ 30% at end inspiration has a positive predictive value of 91% and a negative predictive value of 63% for extubation success (sensitivity 88% and specificity 91%, respectively), with similar results during both SBT and pressure support tests
Diaphragm excursion (DE) and diaphragm thickening fraction (DTF)	Farghaly et al. [71]	The authors found that cut-off values of DE ≥ 10.5 mm, Te-insp ≥ 21 mm, and DTF > 34.2% during SBT with pressure support were associated with successful weaning; combining a DE ≥ 10.5 mm with a Te-insp. ≥ 21 mm decreased the sensitivity to 64.9%, but increased specificity up to 100% for successful weaning
	Zambon et al. [72]	The authors describe both DE and DTF to be useful weaning predictors, but only DTF is shown to be an accurate index of diaphragmatic contractility workload
	Llamas-Alvarez et al. [73]	This systematic review and metanalysis concludes that diaphragm ultrasound measures (DTF > DE) can help predict weaning outcome. It also suggests that the accuracy of DTF and DE may be overestimated in the current literature depending on the patient subpopulation studied
	Vivier et al. [53]	The authors conducted a multicenter prospective study involving 191 patients where DTF and DE data were collected during T-piece SBTs. They found that diaphragmatic dysfunction as assessed by ultrasound (described as DE < 10 mm and DTF < 30%) was not associated with extubation failure

DUS diaphragm ultrasound, *DE* diaphragm excursion, *DTF* diaphragm thickening fraction, *SBT* spontaneous breathing trial, *Te-insp.* end-inspiratory thickness

Some studies have hypothesized that diaphragmatic excursion or liver/spleen movements could predict extubation failure. DE reflects the sum of the patient's inspiratory activity and mechanical ventilatory support, so it only has real value when assessed during a spontaneous breathing trial. Diaphragm displacement is associated with lung volume during the inspiratory phase [57], but it does not correlate with and does not quantify the patient's inspiratory effort [58]; furthermore, its assessment is influenced by numerous factors (see Table 1) [45]. It should also be noted that diaphragmatic excursion can be influenced by PEEP and levels of ventilator support during mechanical ventilation [55]: by increasing lung expiratory volumes, higher levels of PEEP lower the diaphragmatic domes, resulting in a decreased diaphragmatic excursion; during assisted ventilation, diaphragmatic excursion results from ventilator support plus the patient's inspiratory efforts [56]. Therefore, only diaphragm thickening can provide a reliable indicator of diaphragm function during assisted mechanical ventilation [57].

DTF, also known as the "ejection fraction" of the diaphragm, reflects active diaphragm contraction and inspiratory effort [59, 60]. It is associated with ICU length-of-stay, the duration of mechanical ventilation, and mortality [59, 60]. Whereas diaphragmatic excursion is not able to evaluate the degree of contractile activity of the diaphragm, DTF, on the other hand, has this capacity and can be used both in IMV (assisted or supported) and during an SBT [45].

A number of studies have investigated these two parameters, either individually or in combination, with the aim of identifying cut-off values as predictors of successful weaning (see Table 2) [43, 53, 61–73]. However, the results have been heterogeneous in terms of outcome results and cut-off values due to differences in study protocol design and outcome designation.

Although bilateral anterior magnetic stimulation of the phrenic nerves is considered the gold standard for the assessment of diaphragm function [48], it requires high expertise and expensive machines. By contrast, ultrasonography is a widely available non-invasive tool that provides both structural and functional information about the muscle. Regarding diaphragm evaluation by ultrasonography and the therapeutic and prognostic implications of this measure, more studies are needed to evaluate the accuracy of ultrasound measures of the diaphragm and their therapeutic and prognostic implications and applicability in mechanical ventilation (i.e., diaphragm-protective ventilation and weaning from IMV). Further research is also required to standardize the measurement techniques and teaching programs [74].

Conclusions

In the first section of this review, two of the five factors involved in successful weaning from mechanical ventilation were addressed. The remaining components will be discussed in the second section of this review entitled: "Mechanical ventilation weaning issues can be counted on the fingers of just one hand: part 2".

Abbreviations

IMV: Invasive mechanical ventilation; ICU: Intensive care unit; SBT: Spontaneous breathing trial; PEEP: Positive end-expiratory pressure; GCS: Glasgow Coma Scale; RSBI: Rapid shallow breathing index; PAC: Pulmonary artery catheter; LVEF: Left ventricular ejection fraction; LVEDP: Left ventricular end-diastolic pressure; BNP: Brain natriuretic peptide; DUS: Diaphragm ultrasound; Pdi: Trans-diaphragmatic pressure; DE: Diaphragmatic excursion; DTF: Diaphragm thickening fraction; Te-insp: End-inspiration thickness; Te-exp: End expiration thickness; EAdi: Electrical activity of the diaphragm; NAVA: Neurally adjusted ventilator assist.

Acknowledgements

None.

Authors' contributions

LV, GMG and AB contributed equally in writing this manuscript. All authors read and approved the final manuscript.

Author details

[1] Anesthesiology and Intensive Care Clinic, Department of Medicine, University of Udine, Via Colugna 50, 33100 Udine, Italy. [2] Intensive Care Unit, Department of Medical and Surgical Sciences, University Hospital Mater Domini, Magna Graecia University, Catanzaro, Italy.

References

1. Béduneau G, Pham T, Schortgen F, Piquilloud L, Zogheib E, Jonas M, Grelon F, Runge I, Terzi N, Grangé S, Barberet G, Guitard PG, Frat JP, Constan A, Chretien JM, Mancebo J, Mercat A, Richard JM, Brochard L, WIND (Weaning according to a New Definition) Study Group and the REVA (Réseau Européen de Recherche en Ventilation Artificielle) Network (2017) Epidemiology of weaning outcome according to a new definition. The WIND study. Am J Respir Crit Care Med 195:772–783. https://doi.org/10.1164/rccm.201602-0320OC
2. Thille AW, Cortés-Puch I, Esteban A (2013) Weaning from the ventilator and extubation in ICU. Curr Opin Crit Care 19:57–64. https://doi.org/10.1097/MCC.0b013e32835c5095
3. Boles JM, Bion J, Connors A, Herridge M, Marsh B, Melot C, Pearl R, Silverman H, Stanchina M, Vieillard-Baron A, Welte T (2007) Weaning from mechanical ventilation. Eur Respir J 29:1033–1056. https://doi.org/10.1183/09031936.00010206
4. Peñuelas O, Frutos-Vivar F, Fernández C, Ventila Group et al (2011) Characteristics and outcomes of ventilated patients according to time to liberation from mechanical ventilation. Am J Respir Crit Care Med 184:430–437. https://doi.org/10.1164/rccm.201011-1887oc
5. Levine S, Nguyen T, Taylor N, Friscia ME, Budak MT, Rothenberg P, Zhu J, Sachdeva R, Sonnad S, Kaiser LR, Rubinstein NA, Powers SKSJ (2008) Rapid disuse atrophy of diaphragm fibers in mechanically ventilated humans. N Engl J Med 358:1327–1335
6. Caroleo S, Agnello F, Abdallah K, Santangelo E, Amantea B (2007) Weaning from mechanical ventilation: an open issue. Minerva Anestesiol 73:417–427
7. Bruni A, Garofalo E, Pelaia C, Messina A, Cammarota G, Murabito P, Corrado S, Vetrugno L, Longhini F, Navalesi P (2019) Patient-ventilator asynchrony in adult critically ill patients. Minerva Anestesiol 85:676–688. https://doi.org/10.23736/S0375-9393.19.13436-0
8. Lemaire F, Teboul JL, Cinotti L, Giotto G, Abrouk F, Steg G, Macquin-Mavier I, Zapol WM (1988) Acute left ventricular dysfunction during unsuccessful weaning from mechanical ventilation. Anesthesiology 69:171–179
9. Ouellette DR, Patel S, Girard TD, Morris PE, Schmidt GA, Truwit JD, Alhazzani W, Burns SM, Epstein SK, Esteban A, Fan E, Ferrer M, Fraser GL, Gong MN, Hough CL, Mehta S, Nanchal R, Pawlik AJ, Schweickert WD, Sessler CN, Strøm T, Kress JP (2017) Liberation from mechanical ventilation in critically ill adults: an Official American College of Chest Physicians/American Thoracic Society clinical practice guideline: inspiratory pressure augmentation during spontaneous breathing trials, protocols minimizing sedation, and noninvasive ventilation immediately after extubation. Chest 151:166–180. https://doi.org/10.1016/j.chest.2016.10.036
10. Esteban A, Alia I, Gordo F, Fernandex R, Solsona J, Vallverdu I, Macías S, Allegue JM, Blanco J, Carriedo D, León M, de la Cal MA, Taboada F, Gonzalez de Velasco J, Palazón E, Carrizosa F, Tomás R, Suarez J, Goldwasser RS (1997) Extubation outcome after spontaneous breathing trials with t-tube or pressure support ventilation. Am J Respir Crit Care Med 156:459–465
11. Esteban A, Alía I, Tobin MJ, Gil A, Gordo F, Vallverdú I, Blanch L, Bonet A, Vázquez A, de Pablo R, Torres A, de La Cal MA, Macías S (1999) Effect of spontaneous breathing trial duration on outcome of attempts to discontinue mechanical ventilation. Am J Respir Crit Care Med 159:512–518

12. Frutos-Vivar F, Ferguson ND, Esteban A, Epstein SK, Arabi Y, Apezteguía C, González M, Hill NS, Nava S, D'Empaire G, Anzueto A (2006) Risk factors for extubation failure in patients following a successful spontaneous breathing trial. Chest 130:1664–1671
13. Ouanes-Besbes L, Dachraoui F, Ouanes I, Bouneb R, Jalloul F, Dlala M, Najjar MF, Abroug F (2012) NT-proBNP levels at spontaneous breathing trial help in the prediction of post-extubation respiratory distress. Intensive Care Med 38:788–795
14. Meade M, Guyatt G, Cook D, Griffith L, Sinuff T, Kergl C, Mancebo J, Esteban A, Epstein S (2001) Predicting success in weaning from mechanical ventilation. Chest 120:400S–424S
15. Conti G, Montini L, Pennisi MA, Cavaliere F, Arcangeli A, Bocci MG, Proietti R, Antonelli M (2004) A prospective, blinded evaluation of indexes proposed to predict weaning from mechanical ventilation. Intensive Care Med 30:830–836
16. Thille AW, Richard JC, Brochard L (2013) The decision to extubate in the intensive care unit. Am J Respir Crit Care Med 187:1294–1302. https://doi.org/10.1164/rccm.201208-1523CI
17. Silva S, Ait Aissa D, Cocquet P, Hoarau L, Ruiz J, Ferre F, Rousset D, Mora M, Mari A, Fourcade O, Riu B, Jaber S, Bataille B (2017) Combined thoracic ultrasound assessment during a successful weaning trial predicts postextubation distress. Anesthesiology 127:666–674. https://doi.org/10.1097/ALN.0000000000001773
18. Aybar Türkoğlu M, Topeli Iskit A (2008) Ventilator-associated pneumonia caused by high risk microorganisms: a matched case-control study. Tuberk Toraks 56:139–149
19. Soler Morejón Cde D, Tamargo Barbeito TO (2012) Effect of mechanical ventilation on intra-abdominal pressure in critically ill patients without other risk factors for abdominal hypertension: an observational multicenter epidemiological study. Ann Intensive Care 2(Suppl 1):S22. https://doi.org/10.1186/2110-5820-2-S1-S22
20. Namen AM, Ely EW, Tatter SB, Case LD, Lucia MA, Smith A, Landry S, Wilson JA, Glazier SS, Branch CL, Kelly DL, Bowton DL, Haponik EF (2001) Predictors of successful extubation in neurosurgical patients. Am J Respir Crit Care Med 163:658–664
21. Peñuelas Ó, Thille AW, Esteban A (2015) Discontinuation of ventilatory support: new solutions to old dilemmas. Curr Opin Crit Care 21:74–81. https://doi.org/10.1097/MCC.0000000000000169
22. Burns KEA, Soliman I, Adhikari NKJ, Zwein A, Wong JTY, Gomez-Builes C, Pellegrini JA, Chen L, Rittayamai N, Sklar M, Brochard LJ, Friedrich JO (2017) Trials directly comparing alternative spontaneous breathing trial techniques: a systematic review and meta-analysis. Crit Care 21:127. https://doi.org/10.1186/s13054-017-1698-x
23. MacIntyre NR (2013) The ventilator discontinuation process: an expanding evidence base. Respir Care 58:1074–1086. https://doi.org/10.4187/respcare.02284
24. Malbrain MLNG, Van Regenmortel N, Saugel B, De Tavernier B, Van Gaal PJ, Joannes-Boyau O, Teboul JL, Rice TW, Mythen M, Monnet X (2018) Principles of fluid management and stewardship in septic shock: it is time to consider the four D's and the four phases of fluid therapy. Ann Intensive Care 8:66. https://doi.org/10.1186/s13613-018-0402-x
25. Sakr Y, Rubatto Birri PN, Kotfis K, Nanchal R, Shah B, Kluge S, Schroeder ME, Marshall JC, Vincent JL, Intensive Care Over Nations Investigators (2017) Higher fluid balance increases the risk of death from sepsis: results from a large international audit. Crit Care Med 45:386–394. https://doi.org/10.1097/CCM.0000000000002189
26. Boyd JH, Forbes J, Nakada TA, Walley KR, Russell JA (2011) Fluid resuscitation in septic shock: a positive fluid balance and elevated central venous pressure are associated with increased mortality. Crit Care Med 39:259–265. https://doi.org/10.1097/CCM.0b013e3181feeb15
27. Franchi F, Vetrugno L, Scolletta S (2017) Echocardiography to guide fluid therapy in critically ill patients: check the heart and take a quick look at the lungs. J Thorac Dis 9:477–481. https://doi.org/10.21037/jtd.2017.02.94
28. Vignon P, Repessé X, Viellard-Baron A, Maury E (2016) Critical care ultrasonography in acute respiratory failure. Crit Care 20:228. https://doi.org/10.1186/s13054-016-1400-8
29. Epstein SK (1995) Etiology of extubation failure and the predictive value of the rapid shallow breathing index. Am J Resp Crit Care Med 152:545–549
30. Pandey A, Khera R, Kumar N, Golwala H, Girotra S, Fonarow GC (2016) Use of pulmonary arterial catheterization in US patients with failure, 2001–2012. JAMA Intern Med 176:129–132. https://doi.org/10.1001/jamainternmed.2015.6190
31. Della Rocca G, Vetrugno L, Tripi G, Deana C, Barbariol F, Pompei L (2014) Liberal or restricted fluid administration: are we ready for a proposal of a restricted intraoperative approach? BMC Anesthesiol 14:62. https://doi.org/10.1186/1471-2253-14-62
32. Lamia B, Maizel J, Ochagavia A, Chemla D, Osman D, Richard C, Teboul JL (2009) Echocardiographic diagnosis of pulmonary artery occlusion pressure elevation during weaning from mechanical ventilation. Crit Care Med 37:1696–1701. https://doi.org/10.1097/CCM.0b013e31819f13d0
33. Ommen SR, Nishimura RA, Appleton CP, Miller FA, Oh JK, Redfield MM, Tajik AJ (2000) Clinical utility of Doppler echocardiography and tissue doppler imaging in the estimation of left ventricular filling pressures: a comparative simultaneous Doppler-catheterization study. Circulation 102:1788–1794
34. Moschietto S, Doyen D, Grech L, Dellamonica J, Hyvernat H, Bernardin G (2012) Transthoracic echocardiography with Doppler tissue imaging predicts weaning failure from mechanical ventilation: evolution of the left ventricle relaxation rate during a spontaneous breathing trial is the key factor in weaning outcome. Crit Care 16:R81. https://doi.org/10.1186/cc11339
35. Nagueh S, Smiseth O, Appleton C, Byrd B, Dokainish H, Edvardsen T, Flachskampf FA, Gillebert TC, Klein AL, Lancellotti P, Marino P, Oh JK, Popescu BA, Waggoner AD (2016) Recommendations for the evaluation of left ventricular diastolic function by echocardiography: an update from the American Society of Echocardiography and the European Association of Cardiovascular Imaging. J Am Soc Echocardiogr 29:277–314. https://doi.org/10.1016/j.echo.2016.01.011
36. Ferré A, Guillot M, Lichtenstein D, Mezière G, Richard C, Teboul JL, Monnet X (2019) Lung ultrasound allows the diagnosis of weaning-induced pulmonary oedema. Intensive Care Med 45:601–608. https://doi.org/10.1007/s00134-019-05573-6
37. Mekontso Dessap A, Roche-Campo F, Kouatchet A, Tomicic V, Beduneau G, Sonneville R, Cabello B, Jaber S, Azoulay E, Castanares-Zapatero D, Devaquet J, Lellouche F, Katsahian S, Brochard L (2012) Natriuretic peptide-driven fluid management during ventilator weaning: a randomized controlled trial. Am J Respir Crit Care Med 186:1256–1263. https://doi.org/10.1164/rccm.201205-0939OC
38. Robertson CH Jr, Foster GM, Johnson RL Jr (1977) The relationship of respiratory failure to the oxygen consumption of, lactate production by, and distribution of blood flow among respiratory muscles during increasing inspiratory resistance. J Clin Investig 59:31–42
39. Rochester DF, Pradel-Guena H (1973) Measurement of diaphragmatic blood flow in dogs from Xenon-133 clearance. J Appl Physiol 34:68–74
40. Monod H, Scherrer J (1965) The work capacity of a synergic muscular group. Ergonomics 8:329–338
41. Aubier M, Viires N, Syllie G, Mozes R, Roussos CS (1982) Respiratory muscle contribution to lactic acidosis in low cardiac output. Am Rev Respir Dis 126:648–652
42. Macklem PT, Roussos CS (1977) Respiratory muscle fatigue: a cause of respiratory failure? Clin Sci Mol Med 53:419–422
43. Kim WY, Suh HJ, Hong SB, Koh Y, Lim CM (2011) Diaphragm dysfunction assessed by ultrasonography: influence on weaning from mechanical ventilation. Crit Care Med 39:2627–2630. https://doi.org/10.1097/CCM.0b013e3182266408
44. Powers SK, Kavazis AN, Levine S (2009) Prolonged mechanical ventilation alters diaphragmatic structure and function. Crit Care Med 37:S347–S353. https://doi.org/10.1097/CCM.0b013e3181b6e760
45. Vetrugno L, Guadagnin GM, Barbariol F, Langiano N, Zangrillo A, Bove T (2019) Ultrasound imaging for diaphragm dysfunction: a narrative literature review. J Cardiothorac Vasc Anesth 33:2525–2536. https://doi.org/10.1053/j.jvca.2019.01.003
46. Dres M, Dubé BP, Mayaux J, Delemazure J, Reuter D, Brochard L, Similowski T, Demoule A (2017) Coexistence and impact of limb muscle and diaphragm weakness at time of liberation from mechanical ventilation in medical intensive care unit patients. Am J Respir Crit Care Med

195:57–66. https://doi.org/10.1164/rccm.201602-0367OC
47. Lerolle N, Guérot E, Dimassi S, Zegdi R, Faisy C, Fagon JY, Diehl JL (2009) Ultrasonographic diagnostic criterion for severe diaphragmatic dysfunction after cardiac surgery. Chest 135:401–407. https://doi.org/10.1378/chest.08-1531
48. Watson AC, Hughes PD, Louise Harris M, Hart N, Ware RJ, Wendon J, Green M, Moxham J (2001) Measurement of twitch transdiaphragmatic, esophageal, and endotracheal tube pressure with bilateral anterolateral magnetic phrenic nerve stimulation in patients in the intensive care unit. Crit Care Med 29:1325–1331
49. Dubé BP, Dres M (2016) Diaphragm dysfunction: diagnostic approaches and management strategies. J Clin Med 5:E113
50. Bignami E, Guarnieri M, Saglietti F, Ramelli A, Vetrugno L (2018) Diaphragmatic dysfunction following cardiac surgery: is there a role for pulmonary ultrasound? J Cardiothorac Vasc Anesth 32:e6–e7. https://doi.org/10.1053/j.jvca.2018.04.054
51. Barbariol F, Vetrugno L, Pompei L, De Flaviis A, Rocca GD (2015) Point-of-care ultrasound of the diaphragm in a liver transplant patient with acute respiratory failure. Crit Ultrasound J 7:3. https://doi.org/10.1186/s13089-015-0021-9
52. Cammarota G, Sguazzotti I, Zanoni M, Messina A, Colombo D, Vignazia GL, Vetrugno L, Garofalo E, Bruni A, Navalesi P, Avanzi GC, Della Corte F, Volpicelli G, Vaschetto R (2019) Diaphragmatic ultrasound assessment in subjects with acute hypercapnic respiratory failure admitted to the emergency department. Respir Care. https://doi.org/10.4187/respcare.06803
53. Vivier E, Muller M, Putegnat JB, Steyer J, Barrau S, Boissier F, Bourdin G, Mekontso-Dessap A, Levrat A, Pommier C, Thille AW (2019) Inability of diaphragm ultrasound to predict extubation failure: a multicenter study. Chest 155:1131–1139. https://doi.org/10.1016/j.chest.2019.03.004
54. Boussuges A, Gole Y, Blanc P (2009) Diaphragmatic motion studied by M-mode ultrasonography: methods, reproducibility, and normal values. Chest 135:391–400. https://doi.org/10.1378/chest.08-1541
55. Summerhill EM, El-Sameed YA, Glidden TJ, McCool FD (2008) Monitoring recovery from diaphragm paralysis with ultrasound. Chest 133:737–743. https://doi.org/10.1378/chest.07-2200
56. Wait JL, Nahormek PA, Yost WT, Rochester DP (1989) Diaphragmatic thickness-lung volume relationship in vivo. J Appl Physiol 67:1560–1568. https://doi.org/10.1152/jappl.1989.67.4.1560
57. Cohen E, Mier A, Heywood P, Murphy K, Boultbee J, Guz A (1994) Excursion-volume relation of the right hemidiaphragm measured by ultrasonography and respiratory airflow measurements. Thorax 49:885–889
58. Umbrello M, Formenti P, Longhi D, Galimberti A, Piva I, Pezzi A, Mistraletti G, Marini JJ, Iapichino G (2015) Diaphragm ultrasound as indicator of respiratory effort in critically ill patients undergoing assisted mechanical ventilation: a pilot clinical study. Crit Care 19:161. https://doi.org/10.1186/s13054-015-0894-9
59. Goligher EC, Fan E, Herridge MS, Murray A, Vorona S, Brace D, Rittayamai N, Lanys A, Tomlinson G, Singh JM, Bolz SS, Rubenfeld GD, Kavanagh BP, Brochard LJ, Ferguson ND (2015) Evolution of diaphragm thickness during mechanical ventilation: impact of inspiratory effort. Am J Respir Crit Care Med 192:1080–1088
60. Dubé BP, Dres M, Mayaux J, Demiri S, Similowski T, Demoule A (2017) Ultrasound evaluation of diaphragm function in mechanically ventilated patients: comparison to phrenic stimulation and prognostic implications. Thorax 72:811–818. https://doi.org/10.1136/thoraxjnl-2016-209459
61. Jiang JR, Tsai TH, Jerng JS, Yu CJ, Wu HD, Yang PC (2004) Ultrasonographic evaluation of liver/spleen movements and extubation outcome. Chest 126:179–185
62. Spadaro S, Grasso S, Mauri T, Dalla Corte F, Alvisi V, Ragazzi R, Cricca V, Biondi G, Di Mussi R, Marangoni E, Volta CA (2016) Can diaphragmatic ultrasonography performed during the T-tube trial predict weaning failure? The role of diaphragmatic rapid shallow breathing index. Crit Care 20:305
63. Luo L, Li Y, Chen X, Sun B, Li W, Gu W, Wang S, Zhao S, Lv Y, Chen M, Xia J, Sui F, Mei X, Shi H, Tong Z (2017) Different effects of cardiac and diaphragm function assessed by ultrasound on extubation outcomes in difficult-to-wean patients: a cohort study. BMC Pulm Med 17:161. https://doi.org/10.1186/s12890-017-0501-8
64. Garrido-Aguirre E, Ñamendys-Silva SA, del Moral OR, Cortés-Soto CA, Romero-González JP (2019) Diaphragmatic ultrasonography, a novel approach in critical care. A proposal for a new weaning index. Ultrasound Q. https://doi.org/10.1097/ruq.0000000000000442 **(Volume publish ahead of print)**
65. Palkar A, Narasimhan M, Greenberg H, Singh K, Koenig S, Mayo P, Gottesman E (2018) Diaphragm excursion-time index. A new parameter using ultrasonography to predict extubation outcome. Chest 153:1213–1220. https://doi.org/10.1016/j.chest.2018.01.007
66. Carrie C, Gisbert-Mora C, Bonnardel E, Gauche B, Biais M, Vargas F, Hilbert G (2017) Ultrasonographic diaphragmatic excursion is inaccurate and not better than the MRC score for predicting weaning-failure in mechanically ventilated patients. Anaesth Crit Care Pain Med 36:9–14. https://doi.org/10.1016/j.accpm.2016.05.009
67. Jung B, Moury PH, Mahul M, de Jong A, Galia F, Prades A, Albaladejo P, Chanques G, Molinari N, Jaber S (2016) Diaphragmatic dysfunction in patients with ICU-acquired weakness and its impact on extubation failure. Intensive Care Med 42:853–861. https://doi.org/10.1007/s00134-015-4125-2
68. Samanta S, Singh RK, Baronia AK, Poddar B, Azim A, Gurjar M (2017) Diaphragm thickening fraction to predict weaning—a prospective exploratory study. J Intensive Care 5:62. https://doi.org/10.1186/s40560-017-0258-4
69. Blumhof S, Wheeler D, Thomas K, McCool FD, Mora J (2016) Change in diaphragmatic thickness during the respiratory cycle predicts extubation success at various levels of pressure support ventilation. Lung 194:519–525. https://doi.org/10.1007/s00408-016-9911-2
70. DiNino E, Gartman EJ, Sethi JM, McCool FD (2014) Diaphragm ultrasound as a predictor of successful extubation from mechanical ventilation. Thorax 69:423–427. https://doi.org/10.1136/thoraxjnl-2013-204111
71. Farghaly S, Hasan AA (2017) Diaphragm ultrasound as a new method to predict extubation outcome in mechanically ventilated patients. Aust Crit Care 30:37–43. https://doi.org/10.1016/j.aucc.2016.03.004
72. Zambon M, Greco M, Bocchino S, Cabrini L, Beccaria PF, Zangrillo A (2017) Assessment of diaphragmatic dysfunction in the critically ill patient with ultrasound: a systematic review. Intensive Care Med 43:29–38. https://doi.org/10.1007/s00134-016-4524-z
73. Llamas-Álvarez AM, Tenza-Lozano EM, Latour-Pérez J (2017) Diaphragm and lung ultrasound to predict weaning outcome: systematic review and meta-analysis. Chest 152:1140–1150. https://doi.org/10.1016/j.chest.2017.08.028
74. Garofalo E, Bruni A, Pelaia C, Landoni G, Zangrillo A, Antonelli M, Conti G, Biasucci DG, Mercurio G, Cortegiani A, Giarratano A, Vetrugno L, Bove T, Forfori F, Corradi F, Vaschetto R, Cammarota G, Ma A, Murabito P, Bellini V, Zambon M, Longhini F, Navalesi P, Bignami E (2019) Comparisons of two diaphragm ultrasound-teaching programs: a multicenter randomized controlled educational study. Ultrasound J 11:21. https://doi.org/10.1186/s13089-019-0137-4

Mechanical ventilation weaning issues can be counted on the fingers of just one hand: part 2

Luigi Vetrugno[1*†], Alessandro Brussa[1*†], Giovanni Maria Guadagnin[1], Daniele Orso[1], Francesco De Lorenzo[1], Gianmaria Cammarota[2], Erminio Santangelo[3] and Tiziana Bove[1]

Abstract

Assessing heart and diaphragm function constitutes only one of the steps to consider along the weaning path. In this second part of the review, we will deal with the more systematic evaluation of the pulmonary parenchyma—often implicated in the genesis of respiratory failure. We will also consider the other possible causes of weaning failure that lie beyond the cardio-pulmonary-diaphragmatic system. Finally, we will take a moment to consider the remaining unsolved problems arising from mechanical ventilation and describe the so-called protective approach to parenchyma and diaphragm ventilation.

Keywords: Weaning, Mechanical ventilation, Lung ultrasound, Diaphragm dysfunction, Neurally adjusted ventilation assist

Lung ultrasound score (LUS)

The lung ultrasound (LUS) score is a useful tool that quantifies aerated lung mass and provides real-time information during mechanical ventilation and weaning (Fig. 1) [1]. Specifically, its application in the clinical setting enables optimization of the ventilatory settings in challenging patients by estimating the recruitability of poorly aerated pulmonary mass. This allows clinicians to monitor lung aeration during the weaning process, providing a positive prognostic factor. The LUS score may also help discriminate between a cardiac, parenchymal, or diaphragmatic cause of loss of lung aeration [2] and, in turn, help identify the most appropriate therapeutic approach.

Bouhemad and colleagues (2010) were the first to postulate the potential usefulness of LUS as a tool for monitoring parenchymal reaeration. Their studies involved assigning a positive or negative score to reflect the change occurring in the parenchymal ultrasound pattern as a result of adjustments to medical antibiotic therapy [3] or positive end-expiratory pressure (PEEP) titration [4]. They found that the degree of lung reaeration could be accurately estimated using the LUS reaeration score. However, use of the LUS score to set ventilatory parameters resulted in the inability to predict lung over-inflation—the physiopathological basis for ventilation-induced lung injury. Soon after, Stefanidis et al. reached the same conclusions in a small pilot study, which once again pointed out the reliability of LUS in evaluating parenchymal reaeration in acute respiratory distress syndrome (ARDS) patients during a PEEP trial [5]. In a more recent, prospective, multicenter study, Haddam et al. analyzed changes in LUS score during the prone positioning of patients with severe ARDS. They revealed that even though the LUS score provides a way to consistently monitor changes in regional lung aeration, it does not correlate with improvements in blood gas oxygenation. A number of reasons may explain this, including a short prone-positioning trial before blood gas

*Correspondence: luigi.vetrugno@uniud.it; alessandro.brussa@gmail.com
†Luigi Vetrugno and Alessandro Brussa contributed equally to this work.
[1] Anesthesiology and Intensive Care Clinic, Department of Medicine, University of Udine, Via Colugna 50, 33100 Udine, Italy
Full list of author information is available at the end of the article

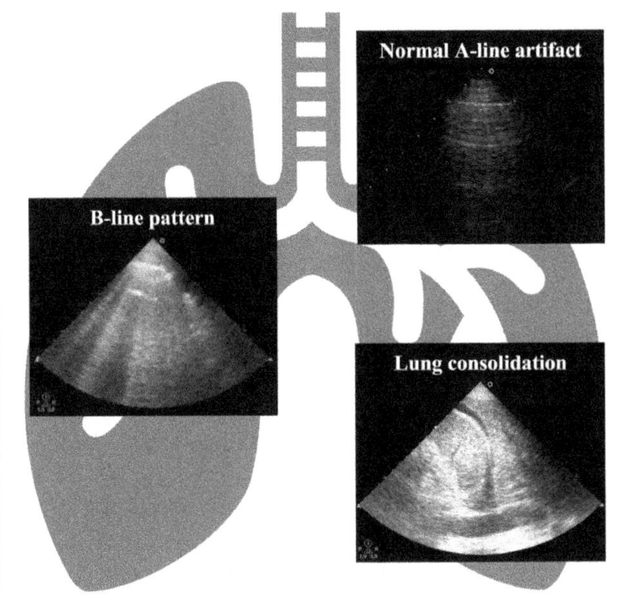

Fig. 1 Different echographic patterns during lung ultrasound evaluation

analysis and a less permissive cut-off in evaluating PaO_2 improvements. Nevertheless, Haddam and colleagues underlined the feasibility and utility of LUS evaluation, practically considering it a routine technique [6]. The capacity of LUS to evaluate lung reaeration was also confirmed by Chinardet et al. who used it to estimate lung reaeration following pleural drainage in ARDS patients [7]. However, a recent randomized crossover study by Chiumello et al. found that variations in the LUS score did not correlate with PEEP-induced lung recruitment due to a still inaccurate definition of consolidation pattern [8]. These results could open up a new line of research aimed at increasing the specificity of ultrasound evaluation.

The monitoring of lung aeration during the weaning process embodies another essential aspect of LUS evaluation since it indirectly leads to successful extubation [9]. Clear evidence of the usefulness of the LUS score in the weaning process is provided in the metanalysis by Llamas-Álvarez et al. in which ultrasound evaluation is concluded to provide valuable information in predicting weaning outcome [10]. Tenza-Lozano et al. also came to this conclusion and went on to propose a new and more reproducible score that only considers the anterior, lateral, and posterior-basal thoracic areas [11]. Soummer et al. showed that an LUS score < 13 after a spontaneous breathing trial (SBT) correlates with successful weaning and safe extubation, whereas a LUS score > 17 predicts weaning failure with post-extubation respiratory distress [12]. The association between lung de-recruitment and weaning failure was emphasized by Jabaudon et al. who found a loss of aerated lung mass to be the only predictor of weaning failure [13]. In addition to corroborating all of the above, Haji et al. also pointed out the clinical relevance of LUS examination in predicting weaning outcome [14].

The role of LUS as a prognostic factor was first suggested by Frassi et al. [15], who showed that the number of B-lines in an ultrasound evaluation correlated with mortality rate in a cardiac subgroup of patients admitted to hospital with dyspnea or chest pain. Extending this concept, Zhao et al. [16] demonstrated how LUS B-line number could be useful in accurately assessing extravascular lung water in ARDS patients. LUS score also correlates with the lung injury score, the PaO_2/FiO_2 ratio, static compliance, and, above all, mortality risk, providing a new and reliable prognostic tool for ARDS patients. More recently, Zou et al. [17] broadened the prognostic value of LUS score to include shock intensive care unit (ICU) patients, and showed that a modified LUS score may act as an independent risk factor for ICU mortality. These data on shock patients were confirmed by Yin et al. [18] in a study involving 175 patients in which the LUS score correlated with 28-day mortality as well as the APACHE II score and lactate serum levels.

Lung ultrasonography, together with its growing role as a prognostic factor, has even been applied in the differential diagnosis of respiratory failure etiology [19]. Jambrik et al. [20] performed the first assessment of extravascular lung water using lung sonography and from these first data LUS has progressed from being the primarily technique to quantify pulmonary interstitial edema, which may derive from different causes, to being developed into a new diagnostic tool for identifying the origin of aerated lung loss. Indeed, over the years, the breadth of application of LUS has expanded, and it is now being applied in the assessment of extravascular lung water in hemodialysis patients [21] and in heart failure patients [22], not to mention the already cited role of the LUS score in predicting a successful SBT [12, 23].

Considering all of the above evidence, the critical role of lung ultrasonography and its various applications in the care of critically ill patients becomes highly evident. The role of the anesthesiologist in the management of this powerful tool is thus paramount in order to provide patients with the best medical treatment.

Out of the box

Neurocritical patients

Mechanical ventilation is often necessary in brain injury patients (i.e., those suffering from ischemic or hemorrhagic stroke, or severe brain trauma, or metabolic brain injury or resulting from alcohol intoxication, and neurosurgery patients) to prevent aspiration, hypoxemia, hypercapnia and further brain injury resulting from reduced/abolished airway protective mechanisms and respiratory drive. Unfortunately, data about mechanical ventilation settings and the weaning process in neurocritical patients are lacking in the literature. A minimal level of arousal should be obtained before weaning and extubation, but neurocritical patients frequently experience prolonged mechanical ventilation periods because of our inability to understand the patient's state of consciousness [24]. The minimal level of arousal necessary to achieve successful extubation also remains controversial. The Glasgow Coma Scale (GCS) has never been validated in intubated patients and, when employed, it has proved to be an inconsistent predictor of successful extubation if used alone [25, 26]. Several scores have been proposed to assess patient arousal, combining airway and neurological statuses, but all lack external validation and often they are not easily applicable at the bedside. In cases of prolonged diminished levels of consciousness, neurocritical patients may never undergo the weaning process, and tracheostomy is commonly employed in the management of these patients, but the timing of this procedure is controversial. Prolonged invasive mechanical ventilation (IMV) in this category of patients can lead to higher rates of ventilator-acquired pneumonia, increased ICU length of stay, and higher mortality rates [24, 25, 27] compared with non-neurological critically ill patients [28].

Intra-abdominal hypertension (IAH)

Intra-abdominal hypertension (IAH) is defined as an abdominal pressure that exceeds 12 mmHg in at least three consecutive assessments performed within a time window of 4–6 h. Abdominal hypertension can transform into abdominal compartment syndrome (ACS) when intra-abdominal pressure (IAP) reaches values above 20 mmHg with associated single or multiple organ dysfunction/failure [29].

The prevalence of IAH varies in the literature according to the different patient populations studied; it stands at around 54% in medical ICU patients, 65% in surgical ICU patients, and 32% in combined medical–surgical ICU patients [30, 31]. IAH is a serious problem that can produce adverse effects involving both abdominal (i.e., bowel, kidney) and extra-abdominal (i.e., cardiovascular, respiratory) organs, and it is recognized as an independent indicator of mortality in critically ill patients [32].

Primary causes of IAH (i.e., pneumoperitoneum, hemoperitoneum, abdominal trauma, pancreatitis, liver transplantation) can lead to ARDS, and primary ARDS may develop into IAH. The primary mechanical effects through which IAH affects respiratory function are a decreased compliance of the thoracic–pulmonary system and an upward displacement of the diaphragm's starting position [33]. As the lower inflection point of the pressure–volume curve shifts to the right, alveolar opening pressure and inspiratory pressures are also increased [33]. All these elements cause an increased respiratory workload for the spontaneously breathing patient, a compensatory increase in frequency, and, if prolonged, muscle exhaustion (Fig. 2). As a result of reduced inspiratory flow and compression of the lung parenchyma, the dependent areas of the lung will tend toward atelectasis [33]. Subsequently, the continued presence of IAH generates secondary acute lung injury [33], i.e., barotrauma, linked to the increase in peak and plateau pressure in the respiratory tract with the activation of a neutrophilic immune response [33]. Atelectasis may trigger the development of pneumonia [33].

Despite some disputes in literature about the effects of mechanical ventilation and PEEP on IAP, ARDS combined with mechanical ventilation is a known risk factor for intra-abdominal hypertension. The use of PEEP

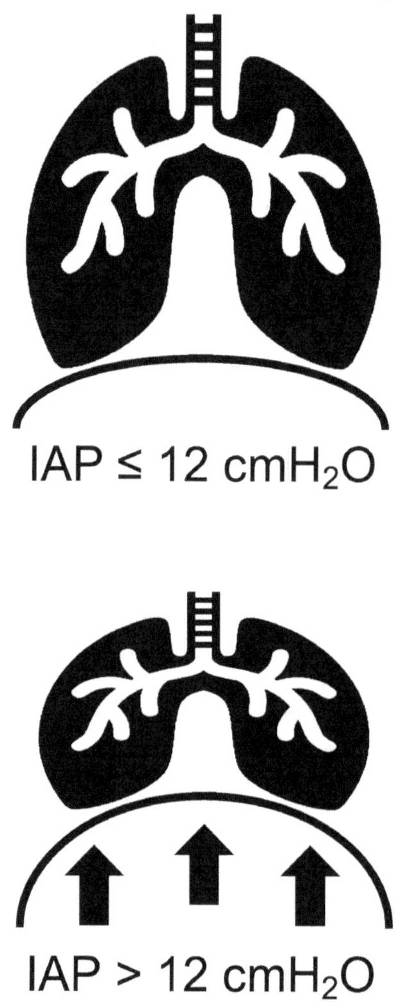

Fig. 2 Effect of intra-abdominal pressure on diaphragmatic dome. *IAP* intra-abdominal pressure

increases alveolar recruitment, in turn, increasing residual functional capacity and oxygenation [34], although it causes a flattening of the diaphragmatic dome and a shift to the right side of the pressure–volume curve with the applied pressure being subsequently directed to the abdominal cavity [35]. As such, PEEP should be employed with caution in ARDS patients with IAH, also because moderate PEEP levels can increase IAP and significantly decrease abdominal perfusion pressure proportionally to the PEEP applied [36].

Given the interdependence of the thoracic and abdominal cavities, it is unsurprising that weaning from mechanical ventilation can be particularly difficult in the presence of IAH [37]. We suggest, therefore, in agreement with various other publications and international recommendations, that IAP is closely monitored in mechanically ventilated patients with ARDS.

Pleural effusion

Pleural effusion (PLEFF) is common in the ICU, although the incidence varies according to the diagnostic technique being used (8% to 60%) [38]. However, its role in weaning failure has never been demonstrated—even though the amount of PLEFF is known to influence diaphragm force [39], but this has never been considered in the context of weaning. PLEFF can exacerbate gas exchange, respiratory dynamics, and hemodynamic stability, whereas pleural drainage can improve oxygenation and respiratory mechanics (Fig. 3). At the time of this review, doubts persist about the effectiveness of pleural drainage. In a previous publication, we addressed the effectiveness of ultrasound-guided placement of a small-bore pleural drain for improving patient respiratory gas exchange in terms of the PaO_2/FiO_2 ratio, but no correlation with the maintenance of spontaneous breathing or with weaning from mechanical ventilation was found, in agreement with the work by Dres et al. [40]. These results support the concept that PLEFF cannot constitute the sole parameter being considered when weaning a patient from the ventilator. However, the inconsistency in PLEFF estimations obtained using ultrasound necessitates the need to standardize the methods used for assessing pleural effusion volume (an issue that is overlooked in the current international recommendations on lung ultrasound) [41, 42]. That said, PLEFF drainage also provides the opportunity to obtain chemical–physical and cytological samples to guide the differential diagnosis of PLEFF and any follow-up therapy.

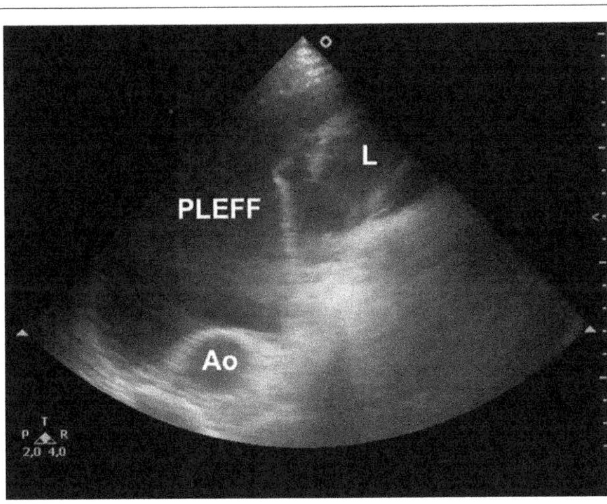

Fig. 3 Massive left-sided pleural effusion with floating fibrin deposition. *PLEFF* pleural effusion, *Ao* aorta, *L* lung

Mechanical ventilation: unsolved issues and possible solutions

Mechanical ventilation itself may cause lung, heart, and diaphragm dysfunction (Table 1). The mechanisms underlying these types of alterations are not entirely known. The concept of lung and heart protection during mechanical ventilation is better established, whereas a significant gap exists in the literature regarding diaphragm protection. In fact, while specific protocols of lung-protective ventilation are available, the diaphragm is very often neglected, despite the fact that it constitutes the primary actor in physiological respiration.

Ventilator-induced lung injury (VILI)

The literature is rich with evidence and explanations regarding how mechanical ventilation can cause lung injury. Excessive pressure (barotrauma) or volume (volutrauma) and cyclic alveolar opening–closing (atelectotrauma) are the components that cause ventilator-induced lung injury (VILI) [43]. The effects of all three mechanisms occur under the broader term of "biotrauma", which defines the inflammatory process that follows the initial injury [44]. Specifically, ventilation pressure and induced tidal volume are closely interconnected in the genesis of parenchymal

Table 1 Benefits and risks deriving from invasive mechanical ventilation

Benefits	Risks
Organ support during acute respiratory illness	VILI
	VAP
Protective ventilation protocols	VIDD
	Overassistance
	Oversedation

VILI ventilation-induced lung injury, *VAP* ventilator-acquired pneumonia, *VIDD* ventilator-induced diaphragm dysfunction

damage. Barotrauma is due to excessive stress applied to the lung, directly proportional to the transpulmonary pressure, while volutrauma is secondary to an excessive parenchymal strain, correlated to the tidal volume [45]. In other words, harmful levels of pressure and volume are the two sides of the same coin. Atelectotrauma refers to the continuous opening and closure of potentially recruitable alveoli, which, mainly due to the poor distribution of the pulmonary surfactant, tend to open in response to increasing pressures during the inspiratory phase and to close in the expiratory phase, in accordance with Laplace's law [46]. In the long run, this mechanism triggers the inflammatory process and progressive alveolar atelectasis.

More recent observations regarding IMV have also considered respiratory flow and frequency among the possible determinants of lung injury. As for the aforementioned relationship between volume and pressure, once again, lung injury can derive from the interdependence between inspiratory flow and respiratory rate. To explain this complicated process in more simple terms: the inspiratory flow conveys a given tidal volume based on the pressure delivered in a unit of time, which is, in turn, determined by the respiratory rate and the I:E ratio (inspiration:expiration ratio). The higher the respiratory rate, the lower the inspiratory time and the higher the flow, resulting in greater pressure applied to the lung parenchyma and an increased risk of VILI [47].

From the fifth day of IMV onward, the risk of ventilator-associated pneumonia increases and its presence is correlated with increased morbidity and mortality [48].

Ventilator-induced diaphragm dysfunction

Mechanical ventilation may also lead to a "...loss of diaphragmatic force-generating capacity" [49], causing ventilator-induced diaphragm dysfunction (VIDD) [49]—an underdiagnosed condition in clinical practice. The causes of this type of diaphragmatic weakness may be prolonged inactivity during mandatory or assisted mechanical ventilation (underloading, i.e., due to the use of myorelaxants or excessive positive pressure support) or an excessive workload (overloading; i.e., due to ventilator asynchrony or inadequate pressure support) [50–53]. Diaphragmatic weakness in critically ill patients in the ICU may also form part of a more general picture of acquired myopathy or polyneuropathy associated with critical illness, or it may present as a single dysfunction in patients who otherwise present no signs of multiple district involvement [54]. Histological changes (oxidative stress and proteolysis phenomena) characterize the pathophysiology of VIDD, which ultimately lead to muscle atrophy [55].

Searching for more protective ventilation

The demonstration that intrinsic damage resulted from mechanical ventilation led to the development of ventilation protocols able to prevent or at least minimize the damage caused by positive pressure ventilation. The search for improved ventilatory protocols commenced at the beginning of the 2000s, with ARDS patients in mind in particular, and it was then that the term protective ventilation was first coined. Protective ventilation initially involved a reduction in the tidal volume, an adjustment of the PEEP values to ensure the highest possible pulmonary recruitment, and a plateau pressure limit set at 30 cm H_2O [56]. Given the clinical relevance of protective ventilation, it was soon extended to the management of mechanical ventilation in the operating room. The daily application of these principles has led to the continuous refinement of lung parenchyma protection protocols—developing the concept of best PEEP, permissive hypercapnia, lung recruitment maneuvers, and, above all, driving pressure [57]. Despite the significant physiopathological rationale, standard protocols for protective ventilation have yet to be identified, mainly due to the ambiguity of the scientific literature [58].

Pressure support ventilation (PSV) is more efficient in limiting ventilator-induced diaphragmatic dysfunction compared with continuous mandatory ventilation (CMV) provided that an adequate level of support pressure and synchronization with the ventilator are maintained [52, 59]. Recently, neurally adjusted ventilator assist (NAVA®) has been introduced as a more "physiological" ventilation method that is, at least potentially, able to prevent both overload and disuse atrophy of to the diaphragm allowing early weaning [60]. NAVA delivers assistance in proportion to and in synchrony with the patient's respiratory efforts, measured as the electrical activity of the diaphragm (EAdi). In this way, it is possible to monitor the force generated by the diaphragm, which is inversely proportional to the amplitude of the electrical stimulus necessary for its contraction [61]. Di Mussi and colleagues, in a recent randomized study on patients in the ICU, compared NAVA with PSV [62]. All the diaphragmatic efficiency indexes, such as the pressure–time produced by the diaphragm, were higher in the group of patients receiving NAVA. Furthermore, episodes of asynchrony were more frequent in the PSV group.

NAVA has the advantage of improving patient–ventilator interaction, synchrony, and diaphragm contractile efficiency [52, 62, 63]; however, the neural component of ventilator-induced diaphragmatic dysfunction remains to be fully understood. Further studies are thus needed to elucidate the mechanisms involved in VIDD with the ultimate aim of developing more effective weaning strategies.

Conclusion

The ideal time and conditions for achieving successful weaning from mechanical ventilation are a hotly debated topic. As such, weaning remains a non-standardized process and an ever growing proportion of the related literature is focused on trying to identify predictive factors. A complete understanding of the underlying mechanisms responsible for weaning failure is still far from being elucidated. Numerous studies are focused on searching for the individual components involved in respiratory function that may determine weaning failure. Progress has been made though, in particular, thanks to the increasing use of ultrasound that provides real-time in vivo visualization of these components and a form of quantification.

With so many questions about the weaning process remaining open, the purpose of this two-part review was to provide a 360° view of this critical procedure, one that observes the integrated vision of both respiratory function and the most state-of-the-art predictive indexes available to date.

Abbreviations

LUS: Lung ultrasound; IMV: Invasive mechanical ventilation; ARDS: Acute respiratory distress syndrome; PEEP: Positive end-expiratory pressure; ICU: Intensive care unit; SBT: Spontaneous breathing trial; GCS: Glasgow Coma Scale; IAH: Intra-abdominal hypertension; IAP: Intra-abdominal pressure; PLEFF: Pleural effusion; VILI: Ventilator-induced lung injury; VIDD: Ventilator-induced diaphragm disfunction; PSV: Pressure support ventilation; EAdi: Electrical activity of the diaphragm; NAVA: Neurally adjusted ventilator assist.

Acknowledgements

None.

Authors' contributions

LV, GMG and AB contributed equally in writing this manuscript. All authors read and approved the final manuscript.

Author details

[1] Anesthesiology and Intensive Care Clinic, Department of Medicine, University of Udine, Via Colugna 50, 33100 Udine, Italy. [2] Department of Anesthesiology and Intensive Care, Maggiore della Carità University Hospital, Corso Mazzini 18, 28100 Novara, Italy. [3] Department of Translational Medicine, University of Eastern Piemonte, via Solaroli, 17, 28100 Novara, Italy.

References

1. Bouhemad B, Mongodi S, Via G, Rouquette I (2015) Ultrasound for "lung monitoring" of ventilated patients. Anesthesiology 122:437–447. https://doi.org/10.1097/ALN.0000000000000558
2. Via G, Storti E, Gulati G, Neri L, Mojoli F, Braschi A (2012) Lung ultrasound in the ICU: from diagnostic instrument to respiratory monitoring tool. Minerva Anestesiol 78:1282–1296
3. Bouhemad B, Liu ZH, Arbelot C, Zhang M, Ferarri F, Le-Guen M, Girard M, Lu Q, Rouby JJ (2010) Ultrasound assessment of antibiotic-induced pulmonary reaeration in ventilator-associated pneumonia. Crit Care Med 38:84–92. https://doi.org/10.1097/CCM.0b013e3181b08cdb
4. Bouhemad B, Brisson H, Le-Guen M, Arbelot C, Lu Q, Rouby JJ (2011) Bedside ultrasound assessment of positive end-expiratory pressure-induced lung recruitment. Am J Respir Crit Care Med 183:341–347. https://doi.org/10.1164/rccm.201003-0369OC
5. Stefanidis K, Dimopoulos S, Tripodaki ES, Vitzilaios K, Politis P, Piperopoulos P, Nanas S (2011) Lung sonography and recruitment in patients with early acute respiratory distress syndrome: a pilot study. Crit Care 15:R185. https://doi.org/10.1186/cc10338
6. Haddam M, Zieleskiewicz L, Perbet S, Baldovini A, Guervilly C, Arbelot C, Noel A, Vigne C, Hammad E, Antonini F, Lehingue S, Peytel E, Lu Q, Bouhemad B, Golmard JL, Langeron O, Martin C, Muller L, Rouby JJ, Constantin JM, Papazian L, Leone M, CAR'Echo Collaborative Network; AzuRea Collaborative Network (2016) Lung ultrasonography for assessment of oxygenation response to prone position ventilation in ARDS. Intensive Care Med 42:1546–1556. https://doi.org/10.1007/s00134-016-4411-7
7. Chinardet B, Brisson H, Arbelot C, Langeron O, Rouby JJ, Lu Q (2016) Ultrasound assessment of lung consolidation and reaeration after pleural effusion drainage in patients with acute respiratory distress syndrome: a pilot study. Acta Anaesthesiol Belg 67:29–35
8. Chiumello D, Mongodi S, Algieri I, Vergani GL, Orlando A, Via G, Crimella F, Cressoni M, Mojoli F (2018) Assessment of lung aeration and recruitment by CT scan and ultrasound in acute respiratory distress syndrome patients. Crit Care Med 46:1761–1768. https://doi.org/10.1097/CCM.0000000000003340
9. Bouhemad B, Mojoli F, Nowobilski N, Hussain A, Rouquette I, Guinot PG, Mongodi S (2020) Use of combined cardiac and lung ultrasound to predict weaning failure in elderly, high-risk cardiac patients: a pilot study. Intensive Care Med. https://doi.org/10.1007/s00134-019-05902-9
10. Llamas-Álvarez AM, Tenza-Lozano EM, Latour-Pérez J (2017) Diaphragm and lung ultrasound to predict weaning outcome: systematic review and meta-analysis. Chest 152:1140–1150. https://doi.org/10.1016/j.chest.2017.08.028
11. Tenza-Lozano E, Llamas-Álvarez AM, Jaimez-Navarro E, Fernandez-Sanchez J (2018) Lung and diaphragm ultrasound as predictors of success in weaning from mechanical ventilation. Crit Ultrasound J 10:12. https://doi.org/10.1186/s13089-018-0094-3
12. Soummer A, Perbet S, Brisson H, Arbelot C, Constantin JM, Lu Q, Rouby JJ, Lung Ultrasound Study Group (2012) Ultrasound assessment of lung aeration loss during a successful weaning trial predicts postextubation distress. Crit Care Med 40:2064–2072. https://doi.org/10.1097/CCM.0b013e31824e68ae
13. Jabaudon M, Perbet S, Pereira B, Soummer A, Roszyk L, Guérin R, Futier E, Lu Q, Bazin JE, Sapin V, Rouby JJ, Constantin JM (2013) Plasma levels of sRAGE, loss of aeration and weaning failure in ICU patients: a prospective observational multicenter study. PLoS ONE 8:e64083. https://doi.org/10.1371/journal.pone.0064083
14. Haji K, Haji D, Canty DJ, Royse AG, Green C, Royse CF (2018) The impact of heart, lung and diaphragmatic ultrasound on prediction of failed extubation from mechanical ventilation in critically ill patients: a prospective observational pilot study. Crit Ultrasound J 10:13. https://doi.org/10.1186/s13089-018-0096-1
15. Frassi F, Gargani L, Tesorio P, Raciti M, Mottola G, Picano E (2007) Prognostic value of extravascular lung water assessed with ultrasound lung comets by chest sonography in patients with dyspnea and/or chest pain. J Card Fail 13:830–835. https://doi.org/10.1016/j.cardfail.2007.07.003
16. Zhao Z, Jiang L, Xi X, Jiang Q, Zhu B, Wang M, Xing J, Zhang D (2015) Prognostic value of extravascular lung water assessed with lung ultrasound score by chest sonography in patients with acute respiratory distress syndrome. BMC Pulm Med 15:98. https://doi.org/10.1186/s12890-015-0091-2
17. Zou TJ, Yin MG, Qin Y, Li Y, Zeng XY, Kang Y (2017) Prognostic value of modified lung ultrasound aeration loss score in shock patient in intensive care unit. Zhonghua Yi Xue Za Zhi. 97:2244–2247. https://doi.org/10.3760/cma.j.issn.0376-2491.2017.29.002
18. Yin W, Zou T, Qin Y, Yang J, Li Y, Zeng X, Kang Y, Chinese Critical Ultrasound Study Group (CCUSG) (2019) Poor lung ultrasound score in shock patients admitted to the ICU is associated with worse outcome. BMC Pulm Med 19:1. https://doi.org/10.1186/s12890-018-0755-9
19. Lichtenstein DA, Meziere GA (2008) Relevance of lung ultrasound in the diagnosis of acute respiratory failure: the BLUE protocol. Chest 134:117–125. https://doi.org/10.1378/chest.07-2800
20. Jambrik Z, Monti S, Coppola V, Aqricola E, Mottola G, Miniati M (2004) Usefulness of ultrasound lung comets as a nonradiologic sign of extravascular lung water. Am J Cardiol 93:1265–1270. https://doi.org/10.1016/j.amjcard.2004.02.012

21. Noble VE, Murray AF, Capp R, Syivia-Reardon MH, Steele DJ, Liteplo A (2009) Ultrasound assessment for extravascular lung water in patients undergoing hemodialysis. Time course for resolution. Chest 135:1433–1439. https://doi.org/10.1378/chest.08-1811
22. Agricola E, Bove T, Oppizzi M, Marino G, Zangrillo A, Margonato A, Picano E (2005) "Ultrasound comet-tail images": a marker of pulmonary edema: a comparative study with wedge pressure and extravascular lung water. Chest 127:1690–1695. https://doi.org/10.1378/chest.127.5.1690
23. Silva S, Ait Aissa D, Cocquet P, Hoarau L, Ruiz J, Ferre F, Rousset D, Mora M, Mari A, Fourcade O, Riu B, Jaber S, Bataille B (2017) Combined thoracic ultrasound assessment during a successful weaning trial predicts postextubation distress. Anesthesiology 127:666–674. https://doi.org/10.1097/ALN.0000000000001773
24. Coplin WM, Pierson DJ, Cooley KD, Newell DW, Rubenfeld GD (2000) Implications of extubation delay in brain-injured patients meeting standard weaning criteria. Am J Respir Crit Care Med 161:1530–1536. https://doi.org/10.1164/ajrccm.161.5.9905102
25. Godet T, Chabanne R, Marin J, Kauffmann S, Futier E, Pereira B, Constantin JM (2017) Extubation failure in brain-injured patients: risk factors and development of a prediction score in a preliminary prospective cohort study. Anesthesiology 126:104–114. https://doi.org/10.1097/ALN.0000000000001379
26. McCredie VA, Ferguson ND, Pinto RL, Adhikari NK, Fowler RA, Chapman MG, Burrell A, Baker AJ, Cook DJ, Meade MO, Scales DC, Canadian Critical Care Trials Group (2017) Airway management strategies for brain-injured patients meeting standard criteria to consider extubation. A prospective cohort study. Ann Am Thorac Soc 14:85–93. https://doi.org/10.1513/AnnalsATS.201608-620OC
27. Asehnoune K, Seguin P, Lasocki S, Roquilly A, Delater A, Gros A, Denou F, Mahé PJ, Nesseler N, Demeure-Dit-Latte D, Launey Y, Lakhal K, Rozec B, Mallédant Y, Sébille V, Jaber S, Le Thuaut A, Feuillet F, Cinotti R, ATLANREA group (2017) Extubation success prediction in a multicentric cohort of patients with severe brain injury. Anesthesiology 127:338–346. https://doi.org/10.1097/ALN.0000000000001725
28. Pelosi P, Ferguson ND, Frutos-Vivar F, Anzueto A, Putensen C, Raymondos K, Apezteguia C, Desmery P, Hurtado J, Abroug F, Elizalde J, Tomicic V, Cakar N, Gonzalez M, Arabi Y, Moreno R, Esteban A, for the Ventila Study Group (2011) Management and outcome of mechanically ventilated neurologic patients. Crit Care Med 39:1482–1492. https://doi.org/10.1097/CCM.0b013e31821209a8
29. Kirkpatrick AW, Sugrue M, McKee JL, Pereira BM, Roberts DJ, De Waele JJ, Leppaniemi A, Ejike JC, Reintam Blaser A, D'Amours S, De Keulenaer B, Malbrain MLNG (2017) Update from the abdominal compartment society (WSACS) on intra-abdominal hypertension and abdominal compartment syndrome: past, present, and future beyond Banff 2017. Anaesthesiol Intensive Ther 49:83–87. https://doi.org/10.5603/AIT.a2017.0019
30. Malbrain ML, Cheatham ML, Kirkpatrick A, Sugrue M, De Waele J, Ivatury R (2006) Abdominal compartment syndrome: it's time to pay attention! Intensive Care Med 32:1912–1914. https://doi.org/10.1007/s00134-006-0303-6
31. Malbrain ML, Chiumello D, Pelosi P, Bihari D, Innes R, Ranieri VM (2005) Incidence and prognosis of intraabdominal hypertension in a mixed population of critically ill patients: a multiple-center epidemiological study. Crit Care Med 33:315–322. https://doi.org/10.1097/01.ccm.0000153408.09806.1b
32. Cheatham ML, Safcsak K (2010) Is the evolving management of intra-abdominal hypertension and abdominal compartment syndrome improving survival? Crit Care Med 38:402–407. https://doi.org/10.1097/ccm.0b013e3181b9e9b1
33. Pelosi P, Quintel M, Malbrain ML (2007) Effect of intra-abdominal pressure on respiratory mechanics. Acta Clin Belg Suppl 1:78–88
34. Gattinoni L, Carlesso E, Brazzi L, Caironi P (2010) Positive end expiratory pressure. Curr Opin Crit Care 16:39–44. https://doi.org/10.1097/MCC.0b013e3283354723
35. Malbrain ML, DeWaele J (2013) Intra-abdominal Hypertension. Cambridge University Press, Cambridge
36. Verzilii D, Constantin JM, Sebbane M, Chanques G, Jung B, Perrigault PF, Malbrain ML, Jaber S (2010) Positive end expiratory pressure effects the value of intra-abdominal pressure in acute lung injury/acute respiratory distress syndrome patients: a pilot study. Crit Care 14:137–142. https://doi.org/10.1186/cc9193
37. Murtaza G, Inam PI KM, Nawaz Jajja MR, Nawaz Z, Koondhar R, Nasim S (2015) Intra abdominal hypertension; incidence, prevalence and outcomes in a mixed intensive care unit: prospective cohort study. Int J Surg 19:67–71. https://doi.org/10.1016/j.ijsu.2015.05.014
38. Brogi E, Gargani L, Bignami E, Barbariol F, Marra A, Forfori F, Vetrugno L (2017) Thoracic ultrasound for pleural effusion in the intensive care unit: a narrative review from diagnosis to treatment. Crit Care 21:325. https://doi.org/10.1186/s13054-017-1897-5
39. Vetrugno L, Bignami E, Orso D, Vargas M, Guadagnin GM, Saglietti F, Servillo G, Volpicelli G, Navalesi P, Bove T (2019) Utility of pleural effusion drainage in the ICU: an updated systematic review and META-analysis. J Crit Care 52:22–32. https://doi.org/10.1016/j.jcrc.2019.03.007
40. Dres M, Roux D, Pham T, Beurton A, Ricard JD, Fartoukh M, Demoule A (2017) Prevalence and impact on weaning of pleural effusion at the time of liberation from mechanical ventilation: a multicenter prospective observational study. Anesthesiology 126(6):1107–1115. https://doi.org/10.1097/ALN.0000000000001621
41. Vetrugno L, Guadagnin GM, Barbariol F, D'Incà S, Delrio S, Orso D, Girometti R, Volpicelli G, Bove T (2019) Assessment of pleural effusion and small pleural drain insertion by resident doctors in an intensive care unit: an observational study. Clin Med Insights Circ Respir Pulm Med 13:1179548419871527. https://doi.org/10.1177/1179548419871527
42. Vetrugno L, Guadagnin GM, Orso D, Boero E, Bignami E, Bove T (2018) An easier and safe affair, pleural drainage with ultrasound in critical patient: a technical note. Crit Ultrasound J. 10:18. https://doi.org/10.1186/s13089-018-0098-z
43. Albert RK (2012) The role of ventilation-induced surfactant dysfunction and atelectasis in causing acute respiratory distress syndrome. Am J Respir Crit Care Med 185:702–708. https://doi.org/10.1164/rccm.201109-1667PP
44. Tremblay LN, Slutsky AS (1998) Ventilator-induced injury: from barotrauma to biotrauma. Proc Assoc Am Physicians 110:482–488
45. Parker JC, Hernandez LA, Peevy KJ (1993) Mechanisms of ventilator-induced lung injury. Crit Care Med 21:131–143. https://doi.org/10.1097/00003246-199301000-00024
46. Taskar V, John J, Evander E, Robertson B, Jonson B (1997) Surfactant dysfunction makes lungs vulnerable to repetitive collapse and reexpansion. Am J Respir Crit Care Med 155:313–320. https://doi.org/10.1164/ajrccm.155.1.9001330
47. Tonetti T, Vasques F, Rapetti F, Maiolo G, Collino F, Romitti F, Camporota L, Cressoni M, Cadringher P, Quintel M, Gattinoni L (2017) Driving pressure and mechanical power: new targets for VILI prevention. Ann Transl Med. 5:286. https://doi.org/10.21037/atm.2017.07.08
48. Heyland DK, Cook DJ, Griffith L, Keenan SP, Brun-Buisson C (1999) The attributable morbidity and mortality of ventilator associated pneumonia in the critically ill patient. The canadian critical care trials group. Am J Respir Crit Care Med 159:1249–1256. https://doi.org/10.1164/ajrccm.159.4.9807050
49. Vassilakopoulos T, Petrof BJ (2004) Ventilator-induced diaphragmatic dysfunction. Am J Respir Crit Care Med 169:336–341. https://doi.org/10.1164/rccm.200304-489CP
50. Cammarota G, Sguazzotti I, Zanoni M, Messina A, Colombo D, Vignazia GL, Vetrugno L, Garofalo E, Bruni A, Navalesi P, Avanzi GC, Della Corte F, Volpicelli G, Vaschetto R (2019) Diaphragmatic ultrasound assessment in subjects with acute hypercapnic respiratory failure admitted to the emergency department. Respir Care 64:1469–1477. https://doi.org/10.4187/respcare.06803
51. Goligher EC, Dres M, Fan E, Rubenfeld GD, Scales DC, Herridge MS, Vorona S, Sklar MC, Rittayamai N, Lanys A, Murray A, Brace D, Urrea C, Reid WD, Tomlinson G, Slutsky AS, Kavanagh BP, Brochard LJ, Ferguson ND (2018) Mechanical ventilation-induced diaphragm atrophy strongly impacts clinical outcomes. Am J Respir Crit Care Med 197:204–213. https://doi.org/10.1164/rccm.201703-0536OC
52. Bruni A, Garofalo E, Pelaia C, Messina A, Cammarota G, Murabito P, Corrado S, Vetrugno L, Longhini F, Navalesi P (2019) Patient-ventilator asynchrony in adult critically ill patients. Minerva Anestesiol 85:676–688. https://doi.org/10.23736/S0375-9393.19.13436-0

53. Vetrugno L, Guadagnin GM, Barbariol F, Langiano N, Zangrillo A, Bove T (2019) Ultrasound imaging for diaphragm dysfunction: a narrative literature review. J Cardiothorac Vasc Anesth 33:2525–2536. https://doi.org/10.1053/j.jvca.2019.01.003
54. Santos PD, Teixeira C, Savi A, Maccari JG, Neres FS, Machado AS, de Oliveira RP, Ribeiro M, Rotta FT (2012) The critical illness polyneuropathy in septic patients with prolonged weaning from mechanical ventilation: is the diaphragm also affected? A pilot study. Respir Care 57:1594. https://doi.org/10.4187/respcare.01396
55. Levine S, Nguyen T, Taylor N, Friscia ME, Budak MT, Rothenberg P, Zhu J, Sachdeva R, Sonnad S, Kaiser LR, Rubinstein NA, Powers SK, Shrager JB (2008) Rapid disuse atrophy of diaphragm fibers in mechanically ventilated humans. N Engl J Med 358:1327–1335. https://doi.org/10.1056/NEJMoa070447
56. Network The Acute Respiratory Distress Syndrome, Brower RG, Matthay MA, Morris A, Schoenfeld D, Thompson BT, Wheeler A (2000) Ventilation with lower tidal volumes as compared with traditional tidal volumes for acute lung injury and the acute respiratory distress syndrome. N Engl J Med 342:1301–1308. https://doi.org/10.1056/NEJM200005043421801
57. Neto AS, Hemmes SN, Barbas CS, Beiderlinden M, Fernandez-Bustamante A, Futier E, Gajic O, El-Tahan MR, Ghamdi AA, Günay E, Jaber S, Kokulu S, Kozian A, Licker M, Lin WQ, Maslow AD, Memtsoudis SG, Reis Miranda D, Moine P, Ng T, Paparella D, Ranieri VM, Scavonetto F, Schilling T, Selmo G, Severgnini P, Sprung J, Sundar S, Talmor D, Treschan T, Unzueta C, Weingarten TN, Wolthuis EK, Wrigge H, Amato MB, Costa EL, de Abreu MG, Pelosi P, Schultz MJ, PROVE Network Investigators (2016) Association between driving pressure and development of postoperative pulmonary complications in patients undergoing mechanical ventilation for general anaesthesia: a meta-analysis of individual patient data. Lancet Respir Med. 4:272–280. https://doi.org/10.1016/S2213-2600(16)00057-6
58. Writing Group for the Alveolar Recruitment for Acute Respiratory Distress Syndrome Trial (ART) Investigators, Cavalcanti AB, Suzumura ÉA, Laranjeira LN, Paisani DM, Damiani LP, Guimarães HP, Romano ER, Regenga MM, Taniguchi LNT, Teixeira C, Pinheiro de Oliveira R, Machado FR, Diaz-Quijano FA, Filho MSA, Maia IS, Caser EB, Filho WO, Borges MC, Martins PA, Matsui M, Ospina-Tascón GA, Giancursi TS, Giraldo-Ramirez ND, Vieira SRR, Assef MDGPL, Hasan MS, Szczeklik W, Rios F, Amato MBP, Berwanger O, Ribeiro de Carvalho CR (2017) Effect of lung recruitment and titrated positive end-expiratory pressure (PEEP) vs low PEEP on mortality in patients with acute respiratory distress syndrome: a randomized clinical trial. JAMA 318:1335–1345. https://doi.org/10.1001/jama.2017.14171
59. Hudson MB, Smuder AJ, Nelson WB, Bruells CS, Levine S, Powers SK (2012) Both high level pressure support ventilation and controlled mechanical ventilation induce diaphragm dysfunction and atrophy. Crit Care Med 40:1254–1260. https://doi.org/10.1097/CCM.0b013e31823c8cc9
60. Lamouret O, Crognier L, Vardon Bounes F, Conil JM, Dilasser C, Raimondi T, Ruiz S, Rouget A, Delmas C, Seguin T, Minville V, Georges B (2019) Neurally adjusted ventilator assist (NAVA) versus pressure support ventilation: patient-ventilator interaction during invasive ventilation delivered by tracheostomy. Crit Care 23:2. https://doi.org/10.1186/s13054-018-2288-2
61. Barwing J, Pedroni C, Olgemöller U, Quintel M, Moerer O (2013) Electrical activity of the diaphragm (EAdi) as a monitoring parameter in difficult weaning from respirator: a pilot study. Crit Care 17:R182. https://doi.org/10.1186/cc12865
62. Di Mussi R, Spadaro S, Mirabella L, Volta CA, Serio G, Staffieri F, Dambrosio M, Cinnella G, Bruno F, Grasso S (2016) Impact of prolonged assisted ventilation on diaphragmatic efficiency: NAVA versus PSV. Crit Care 20:1. https://doi.org/10.1186/s13054-015-1178-0
63. Garofalo E, Bruni A, Pelaia C, Liparota L, Lombardo N, Longhini F, Navalesi P (2018) Recognizing, quantifying and managing patient-ventilator asynchrony in invasive and noninvasive ventilation. Expert Rev Respir Med 12:557–567. https://doi.org/10.1080/17476348.2018.1480941

21

Longitudinal remotely mentored self-performed lung ultrasound surveillance of paucisymptomatic Covid-19 patients at risk of disease progression

Andrew W. Kirkpatrick[1,2,4,5,6*], Jessica L. McKee[5,6] and John M. Conly[3,4]

Abstract

COVID-19 has impacted human life globally and threatens to overwhelm health-care resources. Infection rates are rapidly rising almost everywhere, and new approaches are required to both prevent transmission, but to also monitor and rescue infected and at-risk patients from severe complications. Point-of-care lung ultrasound has received intense attention as a cost-effective technology that can aid early diagnosis, triage, and longitudinal follow-up of lung health. Detecting pleural abnormalities in previously healthy lungs reveal the beginning of lung inflammation eventually requiring mechanical ventilation with sensitivities superior to chest radiographs or oxygen saturation monitoring. Using a paradigm first developed for space-medicine known as Remotely Telementored Self-Performed Ultrasound (RTSPUS), motivated patients with portable smartphone support ultrasound probes can be guided completely remotely by a remote lung imaging expert to longitudinally follow the health of their own lungs. Ultrasound probes can be couriered or even delivered by drone and can be easily sterilized or dedicated to one or a commonly exposed cohort of individuals. Using medical outreach supported by remote vital signs monitoring and lung ultrasound health surveillance would allow clinicians to follow and virtually lay hands upon many at-risk paucisymptomatic patients. Our initial experiences with such patients are presented, and we believe present a paradigm for an evolution in rich home-monitoring of the many patients expected to become infected and who threaten to overwhelm resources if they must all be assessed in person by at-risk care providers.

Introduction

COVID-19 has fundamentally impacted all aspects of human life in 2020. As of December 6 2020, the World Health Organization reported that there had been over 66 million confirmed cases of COVID-19, including 1,523,583 deaths [1], although there may be many more fold cases globally. Globally, various countries and health systems are facing uncertain resource challenges that threaten to overwhelm the capacity to properly care for all citizens. Although very infectious, COVID-19 is very variable in its virulence, being most harmful in older patients, especially those residing in long-term care facilities and having co-morbidities such as hypertension, heart disease, diabetes, and chronic respiratory and kidney diseases [2]. Statistically, young healthy people are still at low risk for progression to severe life-threatening disease and most will experience only mild symptoms and recover by self-isolating at home. However, a small number of such people will deteriorate and become precipitously sick often presenting with advanced pneumonia despite the absence of severe dyspnea due to unique features of the COVID-19 virus. The key to balancing not overwhelming hospital resources, yet still avoiding

*Correspondence: andrew.kirkpatrick@ahs.ca

[1] Department of Critical Care Medicine, Foothills Medical Centre, Calgary, Alberta, Canada

Full list of author information is available at the end of the article

tragedies, has been stated to employ outreach resources, and being quickly recognizing those few isolated patients who are at risk of deterioration, and "rescuing" them quickly with an aggressive and comprehensive response [3, 4].

The diagnosis of COVID-19 typically relies upon PCR-testing, which unfortunately may have significant false-negative test characteristics. Thus early chest computed tomography (CT) has been recommended as a screening tool for suspected COVID-19 patients with better sensitivity than PCR [5], but this is clearly an impractical solution for home-monitoring. However, interest in using lung ultrasound to diagnose, risk stratify, and manage COVID-19 pneumonia has exploded in the emergency and in-hospital settings, as the distinctive pathological findings of an irregular pleural interface, interstitial "comet-tail" artifacts, and sub-pleural consolidations, are typically peripheral and well seen and quantified by ultrasound [3, 6–9]. An International Panel of Experts recently recommended using tele-ultrasound for remote guidance and consultations in COVID-19 [10]. We fully agree, and further believe that lung ultrasound examinations can be provided to willing self-isolating infected and at-risk patients using informatic technologies to facilitate self-lung ultrasound surveillance [3, 11].

Remotely telementored self-performed ultrasound (RTSPUS)

Remotely Telementored Self-Performed Ultrasound (RTSPUS) is an innovative technique that was first described as a solution to providing medical imaging onboard the International Space Station, wherein astronauts were guided from earth to image their own bodies under the direction of terrestrial ultrasound experts [12]. We believe that RTSPUS may be an invaluable tool to monitor those at risk of COVID-19 progression while maintaining self-isolation and quarantine, thus preventing any viral transmission and protecting health-care workers and other members of the community. We further believe that almost any anatomical body location that can be reached by a person is amenable to mentored self-ultrasound. In the context of screening for complications of COVID however, infected and at-risk patients are guided to attempt the standardized COVID-19 lung ultrasound examination protocol of Soldati [6]. This examination involves 14 distinct locations (7 per lung; 3 posterior, 2 lateral, and 2 anterior) and is more detailed than many standard examinations that focus solely on the anterolateral chest. As with any ultrasound examination, the exam does not have to be limited to these anatomic locations and may be tailored as a user sees fit. It has also been suggested that the baseline LUS examination includes as many rib spaces as possible so that comparisons can be made as a change from the baseline. Using the RTSPUS technique, the patient is asked to demonstrate the visceral–parietal pleural interface which is viewed and evaluated remotely by the expert clinician, which allows the clinician to detect early deterioration in lung health. For each of the anatomic lung locations, the patient was guided to self-image until the remote mentor was confident that the adequate pleural imaging was captured [13], which included additional imaging with M-mode and Color Power Doppler capturing both the "Seashore [14]" and "Powerslide signs [15]". While pneumothorax has been reported as a primary complication of COVID-19 [16], they are still rare in a healthy paucisymptomatic population, and these additional signs may not be necessary or practical for widespread adoption of RTSPUS. It should be emphasized that the use of both M-mode and color power Doppler are not typically required to diagnose COVID-19 pneumonia, but were the personal preference of the remote mentor who easily controlled the knobology of the exam remotely.

Technology

Sterilized ultra-portable economical ultrasound probes interfacing with the patients own smartphones or computing devices can be delivered to patients by any means including commercial couriers and even unmanned aerial vehicles. Thereafter, the informatics can be easily provided using off-the-shelf technologies widely available on a global basis. For example, in our experience, the ultra-portable Philips L12-4 broadband linear array transducer (Philips Company, Eindhoven, Netherlands), attached to a Samsung Galaxy Tablet A (Samsung Corporation, Suwon, Korea), communicating with a remote expert using Zoom Teleconferencing (Zoom, Hillsboro, OH) through a standard smartphone (Samsung Galaxy S20 5G, Samsung Corporation, Suwon, Korea) and with remote mentor control of the ultrasound knobology using the Teamviewer real-time remote access and support software (Teamviewer, Göppingen, Germany), provided a simple off-the-shelf communications package to readily facilitate RTSPUS.

Patient eligibility

Any conscious motivated patient who is not in severe respiratory distress and able and willing to follow instructions from a remote mentor is a candidate to participate in a remotely guided self-performed home-surveillance lung program. Musculoskeletal limitations of the arms may be a relative contraindication to performing a complete thoracic evaluation of the back, although recent studies have emphasized examinations limited to the anterior chest, with the most relevant areas of surveillance being the most accessible anterior lung segments in a study performed on hospitalized patients [17].

Current experience

We are currently conducting a prospective study describing the accuracy and logistics of augmenting RTSPUS to the routine surveillance of paucisymptomatic and at-risk COVID-19 patients. However, the practicality of this approach became dramatically apparent during the recent re-evaluation of our initial self-isolating and healthy volunteers after one of these subjects became infected with COVID-19. Neither subject had ever held an ultrasound prior to agreeing to be remotely mentored. Nevertheless, multiple and complete longitudinal RTSPUS examinations were easily accomplished using widely available cellular phone services, with seamless demonstrations of the pleural anatomy of both the infected patient, and the at-risk partner, during pre- and post-COVID infection examinations (Figs. 1, 2, 3, 4 and 5; Additional files 1, 2, 3, 4 and 5). Fortunately, the infected patient made a complete recovery without requiring hospitalization and testing negative by PCR, and the spouse remained well and PCR negative corresponding to their normal lung ultrasound examinations.

Potential limitations

It should be understood that at all times this is an additive adjunct to home surveillance which otherwise consists of symptom and standard vital signs monitoring [4]. At all times the responsible supervising clinician may decide to request formal hospital evaluation of a self-isolating patient and the remote lung ultrasound expert is responsible for quality control in interpretation of the self-generated images. Studies have shown, however, that lung ultrasound is superior to either O_2 saturation or CXR in predicting the future occurrence of adverse outcomes including a requirement for mechanical ventilation and death [17]. The only potential harm envisioned would be if pleural ultrasound findings were falsely interpreted as normal when they were not, but lung ultrasound for COVID has demonstrated an extremely high sensitivity for detecting such abnormalities, which is information that would be unknown if this paradigm was not considered. The high-frequency linear probe utilized optimized the ultrasound images from the pleural interface, but may not be ideal for deeper penetration to detect pathology

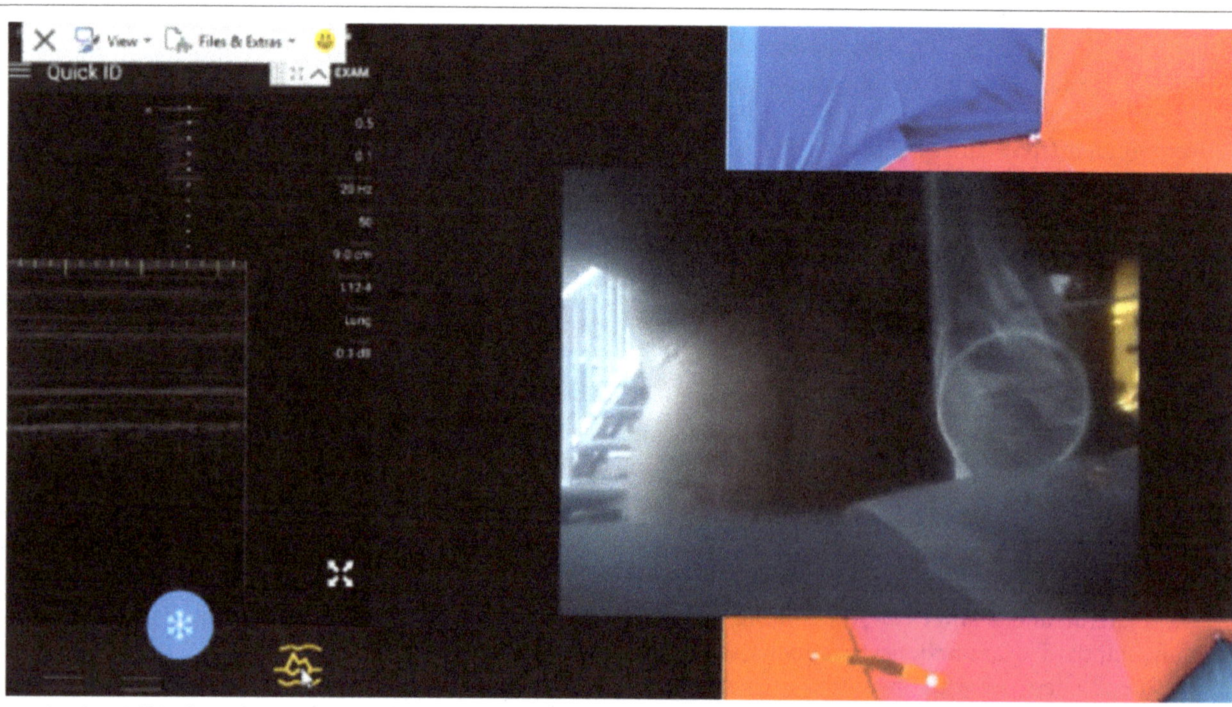

Fig. 1 Baseline Self-Performed Lung Ultrasound Study of 32-year-old patient 6 months prior to COVID-19 diagnosis. Screenshot of the Remote Mentors Computer Screen that shows the patient imaging himself to the right of the screen and the resultant ultrasound image showing the "seashore" sign to the left. As lung ultrasound is a dynamic real-time examination hard to capture in any single image, readers are strongly encouraged to view the accompanying supplemental videos of the entire examination online to gain a true appreciation of the technique

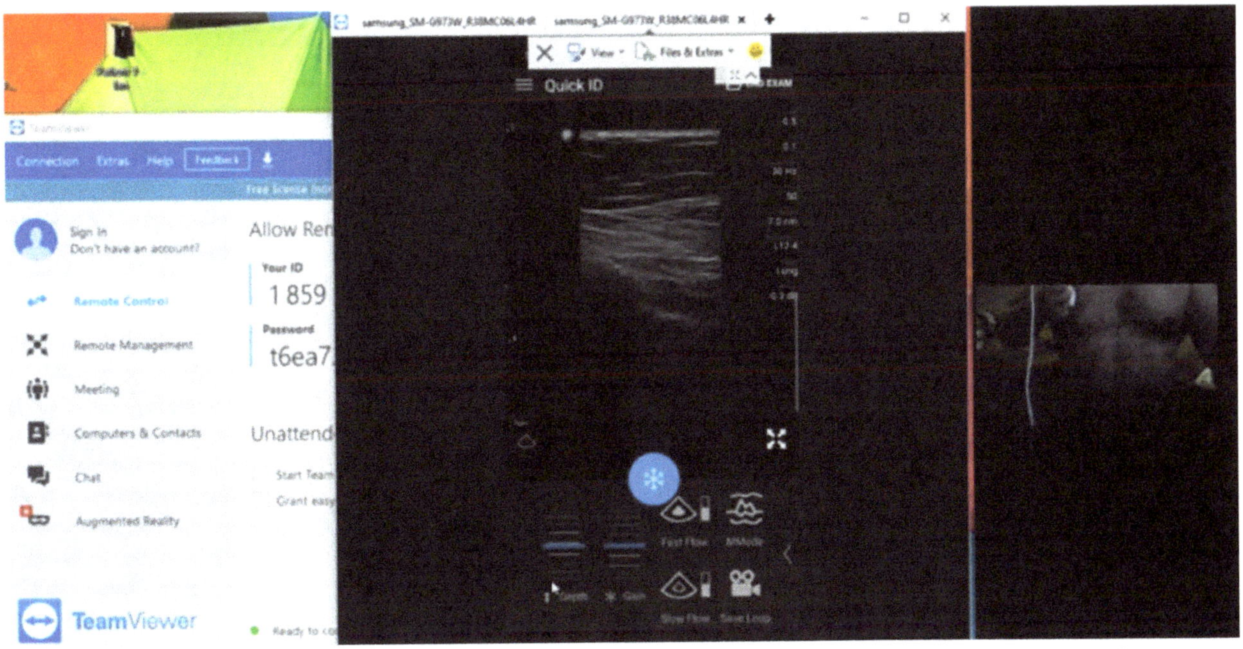

Fig. 2 First follow-up Self-Performed Lung Ultrasound Study of 32-year-old patient 2 weeks after COVID-19 diagnosis. Screenshot of the Remote Mentors Computer Screen that shows the patient imaging himself to the right of the screen and the resultant ultrasound image showing the "batwing" sign to the left. As lung ultrasound is a dynamic real-time examination hard to capture in any single image, readers are strongly encouraged to view the accompanying supplemental videos of the entire examination online to gain a true appreciation of the technique

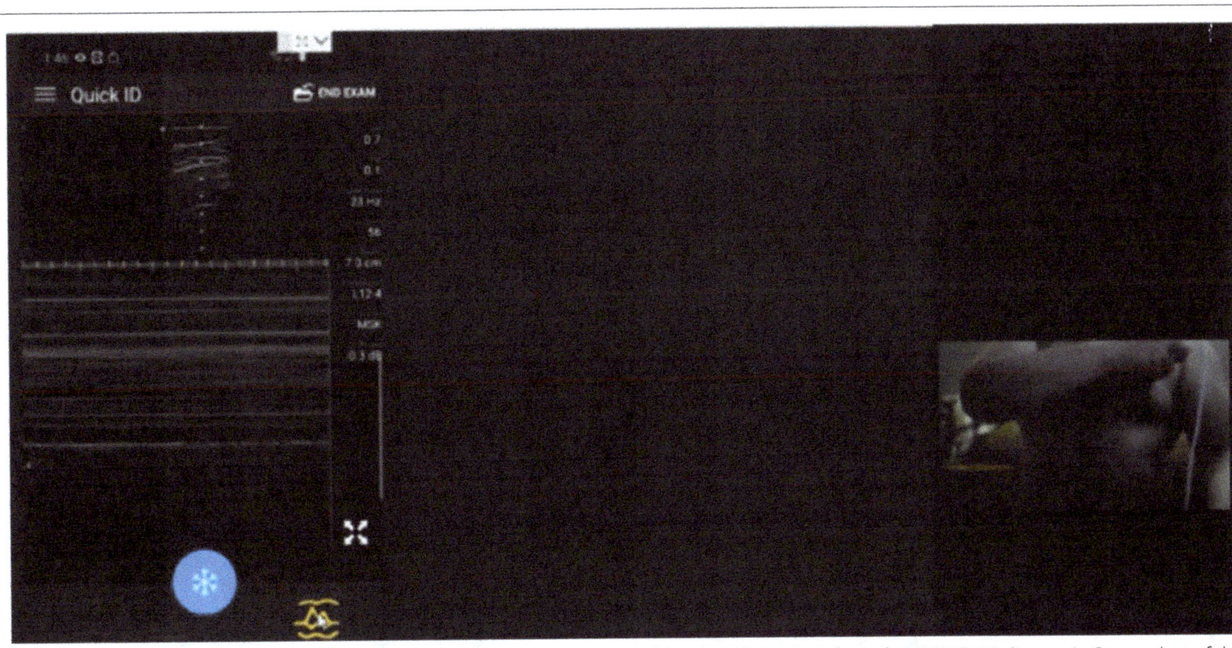

Fig. 3 Second follow-up Self-Performed Lung Ultrasound Study of 32-year-old patient 2 weeks 2 days after COVID-19 diagnosis. Screenshot of the Remote Mentors Computer Screen that shows the patient imaging himself to the right of the screen and the resultant ultrasound image showing the "seashore" sign to the left. As lung ultrasound is a dynamic real-time examination hard to capture in any single image, readers are strongly encouraged to view the accompanying supplemental videos of the entire examination online to gain a true appreciation of the technique

within the lung or pleural effusions. Other probe selection may optimize this and may warrant further evaluation. The suggested protocol used in this study involved self-scanning posteriorly. Other focused ultrasound examinations for COVID-19 do not require a detailed examination of the back and may be easier for people

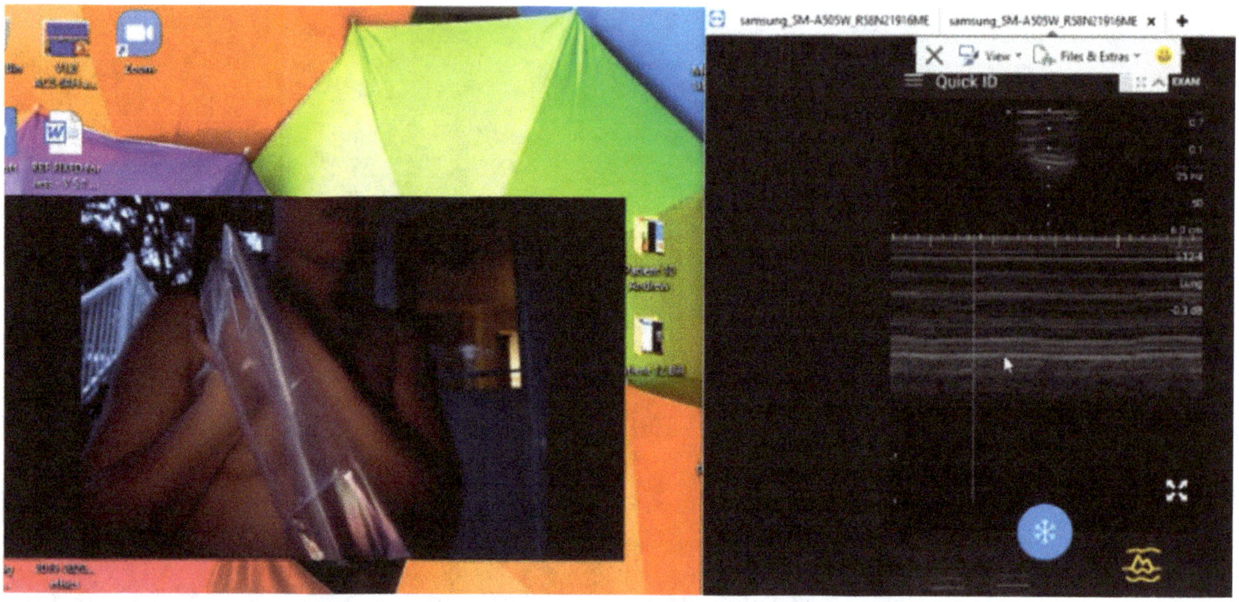

Fig. 4 Baseline Self-Performed Lung Ultrasound Study of 31-year-old potentially exposed patient-spouse 6 months prior to patient COVID-19 Diagnosis. Screenshot of the Remote Mentors Computer Screen that shows the patient imaging herself to the left of the screen and the resultant ultrasound image showing the "seashore" sign to the right. As lung ultrasound is a dynamic real-time examination hard to capture in any single image, readers are strongly encouraged to view the accompanying supplemental videos of the entire examination online to gain a true appreciation of the technique

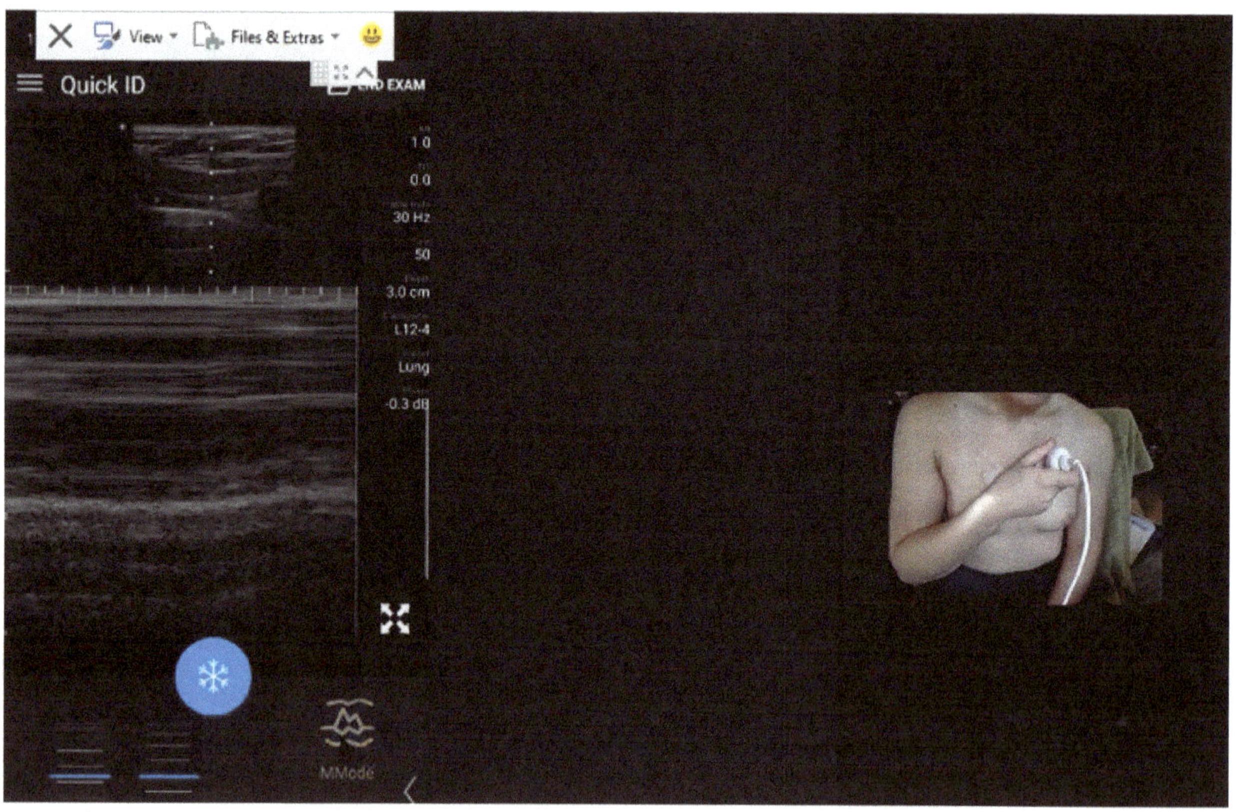

Fig. 5 First follow-up Self-Performed Lung Ultrasound Study of 31-year-old potentially exposed patient-spouse 2 weeks after patients COVID-19 Diagnosis. Screenshot of the Remote Mentors Computer Screen that shows the patient imaging herself to the right of the screen and the resultant ultrasound image showing the "seashore" sign to the left. As lung ultrasound is a dynamic real-time examination hard to capture in any single image, readers are strongly encouraged to view the accompanying supplemental videos of the entire examination online to gain a true appreciation of the technique

to be mentored through [17–19]. Only future detailed studies of test-performance characteristics will inform as to whether there is one ideal lung ultrasound examination protocol, but we suspect any and all use of lung ultrasound will benefit patients versus not using this modality. Finally, while the RTSPUS is an example of a method which a completely self-isolating person or one living alone could perform, we also recognize that other self-isolating family members could be mentored to assist or perform the examination on their partners or family as well.

Future expectations

RTSPUS may potentially revolutionize home-self monitoring for complications of COVID-19. With this paradigm, remote subject matter experts in both infectious diseases and remote tele-ultrasound can easily conference [4, 20], to give at-risk self-isolating patients pleural examinations that will identify those with complicated COVID-19 pneumonia, thus facilitating rapid and early transport to hospital for detailed assessment. Thus, the majority of self-isolating paucisymptomatic infected and asymptomatic at-risk patients can be both better monitored and reassured while completely protecting health-care providers from infection, and reducing the hospital system exposure for these patients to zero until it is deemed necessary that they "enter the hospital".

Supplementary Information

Additional file 1: Video of baseline self-performed lung ultrasound study of 32-year-old patient 6 months prior to COVID-19 Diagnosis.

Additional file 2: Video of first follow-up self-performed lung ultrasound study of 32-year-old patient 2 weeks after COVID-19 Diagnosis.

Additional file 3: Video of second follow-up self-performed lung ultrasound study of 32-year-old patient 2 weeks 2 days after COVID-19 Diagnosis.

Additional file 4: Video of baseline self-performed lung ultrasound study of 31-year-old spouse 6 months prior to patients COVID-19 Diagnosis.

Additional file 5: Video of first follow-up self-performed lung ultrasound study of 31-year-old spouse 6 months prior to patients COVID-19 Diagnosis.

Acknowledgements

The authors would like to thank Ryan and Jill Beuhler for graciously assisting with the collection of data. The authors would also like to acknowledge Dr Douglas R Hamilton and Dr Irene Ma for guidance on background research and advanced paradigms of care on and above the earth.

Authors' contributions

AWK made substantial contributions to the conception and design of the work; and the acquisition, analysis, and interpretation of data; and drafted the work and substantively revised it and approved the submitted version and agreed both to be personally accountable for the author's own contributions and to ensure that questions related to the accuracy or integrity of any part of the work, even ones in which the author was not personally involved, are appropriately investigated, resolved, and the resolution documented in the literature. JLM made substantial contributions to the conception and design of the work; and the acquisition, analysis, and interpretation of data; and approved the submitted version and agreed both to be personally accountable for the author's own contributions and to ensure that questions related to the accuracy or integrity of any part of the work, even ones in which the author was not personally involved, are appropriately investigated, resolved, and the resolution documented in the literature. JMC made substantial contributions to the conception and design of the work and interpretation of data and approved the submitted version and agreed both to be personally accountable for the author's own contributions and to ensure that questions related to the accuracy or integrity of any part of the work, even ones in which the author was not personally involved, are appropriately investigated, resolved, and the resolution documented in the literature. All authors read and approved the final manuscript.

Authors' information

Andrew W Kirkpatrick, is a Professor of Critical Care Medicine and Surgery at the University of Calgary. He is also the Director of the TeleMentored Ultrasound Supported Medical Interventions (TMUSMI) Research Group. He has been performing lung ultrasound for over 20 years initiated in collaboration with the National Aeronautics and Space Administration, and has published some of the seminal work in this topic.

Jessica L McKee, is the Project Manager for the TMUSMI Research Group at the University of Calgary among many other affiliations and responsibilities, with many years of experience in the efficient conduct and publication of research and an extensive publication record.

John M Conly, is a Professor and former head of the Department of Medicine at the University of Calgary, an Order of Canada Recipient, Medical Director for the W21C Research and Innovation Centre (W21C), and Co-Director for the Snyder Institute for Chronic Diseases at the University of Calgary, and a member of the WHO Advisory Group on Integrated Surveillance of Antimicrobial Resistance among innumerable other honors.

Author details

[1] Department of Critical Care Medicine, Foothills Medical Centre, Calgary, Alberta, Canada. [2] Department of Surgery, Foothills Medical Centre, Calgary, Alberta, Canada. [3] Department of Medicine, Foothills Medical Centre, Calgary, Alberta, Canada. [4]Synder Institute for Chronic Diseases, Foothills Medical Centre, Calgary, Alberta, Canada. [5]Trauma Program, University of Calgary and Alberta Health Services, Foothills Medical Centre, Calgary, Alberta, Canada. [6] Tele-Mentored Ultrasound Supported Medical Interventions (TMUSMI) Research Group, Foothills Medical Centre, Calgary, Alberta, Canada.

References

1. World Health Organization. WHO Coronavirus Disease (COVID-19) Dashboard: World Health Organization; 2020 [updated Dec 6 2020; cited 2020 December 6 2020]. https://covid19.who.int/.
2. Shahid Z, Kalayanamitra R, McClafferty B, Kepko D, Ramgobin D, Patel R et al (2020) COVID-19 and older adults: What we know. J Am Geriatr Soc 68(5):926–929
3. Kirkpatrick AW, McKee JL, Volpicelli G, Ma IWY (2020) The potential for remotely mentored patient-performed home self-monitoring for new onset alveolar-interstitial lung disease. Telemed J E Health 26(10):1304–1307
4. Nacoti M, Ciocca A, Giupponi A, Brambillasca P, Lussana F, Pisano M, et al. At the Epicenter of the Covid-19 Pandemic and Humanitarian Crises in Italy: Changing Perspectives on Preparation and Mitigation. Innovations in Care Delivery. 2020.
5. Fang Y, Zhang H, Xie J, Lin M, Ying L, Pang P et al (2020) Sensitivity of chest CT for COVID-19: comparison to RT-PCR. Radiology 296:E115
6. Soldati G, Smargiassi A, Inchingolo R, Buonsenso D, Perrone T, Briganti DF et al (2020) Proposal for International Standardization of the Use of Lung Ultrasound for Patients With COVID-19: A Simple, Quantitative. Reproducible Method J Ultrasound Med 39(7):1413–1419

7. Gargani L, Soliman-Aboumarie H, Volpicelli G, Corradi F, Pastore MC, Cameli M (2020) Why, when, and how to use lung ultrasound during the COVID-19 pandemic: enthusiasm and caution. Eur Heart J Cardiovasc Imaging 21(9):941–948
8. Volpicelli G, Gargani L (2020) Sonographic signs and patterns of COVID-19 pneumonia. Ultrasound J 12(1):22
9. Volpicelli G, Gargani L, Perlini S, Spinelli S, Barbieri G, Lanotte A et al (2021) Lung ultrasound for the early diagnosis of COVID-19 pneumonia: an international multicenter study. Intensive Care Med 47:444
10. Hussain A, Via G, Melniker L, Goffi A, Tavazzi G, Neri L et al (2020) Multi-organ point-of-care ultrasound for COVID-19 (PoCUS4COVID): international expert consensus. Crit Care 24(1):702
11. Kirkpatrick AW, McKee JL (2020) Lung ultrasonography in a woman with COVID-19: This examination could be remote. CMAJ 192(16):E435
12. Sargsyan AE, Hamilton DR, Jones JA, Melton S, Whitson PA, Kirkpatrick AW et al (2005) FAST at MACH 20: clinical ultrasound aboard the International Space Station. J Trauma 58(1):35–39
13. Volpicelli G, Elbarbary M, Blaivas M, Lichtenstein DA, Mathis G, Kirkpatrick AW et al (2012) International evidence-based recommendations for point-of-care lung ultrasound. Intensive Care Med 38(4):577–591
14. Lichtenstein DA, Meziere GA (2008) Relevance of lung ultrasound in the diagnosis of acute respiratory failure: the BLUE protocol. Chest 134(1):117–125
15. Cunningham J, Kirkpatrick AW, Nicolaou S, Liu D, Hamilton DR, Lawless B et al (2002) Enhanced recognition of "lung sliding" with power color Doppler imaging in the diagnosis of pneumothorax. J Trauma 52(4):769–771
16. Martinelli AW, Ingle T, Newman J, Nadeem I, Jackson K, Lane ND, et al. COVID-19 and pneumothorax: a multicentre retrospective case series. Eur Respir J. 2020.
17. Lichter Y, Topilsky Y, Taieb P, Banai A, Hochstadt A, Merdler I et al (2020) Lung ultrasound predicts clinical course and outcomes in COVID-19 patients. Intensive Care Med 46(10):1873–1883
18. Yang Y, Anstey J, Yastrebov K, Nanjayya VB, Orde S, Nalos M et al (2020) COVID-US: A simplified approach to cardiopulmonary ultrasound in suspected and confirmed COVID-19 patients in surge crisis. Australas J Ultrasound Med 23(2):96–102
19. Lichtenstein DA, Meziere GA (2008) Relevance of lung ultrasound in the diagnosis of acute respiratory distress. Chest 134:117
20. Netzer I, Kirkpatrick AW, Nissan M, McKee JL, McBeth P, Dobron A et al (2019) Rubrum Coelis: The Contribution of real-time telementoring in acute trauma scenarios-a randomized controlled trial. Telemed J E Health 25:1108

22

Mean value of B-mode optic nerve sheath diameter as an indicator of increased intracranial pressure

Lisandro Montorfano[1], Qian Yu[1], Stephen J. Bordes[1], Shankarapryan Sivanushanthan[2], Raul J. Rosenthal[1] and Miguel Montorfano[3*]

Abstract

Objectives: Timely diagnosis and treatment of increased intracranial pressure can decrease morbidity and prevent mortality. The present meta-analysis aims to determine the mean value of the ONSD measured in patients with various elevated ICP etiologies under different clinical settings, as well as comparing the value of ONSD between patients with and without elevated ICP.

Methods: This meta-analysis complied with the Preferred Reporting Items for Systematic Reviews and Meta-analysis Statement8. PubMed, Embase, and Cochrane Library were searched to identify ONSD measured by US for patients with increased ICP from establishment to October 2020.

Results: A total of 779 patients with elevated ICP among 22 studies were included in the present meta-analysis. Studies were published between 2003 and 2020. Eighteen were comparative (18/22, 81.8%), and four were single-armed study (4/22, 18.2%). Twenty were prospective studies (20/22, 90.9%). There was moderate-to-high heterogeneity based on the prediction ellipse area and variance logit of sensitivity and specificity.

Conclusions: The mean value of the ONSD among patients diagnosed with increased ICP was 5.82 mm (95% CI 5.58–6.06 mm). Variations were observed based on etiology of intracranial hypertension, clinical settings where ONSD was measured, and standards for diagnosing intracranial hypertension. The US-ONSD among patient with elevated ICP was significantly higher than the normal control. Although a cut-off value is not clearly determined, these mean values can be implemented to evaluate the sensitivity and specificity of US-ONSD in diagnosing intracranial hypertension in future studies.

Keywords: Trauma, traumatic brain injury, ocular ultrasound, Intracranial pressure, Optic nerve sheath, Optic nerve sheath diameter, Point-of-care ultrasound

Introduction

Increased intracranial pressure (ICP) can arise from a variety of cerebral conditions such as stroke, bleeding, malignancy, and trauma [1]. Timely diagnosis and treatment of elevated ICP could prevent detrimental consequences such herniation and decrease mortality [2, 3]. Although invasive intracranial monitoring has been regarded the "gold-standard", it demands neurosurgical

*Correspondence: miguel.montorfano@winfocus.org
[3] Department of Ultrasound and Vascular Doppler, Hospital de Emergencias "Dr. Clemente Alvarez", Av. Pellegrini 3205, Rosario, Santa Fe, Argentina
Full list of author information is available at the end of the article

expertise and is associated with post-procedural complications including infection, hemorrhage, and misplacement [4]. Signs of elevated ICP could manifest as effacement of ventricles and midline shift on CT and MRI [5], but these imaging modalities are not always available in all medical environment and require time for transfer. Within the last two decades, evidence has proven ultrasound (US) measurement of the optic nerve sheath diameter (ONSD) to be a surrogate for intracranial pressure, a point-of-care procedure that can be conveniently done at bedside [6, 7]. Increased ONSD has been noted in patients with elevated ICP of various etiologies in ICU, clinic, and emergency departments. Despite the currently available literature, there is no consensus regarding the cut-off of ONSD for elevated ICP. The present meta-analysis aims to determine the ONSD measured in patients with various elevated ICP etiologies under different clinical settings, as well as comparing the value of ONSD between patients with and without elevated ICP.

Materials and methods

Literature search

This meta-analysis complied with the Preferred Reporting Items for Systematic Reviews and Meta-analysis Statement [8]. PubMed, Embase, and Cochrane Library were searched to identify ONSD measured by US for patients with increased ICP from establishment to October 2020. The following keywords were used: "optic nerve sheath diameter", "ultrasound", "intracranial", "pressure", and "hypertension".

Inclusion criteria and exclusion criteria

The following inclusion criteria were adopted: (a) patients who underwent US measurement of ONSD; (b) patients with elevated ICP; (c) ONSD must be reported in mean and standard deviation on US; (d) confirmation of elevated ICP must be done in another modality other than ultrasound and clinical exam such as CT, MRI, lumbar puncture (LP), and invasive intracranial monitoring. A study was excluded if any of the following criteria were met: (a) non-clinical studies; (b) sample size less than 6; (c) case-reports; (d) pediatric and animal population, and (e) irrelevant studies that did not focus on the topic of using US to measure ONSD of patients with intracranial HTN.

Endnote X8 (Clarivate Analytics, Philadelphia, Pennsylvanian) was used to identify duplicates. Titles, abstracts, and key words were screened, followed by the review of full texts of the remaining studies.

Data collection and statistical analysis

Baseline characteristics were extracted from each study including author, year of publication, country, study design, sample size, "gold-standard" of increased ICP, optic nerve diameter measured by US, hospital setting, etiology of increased ICP. "Gold-standard" is defined as increased ICP confirmed by CT, MRI, lumbar puncture (LP), or invasive intracranial monitoring. Optic nerve diameter was only included if reported in mean and standard deviation. Two researchers extracted the data from the original studies, and any disagreement was resolved through review and discussion.

Quantitative analysis was performed with Stata 15.1 (STATA Corp., College Station, TX, USA). Meta-analysis was conducted with the *-metan* function. Heterogeneity was assessed with the I^2 statistics. A random-effect model was used for a more conservative estimation due to the quality of included studies. Optic nerve diameters were pooled if reported by original articles. Subgroup analysis was made based on hospital settings, etiology of increased ICP, and "gold-standard" of ICP measurement. Comparison of the increased ICP and normal ICP groups was performed via standard mean difference (SMD) by including comparative studies. Funnel plot and Egger's tests were implemented to assess publication bias.

Results

Baseline characteristics

Among the initial 497 unique search results (Fig. 1), a total of 779 patients with elevated ICP among 22 studies were included in the present meta-analysis. Studies were published between 2003 and 2020. Eighteen were comparative (18/22, 81.8%), and four were single-armed study (4/22, 18.2%). Twenty were prospective studies (20/22, 90.9%). Studies were performed in USA ($n=3$), China ($n=3$), India ($n=3$), Italy ($n=2$), Turkey ($n=1$), Thailand ($n=1$), Spain ($n=1$), Saudi Arabia ($n=1$), Pakistan ($n=1$), Nigeria ($n=1$), Iraq ($n=1$), Finland ($n=1$), and France ($n=1$). The brand of US machine implemented by each study is listed in Table 1. All studies measured ONSD at 3 mm posterior to the globe, with varying transverse and/or sagittal measurements and repetition times (Table 1).

ONSD measured by ultrasound

Based on 743 patients from 22 studies with elevated ICP, the overall pooled ONSD measured by ultrasound was 5.82 mm (95% CI 5.58–6.06). Based on etiology of increased ICP, patients who had trauma, hydrocephalus, and pseudotumor cerebri had ONSD of 6.12 (95% CI 5.88–6.35) mm, 5.80 (95% CI 5.64–5.96) mm, and 6.62 (95% CI 6.45–6.79) mm, respectively. By hospital settings, US ONSD that were measured in the ICU, ED, clinic, and OR had a diameter of 6.25 (95% CI 5.92–6.57) mm, 5.72 (95%CI 5.24–6.19) mm, 5.66 (95%CI 5.60–5.71) mm, and 5.80 (95% CI 5.64–5.96) mm, respectively. According to

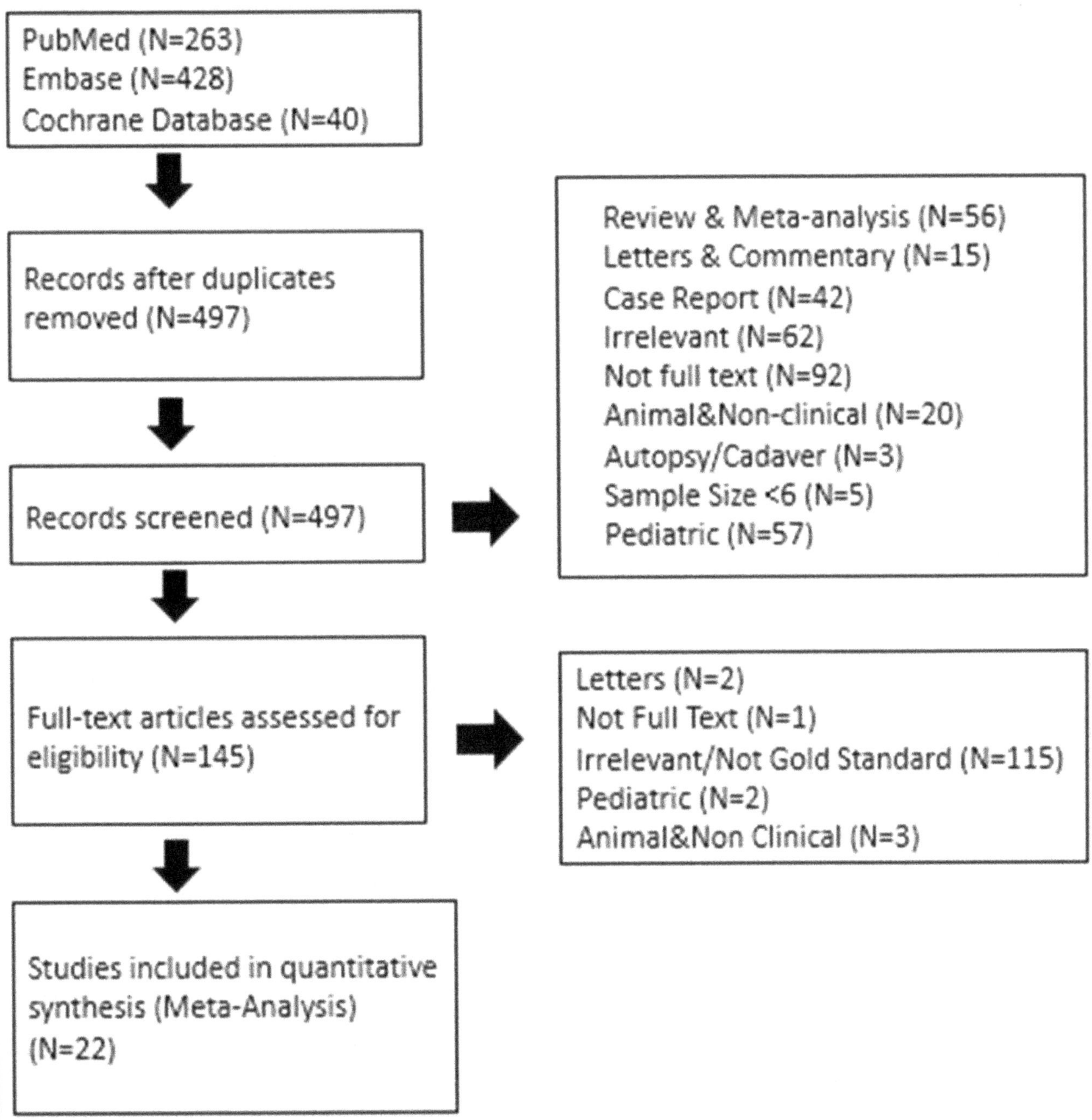

Fig. 1 Flow-diagram of manuscript screening and selection

the diagnosis of increased ICP, patients who were diagnosed by CT, MRI, LP, and invasive intracranial monitoring had ONSD on US of 5.67 (95% CI 5.44–5.91) mm, 5.43 (95% CI 5.25–5.61) mm, 5.75 (95% CI 5.09–6.40) mm, and 6.04 (95% CI 5.76–6.32) mm, respectively.

ONSD between patients with increased ICP and the normal cohort

Among 15 comparative studies, 463 and 609 patients had elevated and normal ICP, respectively. The ONSD measured by US was significantly larger among patients with elevated ICP compared to their normal counterparts (5.6 mm vs 4.1 mm, SMD: 2.44 [95% CI 1.93–2.95]). Similar findings were seen in each subgroup stratified based on gold-standard diagnosis modalities (CT, LP and invasive monitoring). Funnel plot did not show significant asymmetry (Egger's test: $p = 0.145$).

Table 1 Baseline characteristics of included studies

Study/year	Region	Design	Sample size	Mean	Ultrasound brand	Clinical setting	Diagnosis	Etiology	Measurement technique
Aduayi 2015 [9]	Nigeria	Prospective	69	5.7	Mindray DC-6	Mixed	CT	Mixed	3 mm behind the globe; 3 times per eye; averaged
Altayar 2020 [10]	Saudi Arabia	Prospective	28	6.6	Unspecified	ICU	Inv	Trauma	3 mm posterior to the globe in transverse and sagittal planes in both eyes; average diameter was recorded
Bhadari 2019 [11]	India	Prospective	57	5.8	Unspecified	OR	Inv	Hydrocephalus	3 mm behind the posterior sclera
Blaivas 2003 [12]	USA	Prospective	14	6.27	Unspecified	ED	CT	Mixed	3 mm posterior to the globe for both eyes and then averaged.
Bäuerle 2011 [13]	Finland	Prospective	10	6.4	Philips iU22	Mixed	LP	IIH	3 mm behind the papilla. Measured 3 times and then averaged.
Chen 2019 [14]	China	Prospective	29	4.53	Delica MVU-6300	Mixed	LP	Mixed	3 mm behind the globe; averaged two measurements: one sagittal and the other in the transverse plane
del Saz-Saucedo 2016 [15]	Spain	Prospective	19	6.76	Toshiba Aplio XG	Mixed	LP	IIH	Transverse plane
Du 2020 [16]	China	Prospective	49	5.7	Sonosite	ICU	Inv	Trauma	3 mm behind the globe; transverse plane; averaged two eyes.
Geeraerts 2007 [17]	France	Prospective	15	6.3	HP Sonos 5500	ICU	Inv	Trauma	3 mm behind the globe; one sagittal and one transverse
Goel 2008 [18]	India	Prospective	73	5.8	Unspecified	Mixed	CT	Trauma	3 mm behind the globe; one sagittal and one transverse; averaged
Hanafi 2019 [19]	Iran	Prospective	62	6.06	SONOSCAPE-SSI 6000	ED	CT	Trauma	3 mm posterior to the globe; 3 times on each eye in an axial region; averaged.

Table 1 (continued)

Study/year	Region	Design	Sample size	Mean	Ultrasound brand	Clinical setting	Diagnosis	Etiology	Measurement technique
Kimberly 2008 [20]	USA	Prospective	8	5.4	Sonosite Micromaxx	Mixed	Inv	Mixed	3 mm posterior to the orbit; axial image; six measurements; averaged.
Komut 2016 [21]	Turkey	Prospective	50	5.4	Toshiba Aplio 500 Platinum	ED	CT	Mixed	3 mm proximal to the optic disc; in transverse and sagittal planes.
Mohson 2019 [22]	Iraq	Prospective	40	5.6558	Philips HD11XE	Clinic	LP	Mixed	3 mm posterior to the globe; transverse.
Moretti 2009 [23]	Italy	Prospective	19	6.2	Hitachi EUB 405	ICU	Inv	Trauma	3 mm behind the globe; one sagittal and one transverse.
Nash 2015 [24]	USA	Prospective	9	5.8	SonoSite M-Turbo	Mixed	Inv	Trauma	3 mm posterior to the optic disk; longitudinal and transverse.
Rehman 2016 [25]	Pakistan	Cross-sectional	13	6.61	Toshiba Xario 200	Mixed	LP	IIH	3 mm behind the retina; 3 readings were averaged.
Shirodikar 2014 [26]	India	Prospective	35	5.43	Unspecified	Mixed	MRI	Mixed	3 mm behind the globe; averaging three readings from each eye.
Tarzamni 2016 [27]	Iran	Prospective	30	5.48	Aloka Model Prosound 3500	Mixed	CT	Mixed	3 mm posterior to the globe; transverse and sagittal; averaged.
Ussahgij 2020 [28]	Thailand	Prospective	29	5.3	SonoSite M-Turbo	ED	CT	Mixed	3 mm posterior.
Wang 2015 [29]	China	Cross-sectional	101	4.58	Philips iU22	Mixed	LP	Mixed	3 mm posterior to the orbit; transverse and sagittal; repeated twice; averaged
Zoerle 2020 [30]	Italy	Prospective	20	6.44	Phillips iE33	ICU	Inv	Trauma	3 mm behind the globe; transverse and sagittal; repeated twice; averaged

Discussion

The use of ultrasound in the hospital setting has increased drastically in recent years due to multiple factors such as advancements of technology, minimal invasiveness, affordability, ease of use, and increased access to providers [31–37]. Ultrasound is a valuable tool due to its ability to identify or rule-out certain pathologies quickly and efficiently [31–34]. As a result, it has been used in combination with gold standard techniques, which are oftentimes more invasive and require extended time.

The gold standard method to measure intracranial pressure (ICP) is intracranial monitoring with an intraventricular catheter, which typically requires an intraparenchymal catheter to be passed through a cranial burr hole into the ventricle. However, this test has multiple downsides even though it can determine the most accurate value [4, 38], including complications such as infection, post-procedural hemorrhage (due to device placement), parenchymal destruction, and misplacement in addition to other factors such as increased time for device placement and requirement for skilled in-house personnel, typically neurosurgeons [4]. Other less invasive tests that can identify increased ICP include radiological means such as CT and MRI, transcranial Doppler, ophthalmoscopy, tympanic displacement, and optic nerve sheath diameter [38]. As a result, these less invasive tests, especially those involving ultrasound, are frequently used as adjuncts or alternatives to more invasive monitoring. Recently, the use of optic nerve ultrasound as a noninvasive, accurate, safe, reproducible, and cost-effective tool for ICP via the measurement of optic nerve sheath diameter (ONSD) has been validated, thereby decreasing the potentially detrimental consequences of invasive transcranial measurements [6, 9–30].

The anatomical relationship between the optic nerve and subarachnoid space results in an expansion of the optic nerve sheath in states of increased intracranial pressure [9, 12]. Thus, optic nerve sheath diameter can provide information regarding ICP. Ultrasound enables a noninvasive measurement to be taken 3 mm behind the globe, in a retro bulbar position, with a high frequency linear ultrasound probe, which allows for appropriate contrast between the optic nerve and retro bulbar fat to ensure accurate reference points [9, 12, 16]. Normally, three measures for each eye are taken and then averaged. Based on comparative studies, the US-ONSD among patients with elevated ICP was significantly greater than their normal ICP counterparts (Fig. 2A).

Nonetheless, the definitive mean value for ONSD in states of increased ICP has been a point of contention and controversy for many years due lack of meta-analysis and the inability to place an intracranial monitor in all patients where ICP is monitored to correlate this measurements in a more reliable way, though this value approximately lies between 5 and 6 mm based on prior literature [6, 9, 11, 16–18, 20–24, 26, 28]. In order to narrow this range to a more specific value, the present meta-analysis increases the power of the study by pooling available evidence in the literature. According to 22 unique studies over the past 17 years, the overall pooled ONSD measured by ultrasound was found to be 5.82 (95% CI 5.58–6.06) mm, consistent with previously reported MRI measurements (5.81–5.82 mm) [31, 32]. Subtle variations in mean values may be attributed to study site variation in diagnostic control (i.e., CT vs. MRI vs. LP vs. ICP monitor), patient variation such as anatomical differences or severity of illness (i.e., ICU status, etc.), and user variation such as ultrasound probe placement, reference points used for measurements, and the inter equipment variation related with ultrasound devices themselves (i.e., probe frequency, image quality, etc.). Widespread training in this practice is expected to increase precision and accuracy of measurements, and thus sensitivity and specificity of the exam findings.

Due to the easy accessibility of US compared to other imaging modality such as CT and MRI, it can be implemented by physicians in a variety of clinical settings, such as the ED, OR, ICU, clinic, wards, etc. (Table 1). US-ONSD measured in ICU patients demonstrated the largest value 6.25 (95% CI 5.92–6.57) mm (Fig. 3), reflecting the critically ill nature of this patient population and higher ICP requiring ICU care. Because the use of US is operator-dependent, the accuracy and precision of US-ONSD can be influenced by type of clinical setting where measurement takes place. For instance, measuring US-ONSD in a busy ED can be more technically challenging compared to in a controlled environment such as OR or ICU where patients are sedated. Further matched-comparative studies are warranted to compare its use in different clinical settings.

Previous studies indicated a strong correlation between increased ONSD and radiologic findings with CT and MRI [6, 9, 39, 40]. Patients diagnosed with increased ICP by CT or MRI had lower ONSDs on ultrasound (5.67 mm; 95% CI 5.44–5.91 mm and 5.43 mm; 95% CI 5.25–5.61 mm) than patients diagnosed with invasive ICP monitoring (6.04 mm; 95% CI 5.76–6.32 mm). Brain Trauma Foundation recommends considering invasive ICP monitoring under the setting of severe head injury [41]; the longer pooled ONSD of these patients in the present meta-analysis might be related to the severity of increased ICP prompted invasive monitoring.

The present meta-analysis also found variations of ONSD among different etiologies of intracranial hypertension (Fig. 4), though there were only three study dedicated to IIT and one focusing on hydrocephalus.

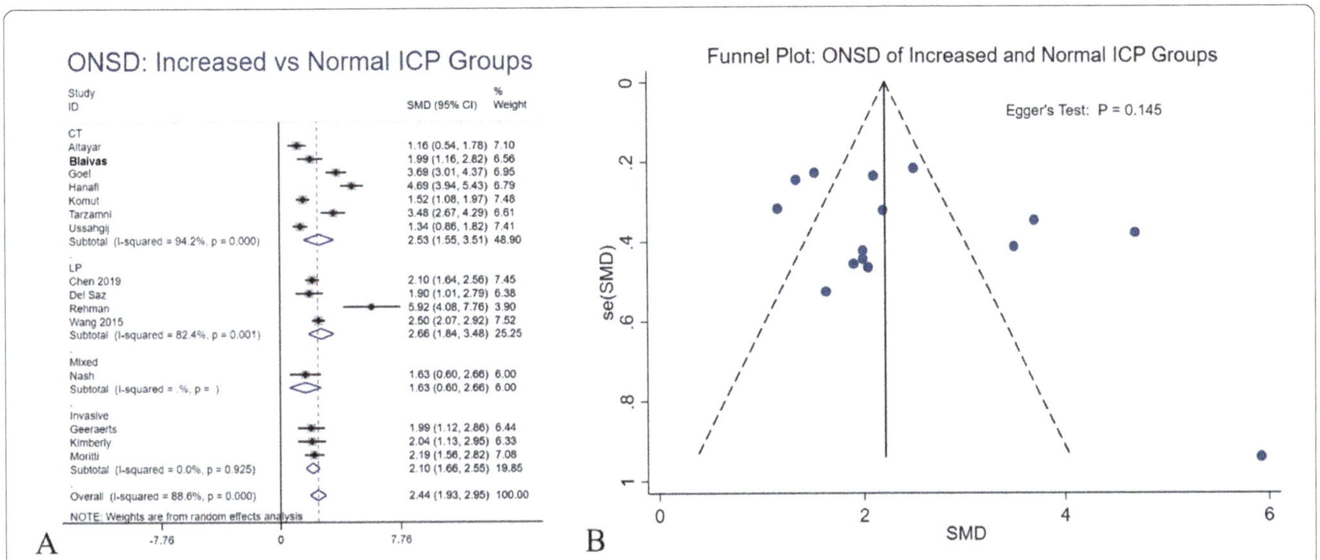

Fig. 2 Optic nerve sheath diameter (ONSD) measured by ultrasound (US) between patients with elevated intracranial pressure (ICP) and normal cohort (**A**). Funnel plot and Egger's test evaluating publication bias (**B**)

Compared to hydrocephalus, values for traumatic etiologies were greater than hydrocephalus (6.12 [95%CI 5.88–6.35] vs 5.8 [95%CI 5.64–5.96] mm), which may be explained by the rapid increase in ICP due to mass effect from head injury. However, the pooled pressure of idiopathic intracranial hypertension was the highest (6.62 [95%CI 6.45–6.79)] mm), which is possibly due to chronic change. Such observation could be affected by the etiology of the disease. Based on the modified Dandy criteria, papilledema is one criterion of diagnosing idiopathic intracranial hypertension [42]. Because papilledema is optic disc edema resulted from elevated ICP transmitted through optic nerve sheath [43], increase of ONSD should takes precedence prior to the development of papilledema. Because of under powering of the number of included studies, these speculation warrants further research (Fig. 5).

Fifteen studies compared the ONSD between patients with increased ICP and a normal cohort (Fig. 2). The ONSD measured by US was significantly larger among patients with elevated ICP compared to their normal counterparts (5.6 mm vs 4.1 mm, SMD: 2.44 [95% CI 1.93–2.95]).

The present study should be interpreted with several caveats. Despite most studies being prospective in nature, baseline patient characteristics can be heterogeneous such as the etiology of increased ICP and clinical settings where US-ONSD measurement was taken place. Subgroup analyses were performed and showed variations in terms of the pooled value in each condition. Nonetheless, the majority of studies were reported ONSD among a mixed population. Future study should report outcomes stratified based on these variables to determine the mean value for elevated ICP in each clinical scenario. Further, the present meta-analysis did not analyze the sensitivity and specificity of the pooled US-ONSD value. Such analysis requires each individual study reporting sensitivity and specificity in the original article, but the criteria of US-ONSD for elevated ICP vary among different authors. A number of studies for the ONSD evaluation used the median values rather than the mean value. Although in our analysis we used all the values relevant in the literature to obtained mean values, this could be a potential confounder when trying to establish an accurate value. ONSD values are usually represented as the average of measurements between the eyes. Normally, three measures for each eye are taken and then averaged. However, some studies used only two measures per eye, and some others used one transverse measurement and one on vertical plane per eye (averaged). Furthermore, some studies have suggested an "internal" ONSD (ONSDi) and an "external" ONSD (ONSDe). The two measurements can differ. These factors can produce differences of measurements and potential bias may be created.

Even if there are several limitations about the use of a unique cut-off value of ONSD for detecting elevated ICP, this update may help to clarify which is the value that could be considered as marker of intracranial hypertension.

Thus, the aim of the present study was to pool the US-ONSD using available studies to determine a mean

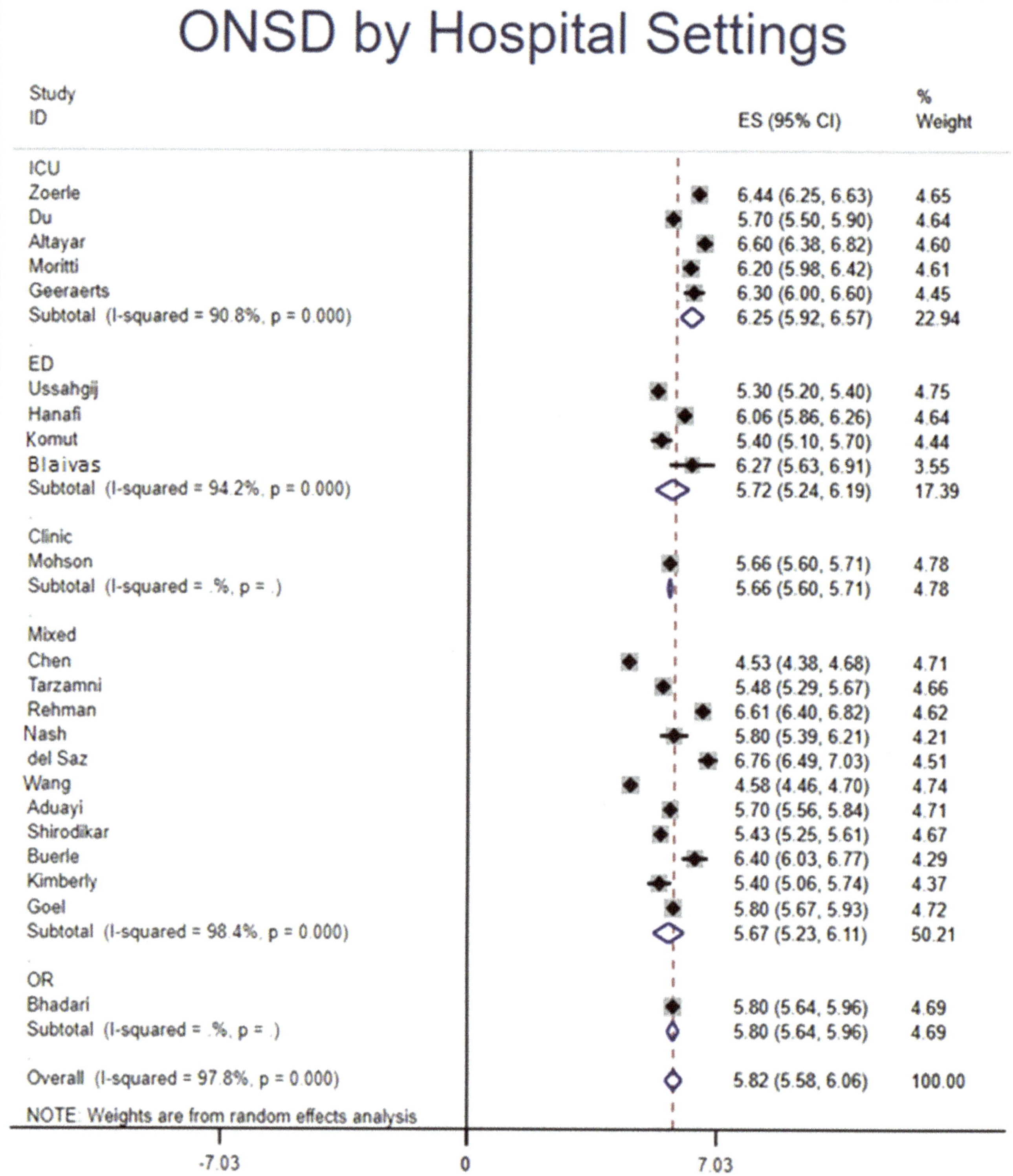

Fig. 3 Optic nerve sheath diameter (ONSD) measured by ultrasound (US) stratified by clinical settings where measurement was taken place. *ICU* Intensive care unit, *ED* Emergency Department, *OR* operating room

value that can be used as a reference for future study to determine its specificity and sensitivity in real-world clinical practice.

Conclusions

Based on available evidence, the mean value of the ONSD among patients diagnosed with increased ICP

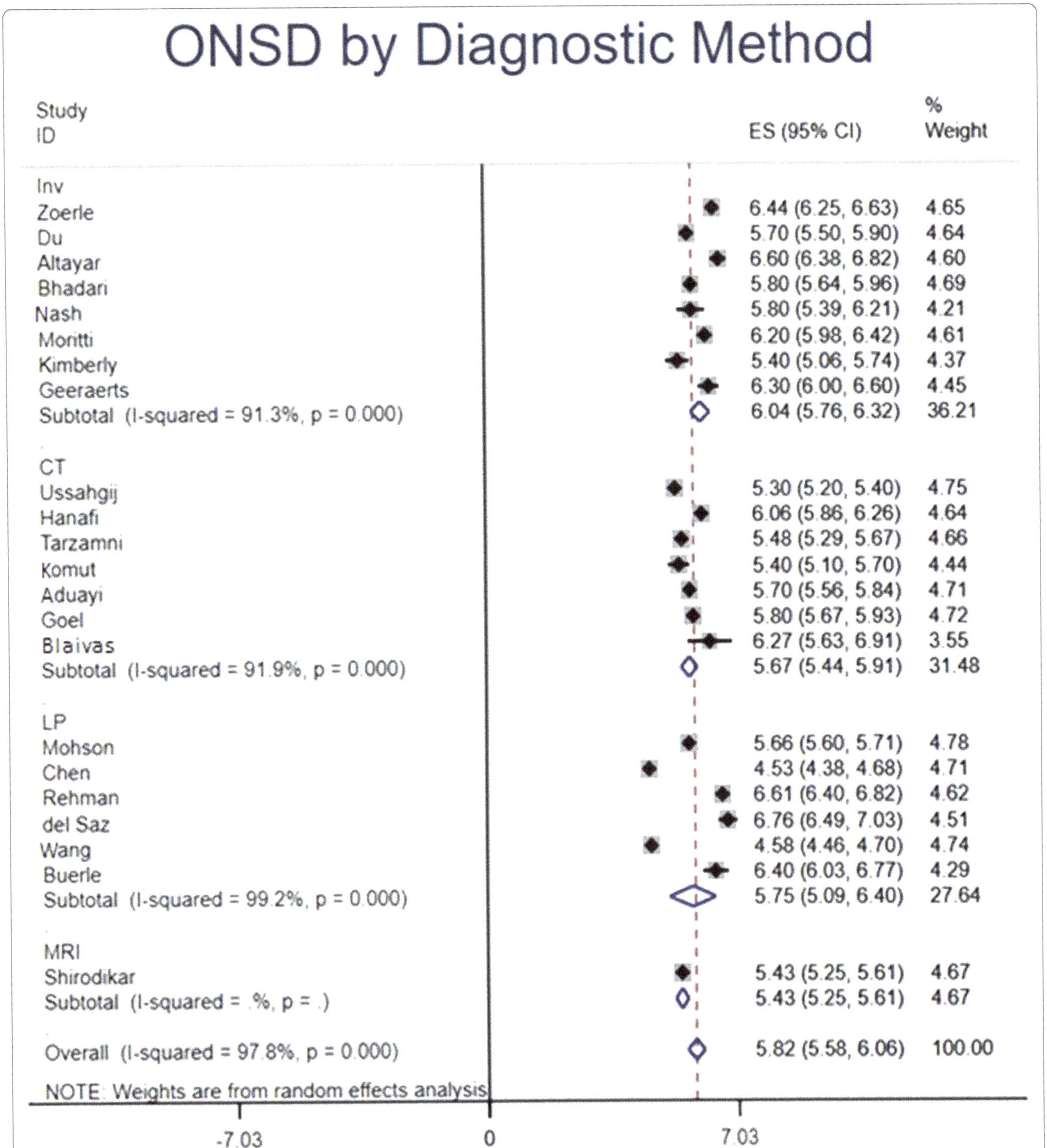

Fig. 4 Optic nerve sheath diameter (ONSD) measured by ultrasound (US) stratified by the diagnostic method of increased intracranial pressure (ICP). *MRI* magnetic resonance imaging, *CT* computed tomography, *LP* lumbar puncture, *Inv* invasive intracranial monitoring

was 5.82 mm (95% CI 5.58–6.06 mm). Variations were observed based on etiology of intracranial hypertension, clinical settings where ONSD was measured, and standards for diagnosing intracranial hypertension. The US-ONSD among patients with elevated ICP was significantly higher than the normal control. Although a cut-off value is not clearly determined these mean values can be implemented to evaluate the sensitivity and specificity of US-ONSD in diagnosing intracranial hypertension in future studies. Larger, stratified,

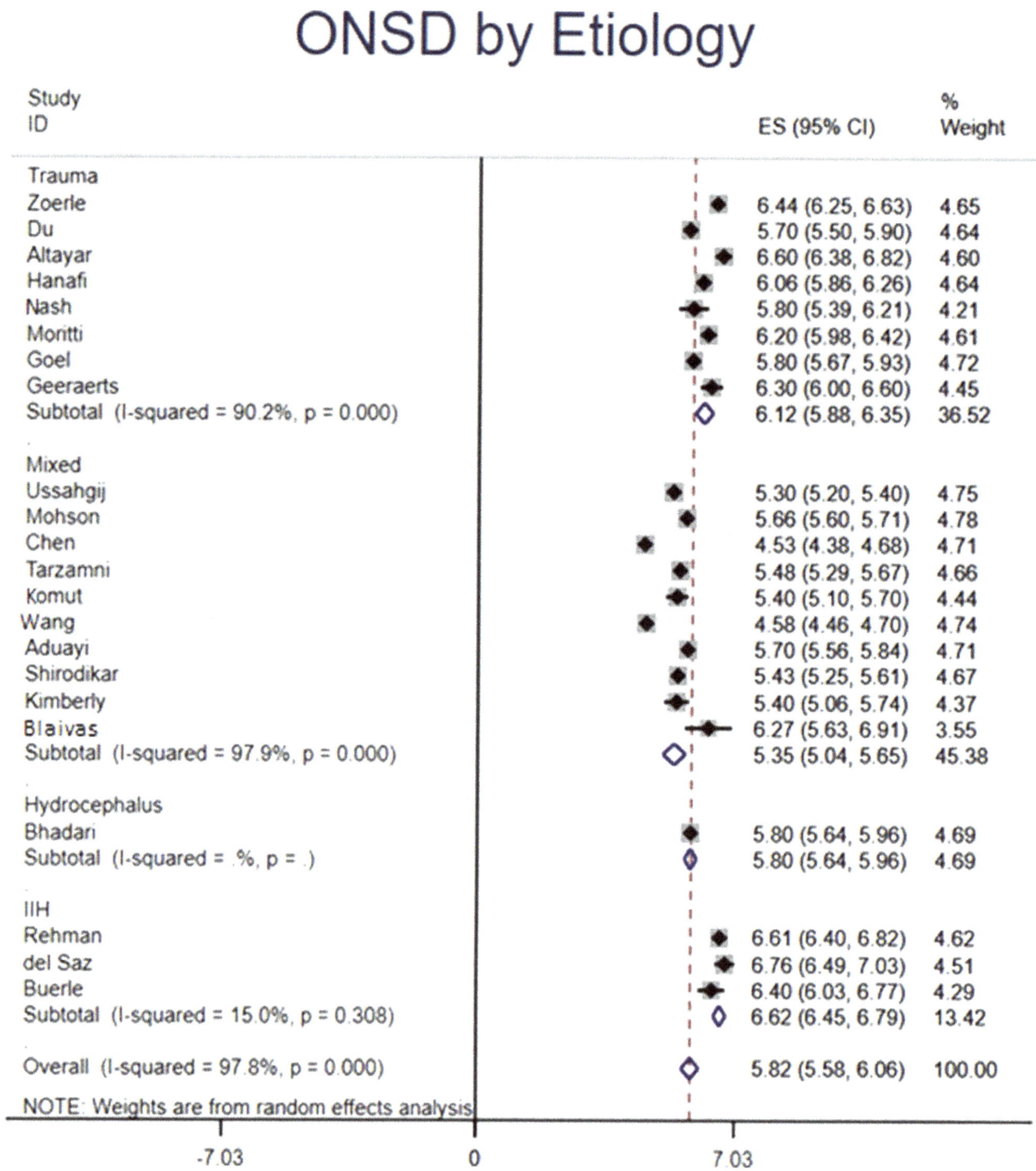

Fig. 5 Optic nerve sheath diameter (ONSD) measured by ultrasound (US) stratified by etiology of elevated intracranial pressure

prospective studies are warranted to determine its value in each clinical setting.

Acknowledgements
Not applicable.

Authors' contributions
LM: manuscript writing, review and final edition. QY: data collection and analysis. SJB: manuscript writing and edition. SS: Data analysis. RJR: manuscript edition. MM: main hypothesis, manuscript final review and edition, advisory input. All authors read and approved the final manuscript.

Author details
[1]Department of General Surgery, Cleveland Clinic Florida, 2950 Cleveland Clinic Blvd, Weston, FL, USA. [2]School of Medicine, Georgetown University, Washington D.C, USA. [3]Department of Ultrasound and Vascular Doppler, Hospital de Emergencias "Dr. Clemente Alvarez", Av. Pellegrini 3205, Rosario, Santa Fe, Argentina.

References

1. Canac N, Jalaleddini K, Thorpe SG, Thibeault CM, Hamilton RB (2020) pathophysiology of intracranial hypertension and noninvasive intracranial pressure monitoring. Fluids Barriers CNS 17(1):1–21
2. Farahvar A, Gerber LM, Chiu Y-L, Carney N, Härtl R, Ghajar J (2012) Increased mortality in patients with severe traumatic brain injury treated without intracranial pressure monitoring. J Neurosurg 117(4):729–734
3. Han J, Yang S, Zhang C, Zhao M, Li A (2016) Impact of intracranial pressure monitoring on prognosis of patients with severe traumatic brain injury: a PRISMA systematic review and meta-analysis. Medicine 95:7
4. Tavakoli S, Peitz G, Ares W, Hafeez S, Grandhi R (2017) Complications of invasive intracranial pressure monitoring devices in neurocritical care. Neurosurg Focus 43(5):E6
5. Kayhanian S, Young AM, Piper RJ et al (2018) Radiological correlates of raised intracranial pressure in children: a review. Front Pediatr 6:32
6. Dubourg J, Javouhey E, Geeraerts T, Messerer M, Kassai B (2011) Ultrasonography of optic nerve sheath diameter for detection of raised intracranial pressure: a systematic review and meta-analysis. Intens Care Med 37(7):1059–1068
7. Montorfano L, Giambartolomei G, Funes DR, Lo Menzo E, Dip F, White KP, Rosenthal RJ (2020) The Cushing reflex and the vasopressin-mediated hemodynamic response to increased intracranial pressure during acute elevations in intraabdominal pressure. Surgery 167(2):478–483
8. Moher D, Shamseer L, Clarke M et al (2015) Preferred reporting items for systematic review and meta-analysis protocols (PRISMA-P) 2015 statement. Syst Control Found Appl 4(1):1
9. Aduayi OS, Asaleye CM, Adetiloye VA, Komolafe EO, Aduayi VA (2015) Optic nerve sonography: a noninvasive means of detecting raised intracranial pressure in a resource-limited setting. J Neurosci Rural Pract 6(4):563
10. Altayar AS, Abouelela AZ, Abdelshafey EE et al (2020) Optic nerve sheath diameter by ultrasound is a good screening tool for high intracranial pressure in traumatic brain injury. Irish J Med Sci 8:254
11. Bhandari D, Udupi Bidkar P, Adinarayanan S, Narmadhalakshmi K, Srinivasan S (2019) Measurement of changes in optic nerve sheath diameter using ultrasound and computed tomography scan before and after the ventriculoperitoneal shunt surgery in patients with hydrocephalus-A prospective observational trial. Br J Neurosurg 33(2):125–130
12. Blaivas M, Theodoro D, Sierzenski PR (2003) Elevated intracranial pressure detected by bedside emergency ultrasonography of the optic nerve sheath. Acad Emerg Med 10(4):376–381
13. Bäuerle J, Nedelmann M (2011) Sonographic assessment of the optic nerve sheath in idiopathic intracranial hypertension. J Neurol 258(11):2014–2019
14. Chen LM, Wang LJ, Shi L, Chen HX, Jiang XH, Chen QQ, Xing YQ (2019) Reliability of assessing non-severe elevation of intracranial pressure using optic nerve sheath diameter and transcranial Doppler parameters. Front Neurol 22(10):1091
15. del Saz-Saucedo P, Redondo-González O, Mateu-Mateu Á, Huertas-Arroyo R, García-Ruiz R, Botia-Paniagua E (2016) Sonographic assessment of the optic nerve sheath diameter in the diagnosis of idiopathic intracranial hypertension. J Neurol Sci 361:122–127
16. Du J, Deng Y, Li H et al (2020) Ratio of optic nerve sheath diameter to eyeball transverse diameter by ultrasound can predict intracranial hypertension in traumatic brain injury patients: a prospective study. Neurocrit Care 32(2):478–485
17. Geeraerts T, Launey Y, Martin L et al (2007) Ultrasonography of the optic nerve sheath may be useful for detecting raised intracranial pressure after severe brain injury. Intensive Care Med 33(10):1704–1711
18. Goel RS, Goyal NK, Dharap SB, Kumar M, Gore MA (2008) Utility of optic nerve ultrasonography in head injury. Injury 39(5):519–524
19. Hanafi MG, Verki MM, Parei SN (2019) Ultrasonic assessment of optic nerve sheath to detect increased intracranial pressure. J Med Ultrasound 27(2):69
20. Kimberly HH, Shah S, Marill K, Noble V (2008) Correlation of optic nerve sheath diameter with direct measurement of intracranial pressure. Acad Emerg Med 15(2):201–204
21. Komut E, Kozaci N, Sönmez BM, et al. Bedside sonographic measurement of optic nerve sheath diameter as a predictor of intracranial pressure in ED. Am J Emerg Med. 2016;34(6):963–7.
22. Mohson KI, Auday N (2019) Role of orbital ultrasound in the assessment of clinically detected papilledema. J Med Ultrasound 27(3):135
23. Moretti R, Pizzi B (2009) Optic nerve ultrasound for detection of intracranial hypertension in intracranial hemorrhage patients: confirmation of previous findings in a different patient population. J Neurosurg Anesthesiol 21(1):16–20
24. Nash JE, O'Rourke C, Moorman ML (2016) Transocular ultrasound measurement of the optic nerve sheath diameter can identify elevated intracranial pressure in trauma patients. Trauma 18(1):28–34
25. Rehman H, Khan MS, Nafees M, Rehman AU, Habib A (2016) Optic nerve sheath diameter on sonography in idiopathic intracranial hypertension versus normal. JCPSP 26(9):758–760
26. Shirodkar CG, Rao SM, Mutkule DP, Harde YR, Venkategowda PM, Mahesh MU (2014) Optic nerve sheath diameter as a marker for evaluation and prognostication of intracranial pressure in Indian patients: an observational study. Ind J Critic Care Med 18(11):728
27. Tarzamni MK, Derakhshan B, Meshkini A et al (2016) The diagnostic performance of ultrasonographic optic nerve sheath diameter and color Doppler indices of the ophthalmic arteries in detecting elevated intracranial pressure. Clin Neurol Neurosurg 141:82–88
28. Ussahgij W, Toonpirom W, Munkong W, Lenghong K, Apiratwarakul K (2020) Optic nerve sheath diameter cutoff point for detection of increased intracranial pressure in the emergency department. J Med Sci 8:62–65
29. Wang L, Feng L, Yao Y, Wang Y, Chen Y, Feng J, Xing Y (2015) Optimal optic nerve sheath diameter threshold for the identification of elevated opening pressure on lumbar puncture in a Chinese population. PLoS ONE 10(2):e0117939
30. Zoerle T, Caccioppola A, D'Angelo E et al (2020) Optic nerve sheath diameter is not related to intracranial pressure in subarachnoid hemorrhage patients. Neurocritic Care. 14:1–8
31. Liao SF, Chen PJ, Chaou CH, Lee CH (2018) Top-cited publications on point-of-care ultrasound: The evolution of research trends. Am J Emerg Med 36(8):1429–1438
32. Kendall JL, Hoffenberg SR, Smith RS (2007) History of emergency and critical care ultrasound: the evolution of a new imaging paradigm. Crit Care Med 35(5 Suppl):S126–S130
33. Carson PL, Fenster A (2009) Anniversary paper: evolution of ultrasound physics and the role of medical physicists and the AAPM and its journal in that evolution. Med Phys 36(2):411–428
34. Montoya J, Stawicki SP, Evans DC, Bahner DP, Sparks S, Sharpe RP, Cipolla J (2016) From FAST to E-FAST: an overview of the evolution of ultrasound-based traumatic injury assessment. Eur J Trauma Emerg Surg 42(2):119–126
35. Cosgrove DO (2017) Evolution of ultrasonography since the 1970s. Ultrasound Med Biol 43(11):2741–2742. https://doi.org/10.1016/j.ultrasmedbio.2017.06.015
36. Goldberg BB, Gramiak R, Freimanis AK (1993) Early history of diagnostic ultrasound: the role of American radiologists. Am J Roentgenol 160(1):189–194. https://doi.org/10.2214/ajr.160.1.8416623
37. Newman PG, Rozycki GS (1998) The history of ultrasound. Surg Clin North Am 78(2):179–195. https://doi.org/10.1016/s0039-6109(05)70308-x
38. Nag DS, Sahu S, Swain A, Kant S (2019) Intracranial pressure monitoring: gold standard and recent innovations. World J Clin Cases 7(13):1535–1553
39. Geeraerts T, Newcombe VF, Coles JP et al (2008) Use of T2-weighted magnetic resonance imaging of the optic nerve sheath to detect raised intracranial pressure. Crit Care 12(5):1–7
40. Abdelrahman AS, Barakat MM (2020) MRI measurement of optic nerve sheath diameter using 3D driven equilibrium sequence as a non-invasive tool for the diagnosis of idiopathic intracranial hypertension. Egypt J Radiol Nuclear Med 51(1):24

23

Transesophageal echocardiography in orthotopic liver transplantation: a comprehensive intraoperative monitoring tool

Luigi Vetrugno[1*], Federico Barbariol[1], Umberto Baccarani[1], Francesco Forfori[2], Giovanni Volpicelli[3] and Giorgio Della Rocca[1]

Abstract

Intraoperative transesophageal echocardiography is a minimally invasive monitoring tool that can provide real-time visual information on ventricular function and hemodynamic volume status in patients undergoing liver transplantation. The American Association for the Study of Liver Diseases states that transesophageal echocardiography should be used in all liver transplant candidates in order to assess chamber sizes, hypertrophy, systolic and diastolic function, valvular function, and left ventricle outflow tract obstruction. However, intraoperative transesophageal echocardiography can be used to "visualize" other organs too; thanks to its proximity and access to multiple acoustic windows: liver, lung, spleen, and kidney. Although only limited scientific evidence exists promoting this comprehensive use, we describe the feasibility of TEE in the setting of liver transplantation: it is a highly valuable tool, not only as a cardiovascular monitoring, but also as a tool to evaluate lungs and pleural spaces, to assess hepatic vein blood flow and inferior vena cava anastomosis and patency, i.e., in cases of modified surgical techniques. The aim of this case series is to add our own experience of TEE as a comprehensive intraoperative monitoring tool in the field of orthotopic liver transplantation (and major liver resection) to the literature.

Keywords: Transesophageal echocardiography, TEE, Liver transplantation, Caval anastomosis, Lung ultrasound

Introduction

The gold standard methods for monitoring cardiac output during liver transplantation surgery are pulmonary arterial catheterization and volumetric device monitoring (PiCCO/EV-1000); nonetheless experts agree that transesophageal echocardiography (TEE) is useful for managing rapid hemodynamic changes [1]. The American Association for the Study of Liver Diseases (AASLD) states that TEE should be used in all liver transplant candidates in order to assess chamber sizes, hypertrophy, systolic and diastolic function, valvular function, and left ventricle outflow tract obstruction [2].

The use of the TEE during liver transplantation to monitor cardiac function and to assess the inferior vena cava patency was described for the first time in 1992. In that case, the TEE probe was used in a patient with a suspected stricture of the suprahepatic inferior vena cava (IVC) anastomosis to evaluate its patency and the subsequent surgical intervention. The authors described how following separation from the venous–venous bypass, the liver appeared swollen, while the Doppler color flow imaging demonstrated marked turbulence in the suprahepatic IVC with narrow jet streaming into the right atrium [3]. With manual elevation of the liver, the pressure gradient disappeared, which allowed them to understand that the obstruction was due to the kinking of the vessel, and the anastomosis was revised. Color Doppler was once again performed and showed a decrease in the turbulence of the IVC blood flow. The case demonstrated that TEE can be used to assess the suprahepatic anastomosis, providing an early, non-invasive assessment of abnormalities that may require prompt correction. After this initial article, reports of TEE for the evaluation of

*Correspondence: luigi.vetrugno@asuiud.sanita.fvg.it; vetrugno.luigi@aoud.sanita.fvg.it
[1] Department of Medicine, University of Udine, P.le S. M. della Misericordia 15, 33100 Udine, Italy
Full list of author information is available at the end of the article

hepatic vein structures have been scarce, despite the fact that TEE is becoming an increasingly popular tool in liver transplant surgery [4, 5].

Study rationale and aim

Unrecognized IVC stenosis, thrombosis, and kinking during liver transplantation can lead to devastating consequences, requiring the patient to undergo further operations, such as surgical repair or re-transplant. The images in Fig. 1 show percutaneous transluminal angioplasty and double stent placement in a 63-year-old cirrhotic patient presenting suprahepatic IVC outflow compromise in the early postoperative period following orthotopic liver transplantation. The American Society of Echocardiography/Society of Cardiovascular Anesthesiologists now recommends that images of the IVC and hepatic veins are obtained as part of a comprehensive perioperative examination [6]. As reported in a recent editorial, although TEE has mainly been used in the context of the heart, it can also be used to "visualize" other

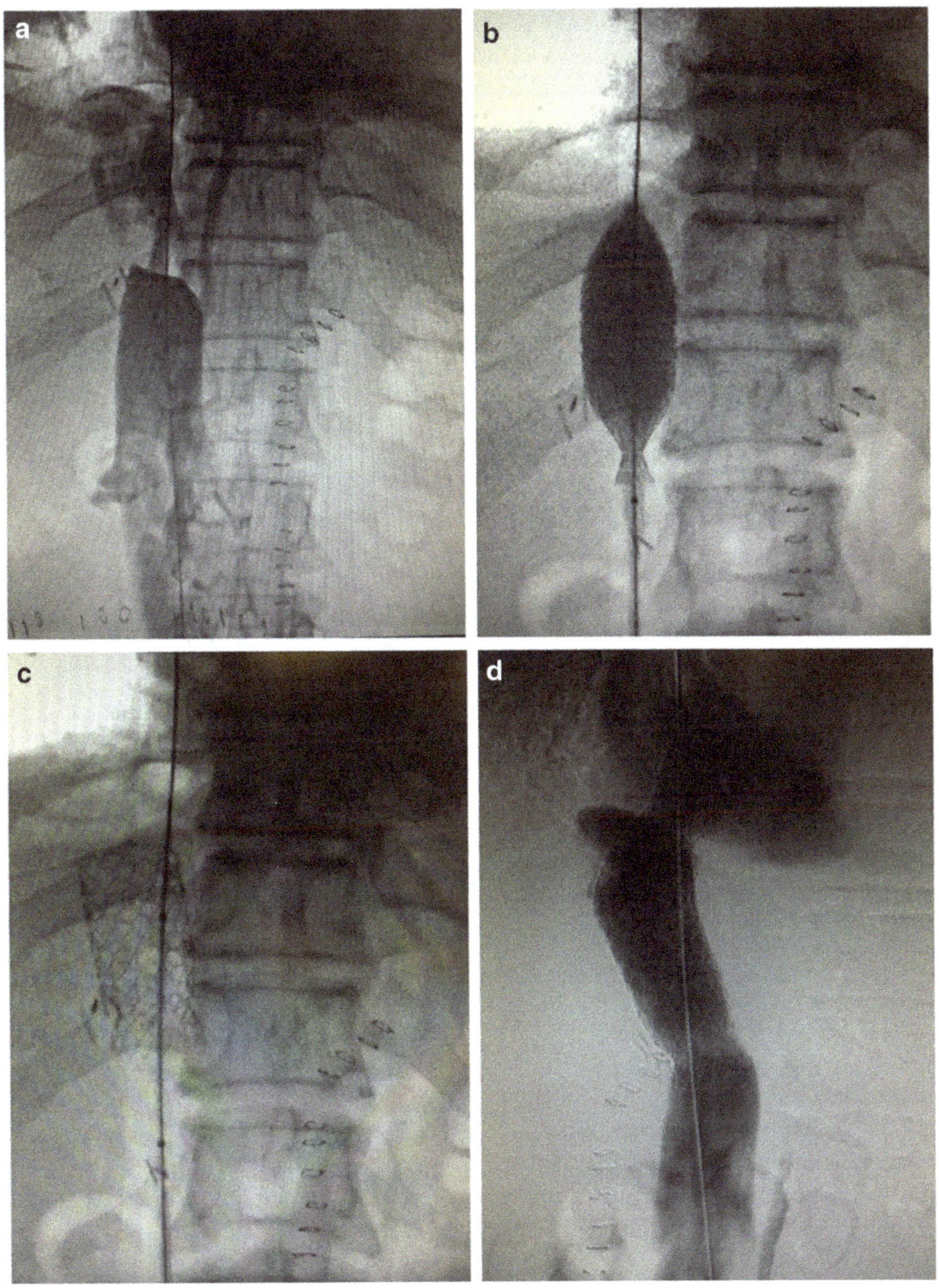

Fig. 1 Percutaneous angioplasty and stent placement in a 63-year-old cirrhotic patient presenting suprahepatic IVC outflow compromise in the early postoperative period following orthotopic liver transplantation. Inferior vena cavogram demonstrates high-grade stenosis of the IVC (**a**); after vena cava angioplasty (**b**) and stent placement, a marked enlargement of IVC lumen is obtained (**c** and **d**)

organs. Inserting the probe beyond the bicaval view is helpful for assessing the IVC, the liver, and the hepatic veins. Furthermore, the literature contains many reports of TEE imaging of the pleura, the kidneys, and even the spinal cord [7–10].

The aim of this case series is to add our own experience of TEE as a comprehensive intraoperative monitoring tool in the field of orthotopic liver transplantation (and major liver resection) to the literature.

Surgical considerations

The orthotopic liver transplantation technique was first described as a complete resection of the recipient's IVC and interposition of the donor intrahepatic vena cava with two end-to-end anastomosis; for hemodynamic stabilization, the procedure also includes a veno-venous bypass, usually from left femoral to left axillary vein. In many centers, this approach still remains the gold standard [11]. In 1989 Tzakis et al. [12] introduced a new modified technique called the 'piggy-back' technique, which consists of preserving the full length of the recipient's vena cava, but with anastomosis of the donor suprahepatic veins to the ostium of the recipient's left and middle suprahepatic veins. The supporters of the piggy-back technique advocate the advantages of this procedure as the shorter operation times with a shorter anhepatic phase and warm ischemia, with one less anastomosis. This could reduce blood loss and give better hemodynamic stability without the use of a venous–venous bypass.

The 'dark side' of the piggy-back technique is the potential for venous outflow obstruction caused by size discrepancy between the donor suprahepatic vena cava and the recipient's hepatic veins' cuff: the associated risk of intra- or postoperative outflow problems of the graft has been reported to be between 1.5 and 8%, leading to major functional problems of the liver graft [13, 14]. For example, Cescon et al. experienced outflow problems in 4.6% of their patients, leading to a re-transplantation rate of 40%; outflow problems were also the cause of death in 23% of cases [15].

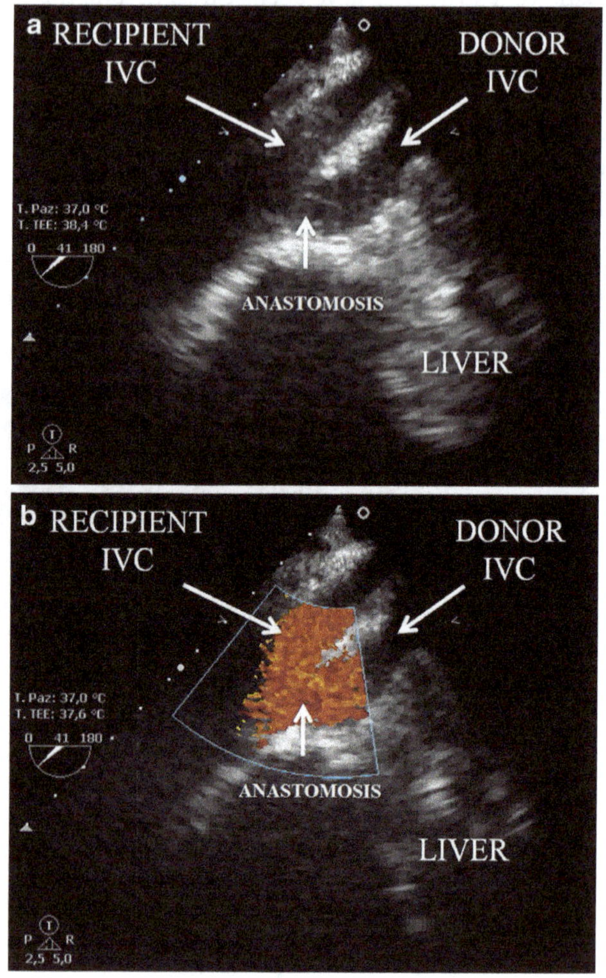

Fig. 2 Transesophageal transgastric view at 41°, showing the double inferior vena cava in parallel manner without (**a**) and with (**b**) Doppler color flow through the patent terminolateral cavo-cavostomy

Case 1

The images presented in Fig. 2 were acquired during liver transplant surgery in a 59-year-old patient with decompensated liver cirrhosis, severe portal hypertension, oesophageal varices (grade F2), and ascites secondary to previous alcohol abuse. After hepatectomy, performed using the piggy-back technique, [4] the donor suprahepatic IVC was anastomized to the hepatic vein cuff of the recipient, but the infrahepatic vena cava of the graft was oversewn. Following portal vein reperfusion, the graft started to swell and indurate in just a few minutes due to insufficient outflow. It is known that this condition, without correction, can lead to acute Budd–Chiari-like syndrome with graft loss in the immediate postoperative period [14]. The surgeons decided to perform a rescue terminolateral cavo-cavostomy by anastomosis of the donor infrahepatic vena cava to the recipient's suprarenal vena cava to correct the inadequate outflow [16], as shown in Fig. 3.

A TEE examination of the liver was performed at the edge of the transesophageal transgastric view at 0 degrees; the probe was rotated clockwise and the phasic array signal emitted transducer moved between 40° and 60°, as previously described, to generate the basic hepatic view [17]. The donor and the recipient IVC were viewed in parallel, together with the flow through the cavocaval anastomosis, as reported in Additional file 1: Video 1, Additional file 2: Video 2, and Fig. 4. At the same time, the liver progressively assumed completely normal dimensions, color, and tissue consistency.

In the same patient, after the first declamping and before the cavo-cavostomy rescue anastomosis, a

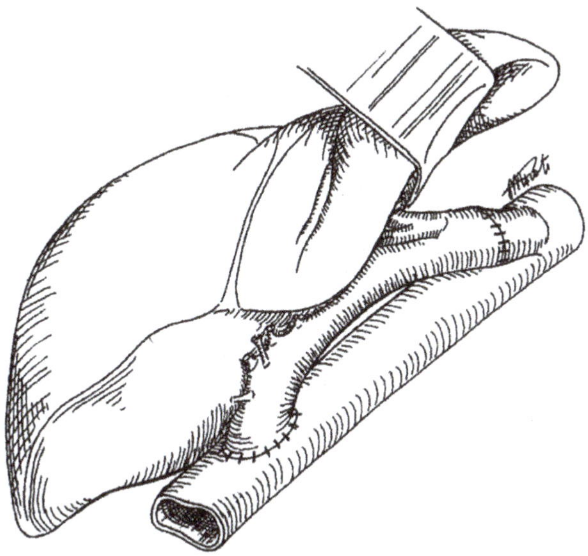

Fig. 3 End-to-end infrahepatic rescue cavo-cavostomy (Reprinted from Transplant Proc. 2001; 33 (1–2):1389 with permission from Elsevier)

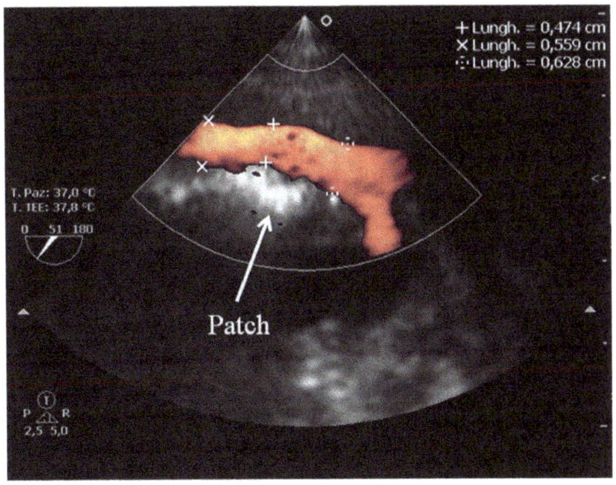

Fig. 5 Color Power Angio Echography of the inferior vena cava blood flow through the patch repair. The Edwards® Bovine Pericardial Patch appears as a hyper echoic structure in the anterior wall of the IVC (as shown by the *white arrow*). Diameters of the ICV before, through, and after the patch are shown

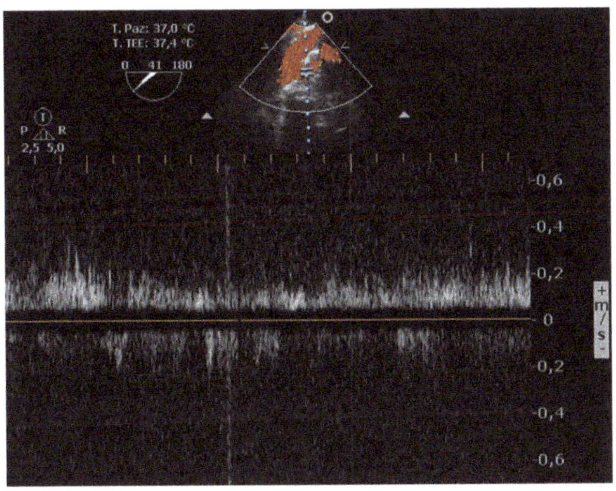

Fig. 4 Doppler analysis of the blood flow through the cavo-cavostomy rescue anastomosis, showing appropriate liver venous drainage

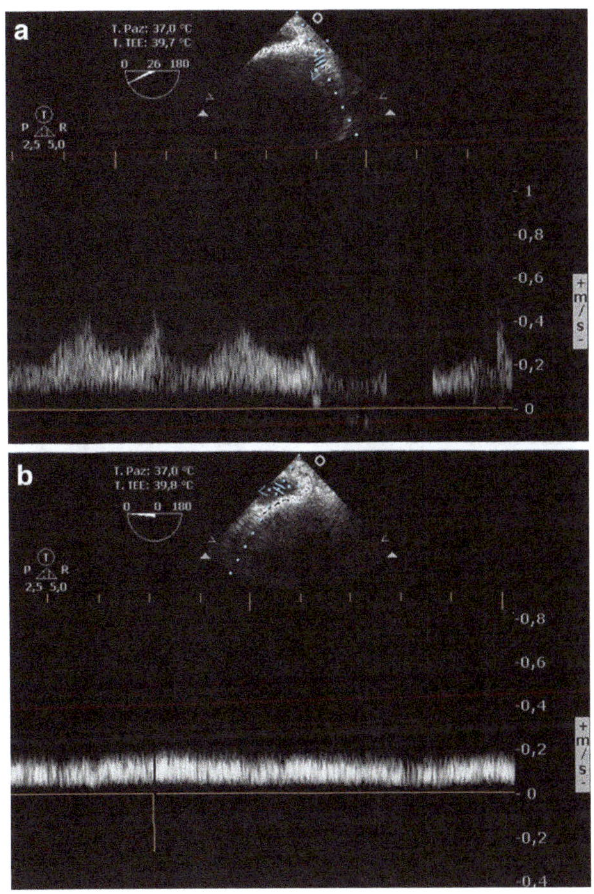

Fig. 6 Pulse Wave Doppler (PW) analysis, measuring adequate blood flow velocity, in the suprahepatic vein (**a**) and inferior vena cava (**b**) after the patch repair

profound reduction in the preload due to the sequestration of blood in the liver and in the splanchnic circulation occurred, and adrenaline boluses were administered to support the hemodynamics. Because of this, the patient developed a transient ballooning syndrome that fortunately recovered after the increase in systolic pressure upon the second declamping following the cavo-cavostomy anastomosis (Additional file 3: Video 3).

Case 2

The images presented in Figs. 5, 6, and the related Additional file 4: Video 4 and Additional file 5: Video 5 were acquired after left lobe liver resection surgery in a

67-year-old woman with a giant hepatic angioma. During the surgical dissection of the tissues, an accidental laceration of the inferior vena cava occurred, which required almost complete clamping. To re-establish blood flow, the surgeons used an Edwards® Bovine Pericardial Patch. After declamping, the surgeon requested that the patency of the inferior vena cava and blood flow in the suprahepatic veins were checked using TEE. A comparison of TEE for visualization of the main hepatic veins with the acquisition of Doppler ultrasound curves using the transabdominal approach was first described by Meierhenrich et al. [18] in their study of 34 patients scheduled for abdominal surgery. Using a multiplane TEE, they were able to identify the three main hepatic veins in all of the patients, and they reported that adequate Doppler tracings of the right and middle hepatic veins could be obtained in 100 and 97% of the patients, respectively, by TEE and in 91 and 50% of the patients by transabdominal sonography (TAS). Doppler tracing of the left hepatic vein could only be acquired in 18% of the patients by TEE, but in 47% of the patients by TAS. Doppler ultrasound and Pulse Wave Doppler (PW) analysis, which measure blood flow velocity (using a correct insonation angle, <60°), play an important role in the assessment of liver vessel patency, resistivity, and flow direction (as already shown in Figs. 5, 6, and Additional file 4: Video 4 and Additional file 5: Video 5).

Usually, the normal hepatic vein waveform has four components: a retrograde A wave (right atrial contraction), an anterograde S wave (right ventricular systolic), a transitional V wave (pulmonary vein closure), and an anterograde D wave (right ventricular diastole)—see

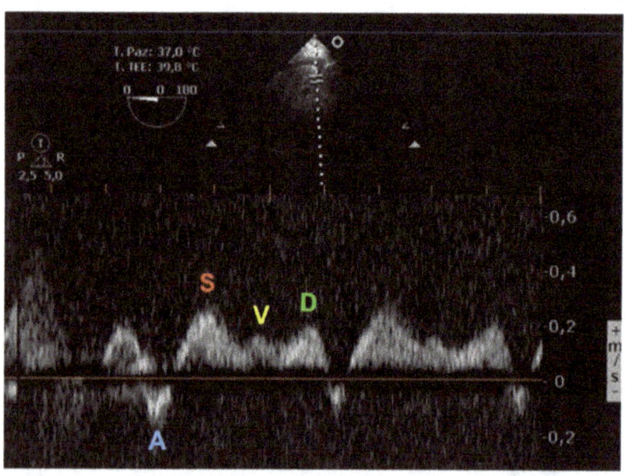

Fig. 7 Normal triphasic hepatic Doppler waveform. The four waveforms constituting the normal spectral Doppler waveform are indicated: the A wave lies below the baseline (retrograde component); the S and D waves peak above the baseline and are caused by anterograde blood flow toward the right heart; and the V wave, a transitional wave, may peak just below or above the baseline

Fig. 7. The Doppler waveform of left hepatic vein blood flow resembles that of the pulmonary vein. It is important for the anesthesiologist to know that flow above the baseline indicates flow toward the transducer and flow below the baseline indicates flow away from the transducer. At least four questions need to be answered: Is there flow? Where it is directed (forward vs. backward)? What is the relationship of magnitude between the S and D waves (normal S>D vs. abnormal S<D)? What is the magnitude of the A wave (normal vs. abnormal)? A detailed explanation has been provided elsewhere [19].

Case 3

During OLTX, the most dangerous phase regarding hemodynamic instability is the reperfusion phase, in which the surgical clamp is removed leading to a sudden release of cold, acidotic, oxidizing, and hyperkalaemic fluid into the circulation [20]. This may also be followed by reperfusion syndrome, occurring in about 42% of patients, which manifests as a temporary myocardial dysfunction with a reduction in heart rate, increased pulmonary arterial pressure, reduced cardiac venous return (preload), and a decrease in mean systemic blood pressure (afterload) of 30% [21]. In such cases, the re-stabilization of the heart becomes priority. In the case of reperfusion syndrome, the patient may experience low preload and afterload. If the patient has left ventricular hypertrophy and long anterior mitral leaflet, left ventricular outflow tract obstruction (LVOTO) may occur: the anterior leaflet of the mitral valve can occlude left ventricle outflow with severe posterolateral mitral regurgitation flow. Without prompt recognition and treatment, the patient could develop a profound cardiovascular collapse. It is important for the anaesthesiologist to be familiar with this possibility and its treatment, which principally consists of giving fluid to the patient, increasing afterload with vasoactive drugs, and reducing cardiac frequency. The images presented in Fig. 7 and the related Additional file 6: Video 6 were acquired in a 57-year-old HCV cirrhotic patient during the reperfusion phase of the liver transplant.

Case 4

After induction of anesthesia in a 69-year-old patient undergoing liver transplantation, the patient suddenly developed desaturation, going from 100 to 90% of peripheral oxygen saturation in 50% oxygen ventilation. The patient did not have any history of hepato-pulmonary syndrome, and the preoperative chest X-ray was normal. Instead of performing recruitment maneuvers blindly, in the hope that the cause of hypoxia was due to the pressure of the diaphragm toward the lungs secondary to the abundant ascites, the TEE probe was inserted and

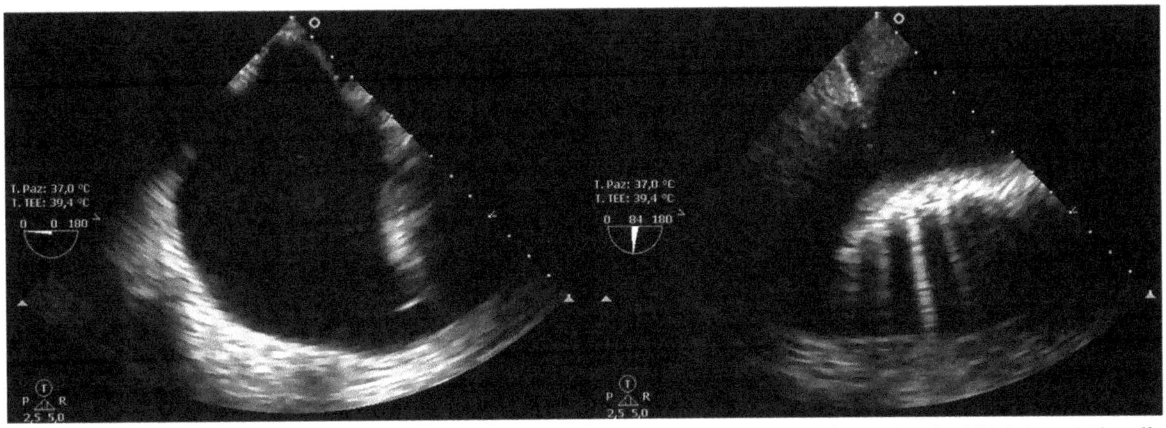

Fig. 8 Pleural effusion in the chest cavity, as seen by trans-esophageal lung ultrasound (TELU) at 0° (*left image*) and 84° (*right image*). The effusion looks anechoic, while the lung parenchyma appears to be compressed, with some B-lines

the lungs explored, leading to a rapid diagnosis of right pleural effusion due to the passage of the ascites into the pleural space.

The reported sensitivity of TEE for the detection of a pleural effusion is 97 with 100% specificity (compared with gold standard computed tomography) [22]. The patient underwent intraoperative pleural drainage and saturation was restored (see Fig. 8; Additional file 7: Video 7). As recently described by Cavayas et al. [23] transesophageal lung ultrasound (TELU) should be performed as a systematic approach. In TELU, the cranio-caudal axis of each lung is divided into apical, middle, and basal regions; the left subclavian artery is used as a landmark to identify the apical regions; the superior pulmonary veins are used to mark the middle regions; and, finally, the inferior vena cava and the right atrial junction are used to identify the basal segments. From each of these landmarks, the lungs are scanned along the longitudinal axis by rotation of the ultrasound plane at 0° and 90°. In this case, the TEE probe was used because it was available as the point-of-care ultrasound methodology.

Discussion

The goal of this paper was to describe how TEE in the setting of OLTX is a highly valuable (but maybe underutilized) tool, as it is important not only for cardiovascular monitoring, but also for evaluating hepatic vein blood flow and inferior vena cava anastomosis and patency. We describe, for the first time, the use of intraoperative TEE for evaluating the patency of a rescue cavo-cavostomy anastomosis in the intraoperative phase. TAS, on the other hand, is impossible to perform during surgery [16–18]. In fact, one of the major advantages of using a TEE probe is its anatomical proximity to the liver, allowing the liver to be studied from the inside without interfering with the surgery. Furthermore, TEE is more sensitive in detecting low blood flow velocity or small changes of blood flow in the hepatic veins [18]. Moreover, the literature reports a case in which intraoperative TEE evaluation of a vena cava tumor resection using the piggy-back technique led to a change in the surgical plain [24]. Thus, our report is not the first to demonstrate the feasibility of obtaining good liver anatomy visualization and acceptable quality images of the IVC through the use of TEE [25].

In patients undergoing liver transplantation, the occurrence of reperfusion syndrome can be dangerous, and visual assessment of the heart is of extreme importance. In the literature, very few reports describe dynamic left ventricular outflow tract obstruction, probably because TEE is used in just 50% of cases and because this condition is difficult to diagnose [26]. No reports describing the use of TEE in association with reperfusion syndrome or ballooning heart are present in the literature and the only case describing its use in liver transplantation is the one reported by Lee HR et al. [27] where it was used in the postoperative period. So our case is probably the first one.

Some limitations should be noted about the present study. First, the liver window is not always easy to obtain or adequate. Second, the presence of esophagus varices or gastric ulcers can limit the extensive use of TEE and its use must, of course, be balanced against the risks associated with performing the procedure [28]. As previously reported, patients with esophageal stricture, esophageal cancer, esophageal diverticulum, and recent esophageal surgery are generally considered to be near absolute contraindications for TEE [29]. Moreover, esophageal varices have been considered a relative contraindication to TEE, depending on the center and/or operator. Third, the anaesthesiologist should be skilled. However, TEE is safe and feasible in liver transplantation candidates. In fact, in a recent study, the major complication rate was just 0.86%, and the overall complication rate was 1.7%—both very low, but just slightly higher than that reported in cardiac literature in terms of morbidity rate of 0.2% [30].

Conclusions

Echocardiography has become an invaluable tool in anesthesia practice and, thanks to its access to multiple acoustic windows, many organs (heart, liver, lung, spleen, kidney) can be explored in many perioperative diagnostic situations. During liver transplantation or major liver surgery, the use of TEE should not just be focused on the heart. It is our opinion that blood flow and patency of the hepatic anastomosis should be studied by TEE with the help of the radiologist before closing the abdomen. If this technique were to become adopted as standard procedure, then it would mirror what happened in cardiovascular surgery before cardiac anaesthesiologists became confident in using this tool.

Additional files

Additional file 1: Video 1. The donor and the recipient IVC, viewed in parallel.

Additional file 2: Video 2. Color Doppler analysis of the blood flow through the cavo-cavostomy rescue anastomosis, showing appropriate liver venous drainage.

Additional file 3: Video 3. Different phases of the a transient ballooning syndrome developed after reperfusion, that recovered after the increase in systolic pressure upon the second de-clamping following a cavo-cavostomy anastomosis.

Additional file 4: Video 4. Color Doppler Echography of the inferior vena cava blood flow through the patch repair. The Edwards® Bovine Pericardial Patch appears as an hyper echoic structure in the anterior wall of the IVC.

Additional file 5: Video 5. Color Power Angio Echography of the inferior vena cava blood flow through the patch repair.

Additional file 6: Video 6. Left ventricular outflow-tract obstruction in a patient with left ventricular hypertrophy and long anterior mitral leaflet: the anterior leaflet of the mitral valve occludes left ventricle outflow with severe posterolateral mitral regurgitation flow.

Additional file 7: Video 7. Pleural effusion in the chest cavity, as seen by trans-esophageal lung ultrasound (TELU) at 0° and subsequently 84°. The effusion looks anechoic, while the lung parenchyma appears to be compressed, with some B-lines.

Abbreviations

IVC: inferior vena cava; TELU: transesophageal lung ultrasound; TTE: transesophageal echocardiography.

Authors' contributions

LV and GDR planned the study and drafted the manuscript. FB and UB collected data, helped develop the bibliography, and drafted the manuscript. FF and GV helped to draft the manuscript. All the authors read and approved the final manuscript.

Author details

[1] Department of Medicine, University of Udine, P.le S. M. della Misericordia 15, 33100 Udine, Italy. [2] Anesthesia and Intensive Care Medicine IV, Pisa University Hospital, Pisa, Italy. [3] Department of Emergency Medicine, San Luigi Gonzaga University Hospital, Turin, Italy.

Acknowledgements

We would like to thank our colleague Stephanie Pearson who provided valuable insight and language expertise that greatly assisted the drafting of our manuscript.

References

1. Shillcutt SK, Ringenberg KJ, Chacon MM, Brakke TR, Montzingo CR, Lyden ER et al (2016) Liver transplantation: intraoperative transesophageal echocardiography findings and relationship to major postoperative adverse cardiac events. J Cardiothorac Vasc Anesth 30:107–114
2. Murray KF, Carithers RL Jr (2005) AASLD practice guidelines: evaluation of the patient for liver transplantation. Hepatology 41:1407–1432
3. Bjerke RJ, Mieles LA, Borsky BJ, Todo S (1992) The use of transesophageal ultrasonography for the diagnosis of inferior vena caval outflow obstruction during liver transplantation. Transplantation 54:939–941
4. Alcaraz G, Meineri M, Dattilo K, Wąsowicz M (2016) Intraoperative transesophageal echocardiographic diagnosis of acute Budd–Chiari syndrome after extended right hepatectomy. A A Case Rep 1(7):13–15
5. Sharma V, Wasowicz M, Brister S, Karski J, Meineri M (2011) Postoperative transesophageal echocardiography diagnosis of inferior vena cava obstruction after mitral valve replacement. Anesth Analg 113:1343–1346
6. Hahn RT, Abraham T, Adams MS, Bruce CJ, Glas KE, Lang RM et al (2013) Guidelines for performing a comprehensive transesophageal echocardiographic examination: recommendations from the American Society of Echocardiography and the Society of Cardiovascular Anesthesiologists. J Am Soc Echocardiogr 26:921–964
7. Lambert AS, Chen R (2016) Transesophageal lung ultrasound: to boldly go.... Can J Anaesth 63:1211–1214
8. Goswami V, Kumar B, Puri GD, Singh H (2016) Utility of transesophageal echocardiography in identifying spinal canal structures and epidural catheter position: a prospective observational study of intraoperative hemodynamics and postoperative analgesia. Can J Anesth 63:911–999
9. Bandyopadhyay S, Kumar Das R, Paul A, Sundar Bhunia K, Roy D (2013) A transesophageal echocardiography technique to locate the kidney and monitor renal perfusion. Anesth Analg 116:549–554
10. Rehfeldt KH, Bruggink SM, Pulido JN (2014) Transesophageal echocardiographic imaging of ultrasound lung rockets. Anesthesiology 121:1335
11. Schmitz V, Schoening W, Jelkmann I, Globke B, Pascher A, Bahra M et al (2014) Different cava reconstruction techniques in liver transplantation: piggyback versus cava resection. Hepatobiliary Pancreat Dis Int 13:242–249
12. Tzakis A, Todo S, Starzl TE (1989) Orthotopic liver transplantation with preservation of the inferior vena cava. Ann Surg 210:649–652
13. Nemes B, Kóbori L, Fehérvári I, Fazakas J, Gerlei Z, Ther G et al (2005) Comparison of the results of conventional, crossclamp and piggyback technique in liver transplantation. Magy Seb 58:155–161
14. Parrilla P, Sànchez-Bueno F, Figueras J, Jaurrieta E, Mir J, Margarit C et al (1999) Analysis of the complications of the piggyback technique in 1112 liver transplants. Transplant Proc 31:2388–2389
15. Cescon M, Grazi GL, Varotti G, Ravaioli M, Ercolani G, Gardini A et al (2005) Venous outflow reconstructions with the piggyback technique in liver transplantation: a single-center experience of 431 cases. Transpl Int 18:318–325
16. Risaliti A, Baccarani U, Cautero N, Donini A, Alessandrini V, Sainz M et al (2001) Infrahepatic cavo-cavostomy as a rescue technique for complicated piggyback liver transplantation. Transplant Proc 33:1388–1389
17. Vetrugno L, Pompei L, Zearo E, Della Rocca G (2014) Could transesophageal echocardiography be useful in selected cases during liver surgery resection? J Ultrasound 19:47–52
18. Meierhenrich R, Gauss A, Georgieff M, Schütz W (2001) Use of multi-plane transoesophageal echocardiography in visualization of the main hepatic veins and acquisition of Doppler sonography curves: comparison with the transabdominal approach. Br J Anaesth 87:711–717
19. Scheinfeld MH, Bilali A, Koenigsberg M (2009) Understanding the spectral Doppler waveform of the hepatic veins in health and disease. Radiographics 29:2081–2098

20. Fung SK, Hui TW, Wong AK, Lei GM (1999) Anaesthesia for liver transplantation: experience at a teaching hospital. Hong Kong Med J 5:27–33
21. Burtenshaw AJ, Isaac JL (2006) The role of trans-oesophageal echocardiography for perioperative cardiovascular monitoring during orthotopic liver transplantation. Liver Transpl 12:1577–1583
22. Tsubo T, Yatsu Y, Okawa H, Ishihara H, Matsuki A (2002) Transesophageal echocardiography is a sensitive method to evaluate pleural effusion. Anesthesiology 96:A322
23. Cavayas YA, Girard M, Desjardins G, Denault AY (2016) Transesophageal lung ultrasonography: a novel technique for investigating hypoxemia. Can J Anesth 63:1266–1276
24. Cywinski JB, O'Hara JF Jr (2009) Transesophageal echocardiography to redirect the intraoperative surgical approach for vena cava tumor resection. Anesth Analg 109:1413–1415
25. Kirkeby-Garstad I, Tromsdal A, Sellevold OFM, Bjørngaard M, Bjella MK, Berg EM et al (2003) Guiding surgical cannulation of the inferior vena cava with transesophageal echocardiography. Anesth Analg 96:1288–1293
26. Essandoh M, Otey AJ, Dalia A, Dewhirst E, Springer A, Henry M (2016) Refractory hypotension after liver allograft reperfusion: a case of dynamic left ventricular outflow tract obstruction. Front Med (Lausanne) 16(3):3
27. Lee HR, Hurst RT, Vargas HE (2007) Transient left ventricular apical ballooning syndrome (Takotsubo cardiomyopathy) following orthotopic liver transplantation. Liver Transpl 13(9):1343–1345
28. Spier B, Larue SJ, Teelin TC, Leff JA, Swize LR, Borkan SH et al (2009) Review of the complications in a series of patients with known gastroesophageal varices undergoing transesophageal echocardiography. J Am Soc Echocardiogr 22:397–401
29. Spencer KT (2009) Transesophageal echocardiography in patients with esophageal varices. J Am Soc Echocardiogr 22:401–403
30. Markin NW, Sharma A, Grant W, Shillcutt SK (2015) The safety of transesophageal echocardiography in patients undergoing orthotopic liver transplantation. J Cardiothorac Vasc Anesth 29:588–593

24

Relationship of spontaneous microembolic signals to risk stratification, recurrence, severity and mortality of ischemic stroke: a prospective study

Rodrigo Bazan[1], Gustavo José Luvizutto[2], Gabriel Pereira Braga[1], Silméia Garcia Zanati Bazan[3], João Carlos Hueb[3], Carlos Clayton Macedo de Freitas[1], Pedro Tadao Hamamoto Filho[1*], Gabriel Pinheiro Módolo[1], André Petean Trindade[4], Marcone Lima Sobreira[5], Hélio Rubens de Carvalho Nunes[1], João Pereira Leite[6] and Octávio Marques Pontes-Neto[6]

Abstract

Introduction: The presence of microembolic signals (MES) during the acute phase of stroke is poorly understood, and its role and clinical application in relation to risk stratification and prognosis in patients remain uncertain. We assessed the prevalence of spontaneous MES in acute stroke and their relationship with risk stratification, stroke recurrence, morbidity, and mortality.

Patients and methods: This was a prospective cohort study conducted in the Stroke Unit. The MES presence was evaluated by transcranial Doppler (TCD) in patients with ischemic stroke within 48 h. The outcomes (risk stratification, morbidity, mortality, and recurrence of a stroke) were followed up for 6 months. The relationship between risk stratification and MES was obtained by odds ratios and that between MES and stroke recurrence, morbidity, and mortality using multiple logistic regression; considering statistical significance at $P < 0.05$.

Results: Of the 111 patients studied, 70 were men (63.1%) and 90 were white (81.1%), with a median age of 68 years. The MES frequency was 7%. There was a significant relationship between MES and symptomatic carotid disease (OR = 22.7; 95% CI 4.1–125.7; $P < 0.001$), a shorter time to monitoring (OR = 12.4; 95% CI 1.4–105.4; $P = 0.02$), and stroke recurrence (OR = 16.83; 95% CI 2.01–141; $P = .009$).

Discussion: It was observed that the stroke recurrence adjusted for prior stroke was higher and earlier among patients with MES detection. In conclusion, MES demonstrated a significant correlation with symptomatic carotid disease and a shorter DELAY until monitoring, and could be a predictor for the early recurrence of stroke in the long term.

Keywords: Brain embolism, Prognosis, Risk factors, Stroke, Transcranial Doppler ultrasonography

Introduction

Transcranial Doppler (TCD) is an important tool used in health care to assess blood flow velocity in brain arteries, with extensive application in neurovascular clinical practice [1, 2]. TCD has potential diagnostic applications in locating embolic sources and long-term risk prediction of ischemic stroke [3]. The detection of embolic signals has

*Correspondence: pthamamotof@hotmail.com
[1] Department of Neurology, Psychology and Psychiatry, Botucatu Medical School, UNESP–Univ Estadual Paulista, Campus de Botucatu, Distrito de Rubião Jr, s/n, Botucatu, Brazil
Full list of author information is available at the end of the article

been observed in a variety of potential embolic sources during patient assessment with TCD. Experimental studies have shown that this technique has a high sensitivity and specificity for the detection of various types of embolic elements [4, 5].

Data from many studies have demonstrated that the detection of spontaneous microembolic signals (MES) can predict the risk of stroke in patients with cardiac emboli or large artery disease, especially in cases of symptomatic internal carotid stenosis [6–10]. TCD is the only method that permits direct identification of embolic phenomena through the detection of an MES [11, 12].

The presence of MES on TCD during the acute phase of stroke is poorly understood, and its role and clinical application in relation to risk stratification and prognosis in patients remain uncertain, with no study having been conducted in the Latin American population. We assessed the hypothesis that investigating MES prevalence in the acute phase of stroke is related to risk stratification, stroke recurrence, disability, and death.

Materials and methods

Ethics approval and consent to participate

This trial was approved by a Committee for Ethics in Research involving human subjects from Ribeirão Preto School of Medicine. Upon inclusion, all patients or legal surrogates provided written informed consent in accordance with the Declaration of Helsinki II.

Study design, setting, and participants

This was a prospective cohort study of consecutive adult patients of both sexes diagnosed with ischemic stroke of the anterior circulation during the first 48 h of ictus. This study was conducted in the Stroke Unit at Botucatu Medical School (UNESP) from January 2015 to March 2016. The inclusion criteria for monitoring included a diagnosis of ischemic stroke of the anterior circulation territory confirmed by neuroimaging examinations (CT or MRI) and by OSCP (The Oxford Community Stroke Project classification) within the first 48 h of ictus, age above 18 years, monitoring with TCD for a minimum duration of 30 min, and performance of phenotypic classification and stroke risk stratification by Trial of Org 10172 in Acute Stroke Treatment (TOAST), preferably in the first 3 months after inclusion in the study [13].

The study excluded patients with a diagnosis of hemorrhagic stroke or with the presence of other types of brain lesions of non-vascular etiology, those who did not have a temporal acoustic window (TAW) to undergo TCD, those who underwent any surgical procedure that impeded the realization of monitoring, or those lost during the 6-month follow-up. Also excluded were examinations of poor technical quality during TCD due to various artifacts during recording.

Variables

Definition of risk factors

The risk factors evaluated were as follows: hypertension, smoking, obesity, diabetes mellitus (DM), at-risk drinkers, dyslipidemia, Chagas' disease, prior stroke, congestive heart failure (CHF), prior acute myocardial infarction (AMI), coronary artery disease (CAD), depression, atrial fibrillation, atrial flutter, patent foramen ovale (PFO, confirmed with transthoracic and/or transesophageal echocardiogram), and extracardiac shunts. These data were collected from the clinical history of patients, such as previous use of antihypertensive medications, oral hypoglycemic agents or parenteral insulin, oral lipid-lowering drugs, or were confirmed clinically and by laboratory tests during hospitalization. Levels considered for confirmation were hypertension with systolic blood pressure $\geq$ 140/90 mmHg, dyslipidemia with cholesterol levels $\geq$ 240 mg/dL, diabetes mellitus with glycated hemoglobin level > 7%, obese patients with a body mass index $\geq$ 30 kg/m^2, and a score > 8 in the Hospital Anxiety and Depression Scale (HADS) [14–17].

TCD examination

A portable TCD device (DWL, Doppler Box model, Compumedics, Singen, Baden-Württemberg, Germany) was placed between the lateral margin of the orbit and the ear, above the zygomatic arch. Low-power pulsed-wave 2-MHz transducers, 1.7 cm in diameter, were used with TCD-8 software (Version 8.00 K) at a pulse repetition frequency of 6500 Hz and a programmable high-pass filter of 50–600 Hz. The transducers were fixed bilaterally to a helmet to monitor both middle cerebral arteries at 45–60 mm.

All patients were initially evaluated by two independent neurologists for the presence of a temporal acoustic window (TAW) by TCD. Patients with bilateral TAWs underwent examination with TCD for at least 30 min. The researchers were single blinded during monitoring to the risk stratification of the patients. By the time of TCD, intravenous solution dripping was interrupted.

Microembolic signals detection

To evaluate MES, the following characteristics were considered according to the microembolus detection consensus [12]: randomly occurring during the cardiac cycle, short (< 0.1 s), high intensity (3–9 dB) above the wave spectrum, and characteristic audible sound. We used the Power Doppler M in all tests to identify the arteries and aid in the identification of microembolic signals (Fig. 1). In general, monitoring took 45 min. Automatic detection

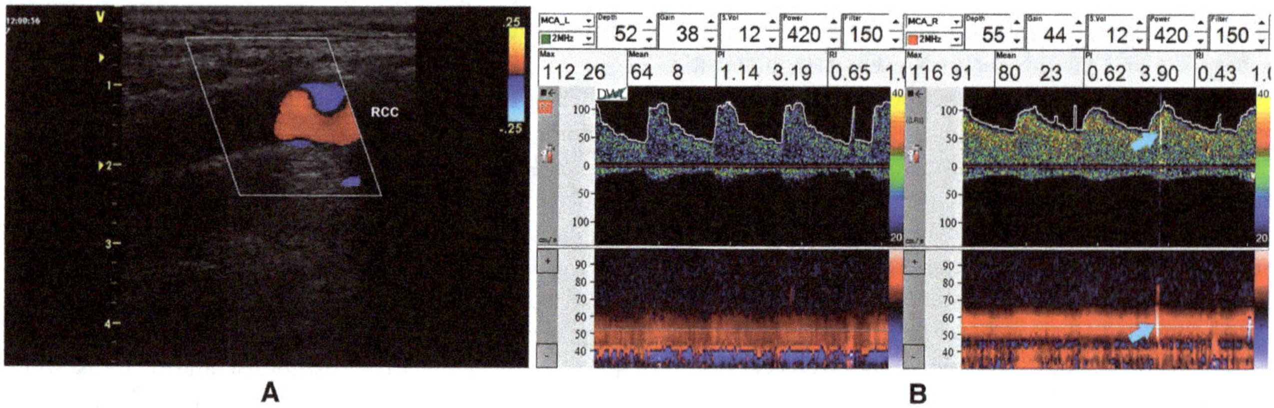

Fig. 1 **a** Suggestive image of a plaque in the right common carotid artery (rcca); **b** in the same patient, spontaneous microembolic signal was detected by transcranial Doppler monitoring in acute phase of stroke. Blue arrows indicate MES in wave spectrum and in Mode M

of microembolic signals was used in association with visual and sound discretion of microemboli. All tests were recorded for at least 30 min, filed, and independently reviewed by two blinded investigators to identify MES [12]. The presence or absence of MES was reported, as well the number of MES for each patient.

Clinical variables and risk stratification

The patients were classified according to TOAST, examination of brain imaging by computed tomography (CT) or magnetic resonance imaging (MRI), extensive laboratory examinations, electrocardiogram (ECG), transthoracic or transesophageal echocardiography, and duplex or CT angiography of the carotid and vertebrobasilar system. All patients underwent hospitalization in the Stroke Unit and received standard care according to the international protocols [18–20]. The degree of carotid stenosis was classified by the NASCET criteria, defined as < 50%, 50–69%, ≥ 70%, or occlusion [21]. TCD examination was performed in all patients to evaluate possible intracranial stenosis. MR angiography, CT angiography, and digital arteriography were performed on the suspicion of stenosis of intracranial or extracranial vessels. The examination of digital 24-h Holter monitoring was conducted in subjects over 55 years and suspected of paroxysmal atrial fibrillation.

Follow-up

Outpatient follow-up time was 6 months after the onset of stroke and was performed by a blinded investigator. Disability was monitored using the modified Rankin Scale (mRS), with mRS 0–2 being classified as favorable and mRS 6 as death, and the recurrence of stroke was monitored throughout the study. Recurrence of stroke was documented by means of clinical and radiological evaluation.

Primary outcome measures

Disability and death in 6 months.

Secondary outcome measures

Recurrence of stroke in 6 months.

Study size and sampling

We needed a minimum of 100 subjects to obtain a maximum sampling error of 7.5% and a confidence level of 95%. Type I and II error probabilities equaled 0.05 and 0.20, respectively, and it was estimated that the power to test the association between the presence of MES with stroke < 48 h post-ictus, atheromatous carotid, and symptomatic carotid artery disease was above 80%. For clinical follow-up data, it was estimated that the power to test the association between the presence of MES and recurrence, disability, and death was below 65%.

Statistical methods

The interobserver agreement of the presence of MES was classified by Cohen's κ coefficient. The risk stratification of patients with acute ischemic stroke and the relationship with MES had point and interval estimations of the odds ratios, depending on the statistically related independent variables calculated by Fisher's exact test, taking into account confounding factors (thrombolysis, level of anticoagulation, and antiplatelet therapies) at monitoring. The selected variables with $P < 0.05$ in the univariate analysis were included in the multiple logistic regression to determine the independent variables associated with the presence of MES.

The relationship between morbidity and mortality in patients and MES (presence or absence and number for patient) during follow-up was evaluated using univariate analysis for potential confounders, such as age, sex, race, hypertension, NIHSS at admission, previous mRS, hemorrhagic transformation, smoking, obesity, diabetes, dyslipidemia, Chagas' disease, prior stroke, prior AMI, CAD, depression, wake-up stroke, carotid dissection, carotid atheroma, symptomatic carotid disease, intracranial stenosis, atrial flutter, atrial fibrillation, cardiac heart failure (CHF), patent foramen ovale (PFO), extracardiac shunt, and thrombolysis. A subsequent multiple logistic regression analysis was performed with backward selection correcting for the effect of potential confounders.

The variables more strongly associated ($P<0.20$) with the incidence rate of stroke recurrence were included in a Cox proportional regression model. Statistical analysis was carried out with SPSS software (Version 21.0, SPSS, Chicago, IL, USA).

Results

A total of 254 patients were screened in this study, with 105 excluded by the exclusion criteria. Only 149 patients were considered for monitoring, and 38 patients (26%) showed no TAW during TCD evaluation (Fig. 2).

A high level of concordance was demonstrated between the two experts who rated the presence of MES ($\kappa=0.95$; $P<0.01$, % agreement = 98%). The total number of patients monitored with TCD was 111; 70 were men (63.1%) and 90 were white (81.1%), with a median age of 68 years. Hypertension was found to be the main risk factor (83.8%). MES were found in eight patients (7%). Participant characteristics are displayed in Table 1.

In relation to MES detection, thrombolytic therapy and the level of use of therapeutic oral anticoagulation (INR > 2) and antiplatelet therapies at the time

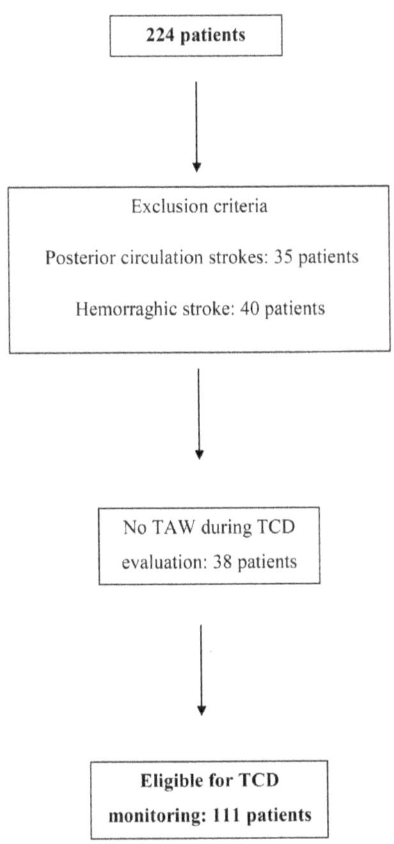

Fig. 2 Flow chart

Table 1 Demographic profile, key risk factors, and clinical and etiological classification of monitored patients

Variables	*n*	%
Demographic profile		
Male	70	63.1
Age (years)	68 (33–97)	
Race		
White	90	81.1
Black/Asian	21	19.9
Risk factors		
Hypertension	93	83.8
Smoking	60	54.1
Obesity	6	5.4
Diabetes	30	27
Dyslipidemia	17	15.3
Chagas disease	8	7.2
Prior stroke	36	32.4
Congestive heart failure	8	7.2
Prior AMI	11	9.9
CAD	12	10.8
Depression	6	5.4
Atrial fibrillation	29	26.1
Atrial flutter	4	3.6
PFO	2	1.8
Extracardiac shunt	1	0.9
Thrombolysis	26	23.4
Antiplatelets	67	60.0
Anticoagulation	3	2.7
Wake-up stroke	18	16.2
NHISS at admission	8 (0–28)	
OSCP		
TACS	25	22.5
PACS	56	50.4
LACS	30	27.0
TOAST		
Small-vessel occlusion	23	21.0
Large-artery atherosclerosis	11	9.9
Cardioembolism	31	28.0
Other determined etiology	5	4.5
Undetermined etiology	41	37

AMI acute myocardial infarction, *CAD* coronary artery disease, *NIHSS* National Institutes of Health Stroke Scale, *OSCP* The Oxford Community Stroke Project classification, *TACS* total anterior circulation syndrome, *PACS* partial anterior circulation syndrome, *LACS* lacunar syndrome

of monitoring were analyzed as potential confounders. There was no statistically significant relationship to these variables. Demographic variables, such as sex and race, were also not statistically significant for MES detection.

MES detection was higher in patients with atherosclerotic carotid (OR=15.5, 95% CI 3.2 to 74.7; P=0.001) and symptomatic carotid artery disease (OR=22.7; 95% CI 4.1 to 125.7; P=0.001). MES were not detected in patients with small vessel disease or atrial fibrillation. MES detection was higher among patients who were monitored earlier in relation to the onset of symptoms of stroke (OR=2.4, 95% CI 1.4 to 105.4; P=0.02) (Table 2).

Table 3 shows the association between MES and outcomes. The chance for favorable outcomes were reduced with increasing age (OR=0.96; 95% CI 0.91 to 1.00, P=0.036), increasing NIHSS at admission (OR=0.80; 95% CI 0.73 to 0.87, P<0.001), and higher prior mRS (OR=0.31; 95% CI 0.14 to 0.66, P=0.002). The probability for favorable outcomes tended to be higher in patients who smoked (OR=2.83; 95% CI 0.98 to 8.15, P=0.054). There was no significant relationship between MES and favorable outcomes (mRS 0–2) (OR=2.4, 95% CI 0.36 to 16.36, P=0.366). The probability of death was higher with increasing age (OR=1.07; 95% CI 1.01 to 1.12, P=0.014) and increasing NIHSS (OR=1.16; 95% CI 1.07 to 1.26, P<0.001). There was no significant relationship between MES and the occurrence of death (mRS 6) (OR=2.27, 95% CI 0.19 to 26.50, P=0.513).

The absence of a statistically significant association was found between favorable outcomes (mRS 0–2) (P=0.429), and death (P=0.154) and positive association between the number of MES for patient and recurrence (P=0.017). However, multivariate analysis was not performed due to the low number of patients with MES (great asymmetry of the sample). The OR for the outcomes as a function of the number of MES was analyzed for the total sample, and the analysis showed no statistical differences in terms of favorable outcomes for lower number of MES for patient (OR=0.85 95% CI 0.56 to 1.30). The mortality (OR=1.41 95% CI 0.92 to 2.16) and recurrence (OR=1.55 95% CI 0.88 to 2.76) increased with the more number of MES for patient, but none of the three associations was statistically significant.

Four patients (3.6%) had a recurrence of stroke within 6 months of follow-up, and the TOAST classifications of these strokes were small vessels, cardioembolic, atherosclerosis of large vessels, and indeterminate nature, respectively. There were no confounding factors for stroke recurrence, and there was a significant relationship between the detection of MES and stroke recurrence during follow-up (OR=16.83, 95% CI 2.01 to 141.08; P=0.009).

Table 2 Relationship between risk factors, etiology, and clinical presentation with MES presence

	MES n (%)	P
Hypertension		
No (n=18)	3 (17%)	0.119
Yes (n=93)	5 (5%)	
Smoking		
No (n=51)	4 (8%)	1.000
Yes (n=60)	4 (7%)	
Obesity		
No (n=105)	7 (7%)	0.369
Yes (n=6)	1 (17%)	
Diabetes		
No (n=81)	6 (7%)	1.000
Yes (n=30)	2 (7%)	
Dyslipidemia		
No (n=94)	6 (6%)	0.354
Yes (n=17)	2 (12%)	
Chagas disease		
No (n=103)	7 (7%)	0.462
Yes (n=8)	1 (12.5%)	
Prior stroke		
No (n=75)	7 (9%)	0.271
Yes (n=36)	1 (3%)	
Cardiac heart failure		
No (n=103)	8 (8%)	1.000
Yes (n=8)	0 (0%)	
Prior AMI		
No (n=100)	8 (8%)	1.000
Yes (n=11)	0 (0%)	
CAD		
No (n=99)	8 (8%)	0.595
Yes (n=12)	0 (0%)	
Depression		
No (n=105)	7 (6%)	0.369
Yes (n=6)	1 (17%)	
TOAST		
Small-vessel occlusion (n=23)	0 (0%)	<0.001
Large-artery atherosclerosis (n=11)	5 (46%)	
Cardioembolism (n=31)	0 (0%)	
Other determined etiology (n=5)	2 (40%)	
Undetermined etiology (n=41)	1 (2%)	
Ictus time<24 h		
No (n=67)	1 (1.5%)	0.006
Yes (n=44)	7 (16%)	
Wake-up stroke		
No (n=93)	6 (7%)	0.614
Yes (n=18)	2 (11%)	
Carotid dissection		
No (n=109)	7 (6%)	0.140
Yes (n=2)	1 (50%)	

Table 2 (continued)

	MES n (%)	P
Carotid atheromatous		
No ($n=96$)	3 (3%)	0.001
Yes ($n=15$)	5 (33%)	
Symptomatic carotid		
No ($n=93$)	2 (2%)	<0.001
Yes ($n=18$)	6 (3%)	
Intracranial stenosis		
No ($n=105$)	8 (7%)	1.000
Yes ($n=6$)	0 (0%)	
Atrial flutter		
No ($n=107$)	8 (8%)	1.000
Yes ($n=4$)	0 (0%)	
Atrial fibrillation		
No ($n=82$)	8 (10%)	0.108
Yes ($n=29$)	0 (0%)	
PFO		
No ($n=109$)	8 (7%)	1.000
Yes ($n=2$)	0 (0%)	
Extracardiac shunt		
No ($n=110$)	8 (7%)	1.000
Yes ($n=1$)	1 (100%)	
Plaques in the aortic arch		
No ($n=109$)	8 (7%)	1.000
Yes ($n=2$)	0 (0%)	

Fisher exact test

Table 4 and Fig. 3 demonstrate the identified factors that were more strongly associated with the incidence rate of stroke recurrence.

It was observed that the stroke recurrence adjusted for prior stroke was higher and earlier among patients with MES detection (RRadjusted = 36 (4–323), $P<0.001$).

During hospitalization and after discharge, 16 patients started using anticoagulant therapy, while all others were given antiplatelet therapies. The treatment of carotid artery disease was performed in 5 patients exclusively with endovascular therapy (stent). No patient was treated with endarterectomy due to an intrinsic characteristic of the hospital.

Discussion

Of the total number of patients involved in this study, 26% did not have a TAW on TCD examination. These results were demonstrated in a previous study with the same sample by our stroke team [22]. The other studies in the literature showed a range of 3–34% absence of acoustic window, including populations from healthy volunteers and patients with cerebrovascular disease [23].

The MES detected by TCD have been described in patients with carotid artery stenosis, dissection of large cervical vessels, atrial fibrillation, catheter-based procedures, and atheromatous plaques in the aortic arch, but their clinical application remains uncertain [24, 25]. The number of patients with MES in this study was 8 patients (7%). Other samples showed variations in the rate of MES detection in the acute phase of stroke ranging between 9.3 and 71%, with most studies demonstrating a relationship with large artery disease and less frequently with cardioembolic disease [26–29]. MES were not detected in cases with intracranial stenosis, in contrast to a prevalence of 22% reported in other studies [3]. The high percentage of patients who underwent thrombolytic treatment or who were using antiplatelet therapies during transcranial Doppler monitoring, despite not presenting a statistically significant correlation with the detection of MES, may have influenced the low detection rate of these MES. However, it must be emphasized that these monitoring conditions in the acute and subacute stages of a stroke correspond to the conditions that most resemble the real world.

A statistically significant relationship between the MES and patients with large vessel disease was found. There was also a significant association between detecting MES and symptomatic carotid artery disease. Of patients with symptomatic carotid disease, two had arterial dissection at the time of monitoring by TCD, and in one of these, MES were found. Some other studies have demonstrated the importance of microembolism in TCD monitoring as a risk factor for stroke in carotid dissection [30–32]. One of the patients examined in the present study was diagnosed with pulmonary thromboembolism and left-to-right shunts could be detected with a simple bubble test, without contrast. This patient had extensive ischemia in the territory of both the middle cerebral arteries with bilateral MES during TCD monitoring, a relatively rare finding in the literature [33]. TCD associated with the use of contrast is a useful tool in the investigation of right-left deviations, such as patent foramen ovale and other rare medical conditions, such as pulmonary fistula.

This study showed a higher chance of MES detection the sooner the monitoring time was in relation to the onset of symptoms of stroke. Studies conducted in the 1990s showed that early monitoring with TCD in acute stroke increases the likelihood of the detection of MES [34].

No relationship was found between the detection of MES and the degree of disability and death; correlations were found with aging, NIHSS, and prior mRS. These findings were similar to other studies in the literature [6, 34]. In this study, smoking seemed to be a protective factor. This paradoxical finding was shown in other studies

Table 3 Simple and multiple regression logistics between confounder factors with outcomes

Variables	Simple regression (univariate analysis)						Multiple regression (multivariate analysis)					
	mRS 0–2		Death		Recurrence		mRS 0–2		Death		Recurrence	
	n (%)	*P*	*n* (%)	*P*	*n* (%)	*P*	*P*	OR (CI95%)	*P*	OR (IC95%)	*P*	OR (CI95%)
Sex		0.548		0.851		1.000						
Male	44 (62.9)		11 (15.7)		3 (2.4)							
Female	23 (56.1)		7 (17.1)		1 (4.3)							
Age (years)	–	0.002	–	0.005	–	0.986	0.036	0.96 (0.92–1.0)	0.014	1.07 (1.01–1.12)		
Race		0.366		0.187		1.000						
Caucasian	52 (57.8)		17 (18.9)		4 (4.4)							
Non-Caucasian	15 (75.7)		1 (5.0)		0							
Hypertension		0.132		0.46		1.000						
Yes ($n=93$)	59 (63.4)		13 (14.0)		4 (4.3)							
No ($n=18$)	8 (44.4)		5 (27.8)		0							
NIHSS at admission	–	< 0.001	–	<0.001	–	0.295	0.000	0.80 (0.73–0.87)	0.000	1.16 (1.07–1.26)		
Prior mRS	–	0.014	–	0.876	NC	–	0.002	0.31 (0.14–0.66)				
Hemorrhagic transformation		0.111		0.317		1.000						
Yes	2 (28.6)		2 (28.6)		0							
No	65 (62.5)		16 (15.4)		4 (3.8)							
Smoking		0.002		0.158		0.623	0.054	2.83 (0.98–8.15)				
Yes ($n=60$)	44 (73.3)		7 (11.7)		3 (5.0)							
No	23 (45.1)		11 (21.6)		1 (2.0)							
Obesity		0.680		1.000		1.000						
Yes ($n=6$)	3 (50.0)		1 (16.7)		0							
No ($n=105$)	64 (61.0)		17 (16.2)		4 (3.8)							
Diabetes		0.206		0.280		0.295						
Yes ($n=30$)	21 (70.0)		3 (18.5)		2 (6.7)							
No ($n=81$)	46 (56.8)		15 (10.0)		2 (2.5)							
Dyslipidemia		0.182		0.298		0.110						
Yes ($n=17$)	13 (76.5)		1 (5.9)		2 (11.8)							
No ($n=94$)	54 (57.4)		17 (18.1)		2 (2.1)							
Chagas disease		0.710		0.350		1.000						
Yes ($n=8$)	4 (50.0)		0		0							
No ($n=103$)	63 (61.2)		18 (17.5)		4 (3.9)							
Prior stroke		0.122		0.523		0.099						

Table 3 (continued)

Variables	Simple regression (univariate analysis)						Multiple regression (multivariate analysis)					
	mRS 0–2		Death		Recurrence		mRS 0–2		Death		Recurrence	
	n (%)	*P*	*n* (%)	*P*	*n* (%)	*P*	*P*	OR (CI95%)	*P*	OR (IC95%)	*P*	OR (CI95%)
Yes ($n=36$)	18 (50.0)		7 (19.4)		3 (8.3)							
No ($n=75$)	49 (65.3)		11 (14.7)		1 (1.3)							
Prior AMI		0.287		1.000		0.345						
Yes ($n=11$)	5 (45.5)		2 (18.2)		1 (9.1)							
No ($n=100$)	62 (62.0)		16 (16.0)		3 (3.0)							
CAD		0.879		0.687		0.057						
Yes ($n=12$)	7 (58.3)		1 (8.3)		2 (16.7)							
No ($n=99$)	60 (60.6)		17 (17.2)		2 (2.0)							
Depression		1.000		0.587		0.202						
Yes ($n=6$)	4 (60.6)		0		1 (16.7)							
No ($n=105$)	63 (50.0)		18 (17.1)		3 (2.9)							
Wake-up stroke		0.943		1.000		0.512						
Yes ($n=18$)	11 (61.1)		3 (16.7)		1 (5.6)							
No ($n=93$)	56 (60.2)		15 (16.1)		3 (3.2)							
Carotid dissection		1.000		1.000		1.000						
Yes ($n=2$)	1 (60.6)		0		0							
No ($n=109$)	66 (50.0)		18 (16.5)		4 (3.7)							
Carotid atheromatous		0.550		0.708		0.445						
Yes ($n=15$)	8 (53.3)		3 (20.0)		1 (6.7)							
No ($n=96$)	59 (61.5)		15 (15.6)		3 (3.1)							
Symptomatic carotid		0.326		1.000		0.512						
Yes ($n=18$)	9 (50.0)		3 (16.7)		1 (5.6)							
No ($n=93$)	58 (62.4)		15 (16.1)		3 (3.2)							
Intracranial stenosis		0.400		1.000		1.000						
Yes ($n=6$)	5 (83.3)		1 (16.7)		0							
No ($n=105$)	62 (59.0)		17 (16.2)		4 (3.8)							
Atrial flutter		0.648		0.512		1.000						
Yes ($n=4$)	2 (50.0)		1 (25.0)		0							
No ($n=107$)	65 (60.7)		17 (15.9)		4 (3.7)							
Atrial fibrillation		0.004		0.012		1.000						
Yes ($n=29$)	11 (37.9)		9 (31.0)		1 (3.4)							

Table 3 (continued)

Variables	Simple regression (univariate analysis)						Multiple regression (multivariate analysis)					
	mRS 0–2		Death		Recurrence		mRS 0–2		Death		Recurrence	
	n (%)	*P*	*n* (%)	*P*	*n* (%)	*P*	*P*	OR (CI95%)	*P*	OR (IC95%)	*P*	OR (CI95%)
No ($n=82$)	56 (68.3)		9 (11.0)		3 (3.7)							
Aortic arch		1.000		0.299		1.000						
Yes ($n=2$)	1 (50.0)		1 (50.0)		0							
No ($n=109$)	66 (60.6)		17 (15.6)		4 (3.7)							
Cardiac heart failure		0.155		0.299		1.000						
Yes ($n=2$)	0		1 (50.0)		0							
No ($n=109$)	67 (61.5)		17 (15.6)		4 (3.7)							
PFO		0.155		1.000		1.000						
Yes ($n=2$)	0		0		0							
No ($n=109$)	67 (61.5)		18 (16.5)		4 (3.7)							
Extracardiac shunt		0.396		0.162		1.000						
Yes ($n=1$)	0		1 (100.0)		0							
No ($n=110$)	67 (61.5)		17 (15.5)		4 (3.6)							
Thrombolysis		0.751		0.021		1.000						
Yes ($n=26$)	21 (70.0)		8 (30.8)		1 (3.8)							
No ($n=85$)	46 (56.8)		10 (11.8)		3 (3.5)							
MES									0.547			16.83 (2.01–141)
Number of MES												
0	62 (60%)	0.429	16 (15.5%)	0,154	2 (1.9%)	0.017						
1	3 (100%)		0 (0%)		1 (33%)							
3	1 (50%)		0 (0%)		1 (50%)							
5	1 (33%)		2 (66%)		0 (0%)							

NIHSS National Institutes of Health Stroke Scale, *AMI* acute myocardial infarction, *CAD* coronary artery disease, *CHF* cardiac heart failure, *PFO* patent foramen ovale, *NC* not confounder for stroke recurrence

Table 4 Simple regression models of Cox adjusted to the incidence rate of stroke recurrence due to each independent variable

Variable	*B* estimate	Standard error	Wald test	*P*	Relative risk	CI95%	
Sociodemographic profile							
Sex, Male	0.57	1.16	0.25	0.620	1.77	0.18	17.0
Age (years)	0.00	0.04	0.00	0.988	1.00	0.93	1.1
Race, Non-white	−3.33	5.48	0.37	0.543	0.04	0.00	1642.1
Risk factors							
Hypertension	3.28	5.85	0.31	0.576	26.47	0.00	3.E+06
Smoking	0.95	1.16	0.67	0.412	2.58	0.27	24.8
Obesity	−3.09	9.75	0.10	0.752	0.05	0.00	9.E+06
Diabetes	0.99	1.00	0.98	0.323	2.69	0.38	19.1
Dyslipidemia	1.72	1.00	2.94	0.086	5.55	0.78	39.4
Chagas disease	−3.12	8.49	0.14	0.714	0.04	0.00	8.E+05
Prior stroke	1.87	1.16	2.62	0.106	6.48	0.67	62.3
Prior CHF	1.48	1.16	1.64	0.200	4.39	0.46	42.2
Prior AMI	1.12	1.16	0.94	0.331	3.07	0.32	29.5
Prior CAD	2.20	1.00	4.82	0.028	9.00	1.27	63.9
Clinical profile							
NIHSS	−0.11	0.10	1.10	0.294	0.90	0.74	1.1
Previous mRS	0.18	0.52	0.12	0.729	1.20	0.44	3.3
Wake-up stroke	0.53	1.16	0.21	0.646	1.70	0.18	16.3
Time to monitoring < 24 h	1.52	1.16	1.73	0.188	4.57	0.48	43.9
Etiologic investigation							
Atrial fibrillation	−0.06	1.16	0.00	0.957	0.94	0.10	9.0
Atrial flutter	−3.06	11.87	0.07	0.797	0.05	0.00	6.E+08
CHF	−3.03	16.69	0.03	0.856	0.05	0.00	8.E+12
PFO	−3.03	16.69	0.03	0.856	0.05	0.00	8.E+12
Extracardiac shunt	−3.01	23.54	0.02	0.898	0.05	0.00	5.E+18
Debris in aortic arch	−3.03	16.69	0.03	0.856	0.05	0.00	8.E+12
Carotid atheromatous	0.74	1.16	0.42	0.519	2.11	0.22	20.2
Carotid dissection	−3.03	16.69	0.03	0.856	0.05	0.00	8.E+12
Symptomatic carotid	0.60	1.16	0.27	0.605	1.82	0.19	17.5
Intracranial stenosis	−3.09	9.75	0.10	0.752	0.05	0.00	9.E+06
Treatment							
Thrombolysis	0.08	1.16	0.01	0.942	1.09	0.11	10.5
MES							
Presence of MES	2.58	1.00	6.65	0.010	13.18	1.86	93.64

CI: confidence interval; CHF: cardiac heart failures; AMI: acute myocardial infarction; CAD: coronary artery disease; NIHSS: National Institutes of Health Stroke Scale; mRS: modified Rankin scale; PFO: patent foramen ovale

and can be explained by the better vascular recanalization in patients who smoke [35].

The presence of MES showed a good correlation with early stroke recurrence. A study that analyzed 467 patients showed that the risk of ischemic stroke occurrence increased 5.57 times over the course of 2 years of follow-up when MES were identified and that when MES were detected, there was a greater chance of new cerebral ischemic events occurring [27, 28]. In a meta-analysis from 2009, the authors found a twofold increase in the chance of new cerebral ischemic events when they identified embolic signals in TCD monitoring [3].

In relation to the recurrence of cerebral ischemic events, the present study showed a relationship between coronary artery disease (CAD) and stroke recurrence, demonstrating the probable role of systemic atherosclerotic disease and the role and coexistence of atherosclerotic cardiac comorbidities in these patients, even though we cannot rule out the presence of hidden atrial fibrillation in patients with high burden of atherosclerotic

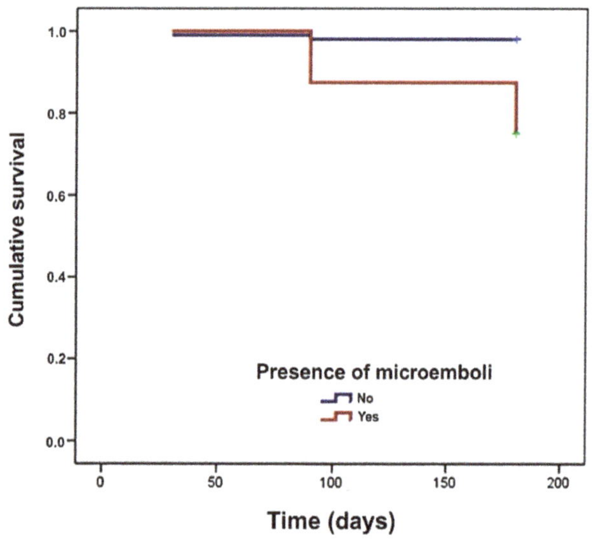

Fig. 3 Survival curves according to the presence of MES corrected by prior stroke

diseases. The low rate of stroke recurrence at 6 months of follow-up may be justified by the clinical and endovascular therapies instituted.

Clinical implications

Early detection of MES in acute phase of stroke may be a clinical indicator to determine carotid disease and recurrences of stroke. This indicator should promptly request a confirmation of possible carotid disease with other methods.

Limitations and strengths

The main limitation of this study is the small number of patients included, as well as the non-inclusion of patients with strokes in the posterior circulation. Also, a limitation of TCD is that the TAW can be obtained from a variable percentage of patients, as well as the fact that this technique is operator dependent. Other limitations of this study are related to the characteristics of the recruited patients (the study was performed in a single center), in addition to technical difficulties with the settings of the monitoring helmet, which generated a greater number of artifacts. The fact that the patients were in the acute phase of stroke and the presence of neurological symptoms, such as unilateral spatial neglect, aphasia, psychomotor agitation, or delirium, made TCD monitoring difficult. In relation to the MES detection points, care must be taken during the examination and the interpretation of the findings due to the need to discriminate MES from possible artifacts.

Conclusion

In conclusion, it was found that MES detection showed a higher correlation with symptomatic carotid disease and a shorter time between ictus and TCD monitoring. In addition, the presence of MES and CAD could be predictors for stroke recurrence.

Acknowledgements

None.

Authors' contributions

Conceptualization: RB, JPL, OMPN. Data curation: RB, GJL, GPB, SGZB, JCH, APT, MLS, GPM. Formal analysis: RB, GJL, SGZB, JCH, PTHF, HRCN. Investigation: RB, GPB, JCH, CCMF, APT, MLS, GPM. Methodology: RB, SGZB, JCH, HRCN. Project administration: RB, PTHF, JPL. Writing-original-draft: RB, GJL. Writing-review and editing: RB, PTHF, JPL, OMPN. Validation: HRCN. Supervision: JPL, OMPN. All authors read and approved the final manuscript.

Author details

[1] Department of Neurology, Psychology and Psychiatry, Botucatu Medical School, UNESP–Univ Estadual Paulista, Campus de Botucatu, Distrito de Rubião Jr, s/n, Botucatu, Brazil. [2] Department of Applied Physical Therapy, Institute of Health Sciences, UFTM–Univ Federal do Triângulo Mineiro, Uberaba, Brazil. [3] Department of Internal Medicine, Botucatu Medical School, UNESP–Univ Estadual Paulista, Botucatu, Brazil. [4] Department of Tropical Diseases and Imaging Diagnosis, Botucatu Medical School, UNESP–Univ Estadual Paulista, Botucatu, Brazil. [5] Department of Surgery and Orthopedics, Botucatu Medical School, UNESP–Univ Estadual Paulista, Botucatu, Brazil. [6] Department of Neuroscience and Behavior, Ribeirão Preto School of Medicine, USP–Univ São Paulo, Ribeirão Preto, Brazil.

References

1. Garami Z, Alexandrov AV (2008) Neurosonology. Neurol Clin 27:89–108
2. Sloan MA, Alexandrov AV, Tegeler CH, Spencer MP, Caplan LR, Feldmann E et al (2004) Therapeutics and technology assessment subcommittee of the American Academy of Neurology. Assessment: transcranial Doppler ultrasonography. Neurology 62:1468–1481
3. King A, Markus HS (2009) Doppler embolic signals in cerebrovascular disease and Prediction of stroke risk: a systematic review and meta-analysis. Stroke 40:3711–3717
4. Markus HS, Brown MM (1993) Differentiation between different pathological cerebral embolic materials using transcranial Doppler in an in vitro model. Stroke 24:1-5
5. Markus HS, Droste DW, Brown MM (1994) Detection of asymptomatic cerebral embolic signals with Doppler ultrasound. Lancet 343:1011–1012
6. Markus HS, MacKinnon A (2005) Asymptomatic embolization detected by Doppler ultrasound predicts stroke risk in symptomatic carotid artery stenosis. Stroke 36:971–975
7. Batista P, Oliveira V, Ferro JM (1999) The detection of microembolic signals in patients at risk of recurrent cardioembolic stroke: possible therapeutic relevance. Cerebrovasc Dis 9:314–319
8. Spence JD, Tamayo A, Lownie SP, Ng WP, Ferguson GG (2005) Absence of microemboli on transcranial Doppler identifies low-risk patients with asymptomatic carotid stenosis. Stroke 36:2373–2378
9. Spence JD (2017) Transcranial Doppler monitoring for microemboli: a marker of a high-risk carotid plaque. Semin Vasc Surg 301:62–66
10. Spence JD, Coates V, Li H, Tamayo A, Hackam DG, DiCicco M et al (2010) Effects of intensive medical therapy on microemboli and cardiovascular risk in asymptomatic carotid stenosis. Arch Neurol 67:180–186
11. Jiang J, Jiang Y, Feng S, Feng S, Sun D, Zhuang A, Zeng Q et al (2013) Microembolic signal monitoring of TOAST-classified cerebral infarction patients. Mol Med Rep 8(4):1135–1142

12. Sliwka U, Job FP, Wissuwa D, Diehl RR, Flachskampf FA, Hanrath P et al (1995) Occurrence of transcranial Doppler high-intensity transient signals in patients with potential cardiac sources of embolism. Stroke 26:2067–2070
13. Adams HP, Bendixen BH, Kappelle LJ, Biller J, Love BB, Gordon DL et al (1993) Classification of subtype of acute ischemic stroke. Definitions for use in a multicenter clinical trial. TOAST. Stroke 24:35–41
14. Mancia G, Fagard R, Narkiewicz K, Redón J, Zanchetti A, Böhm M et al (2013) The task force for the management of arterial hypertension of the European Society of Hypertension (ESH) and of the European Society of Cardiology (ESC). J Hypertens 31:1281–1357
15. Jellinger PS, Smith DA, Mehta AE, Ganda O, Handelsman Y, Rodbard HW et al (2012) American Association of Clinical Endocrinologists' Guidelines for management of dyslipidemia and prevention of atherosclerosis. Endocr Pract 18(Suppl 1):1–78
16. American Diabetes Association (2008) Standards of medical care in diabetes. Diabetes Care 31(Suppl 1):S12–S54
17. Wirth A, Wabitsch M, Hauner H (2014) The prevention and treatment of obesity. Dtsch Arztebl Int 111:705–713
18. Adams HP Jr, Brott TG, Furlan AJ, Gomez CR, Grotta J, Helgason CM et al (1996) Guidelines for thrombolytic therapy for acute stroke: a supplement to the guidelines for the management of patients with acute ischemic stroke. Circulation 94:1167–1174
19. Hacke W, Kaste M, Skyhoj Olsen T, Bogousslavsky J, Orgogozo JM (2000) Acute treatment of ischemic stroke. Cerebrovasc Dis 10(Suppl 3):S22–S33
20. European Stroke Initiative (EUSI): recommendations for stroke management. Cerebrovasc Dis 2000; 10(Suppl 3):S1–S34
21. Barnett HJ, Taylor W, Eliasziw M, Fox AJ, Fergunson GG, Haynes RB et al (1998) Benefit of carotid endarterectomy in patients with symptomatic moderate or severe stenosis North American Symptomatic Carotid Endarterectomy Trial Collaborators. N Engl J Med 339:1415–1425
22. Bazan R, Braga GP, Luvizutto GJ, Hueb JC, Hokama NK, Zanati Bazan SG et al (2015) Evaluation of the temporal acoustic window for transcranial Doppler in a multi-ethnic population in Brazil. Ultrasound Med Biol 41:2131–2134
23. Klotzsch C, Popescu O, Berli P (1998) A new 1 MHz probe for transcranial Doppler sonography in patients with inadequate temporal bone windows. Ultrasound Med Biol 24:101–103
24. Rundek T, Di Tullio MR, Sciacca RR, Titova IV, Mohr JP, Homma S et al (1999) Association between large aortic arch atheromas and high intensity transient signals in elderly stroke patients. Stroke 30:2683–2686
25. Oliveira V, Batista P, Soares F, Ferro JM (2001) HITS in internal carotid dissections. Cerebrovasc Dis 11:330–334
26. Iguchi Y, Kimura K, Kobayashi K, Ueno Y, Shibazaki K, Inoue T (2008) Microembolic signals at 48 hours after stroke onset contribute to new ischaemia within a week. J Neurol Neurosurg Psychiatry 79:253–259
27. Poppert H, Sadikov S, Sander K, Wolf O, Sander D (2006) Embolic signals in unselected stroke patients: prevalence and diagnostic benefit. Stroke 37:2039–2043
28. Markus HS, King A, Shipley M, Topakian R, Cullinane M, Reihill S et al (2010) Asymptomatic embolisation for prediction of stroke in the asymptomatic carotid emboli study (ACES): a prospective observational study. Lancet Neurol 9:663–671
29. Wong KS, Chen C, Fu J, Chang HM, Suwanwela NC, Huang YN, CLAIR study investigators et al (2010) Clopidogrel plus aspirin versus aspirin alone for reducing embolisation in patients with acute symptomatic cerebral or carotid artery stenosis (CLAIR study): a randomised, open-label, blinded-endpoint trial. Lancet Neurol 9(5):489–497
30. Markus HS, Droste DW, Kaps M, Larrue V, Lees KR, Siebler M et al (2005) Dual antiplatelet therapy with clopidogrel and aspirin in symptomatic carotid stenosis evaluated using doppler embolic signal detection: the clopidogrel and Aspirin for Reduction of Emboli in Symptomatic Carotid Stenosis (CARESS) trial. Circulation 111:2233–2240
31. Molina CA, Alvarez-Sabín J, Schonewille W, Montaner J, Rovira A, Abilleira S, Codina A (2000) Cerebral microembolism in acute spontaneous internal carotid artery dissection. Neurology. 55:1738–1740
32. Brunser AM, Lavados PM, Hoppe A, Muñoz-Venturelli P, Sujima E, López J et al (2017) Transcranial Doppler as a predictor of ischemic events in carotid artery dissection. J Neuroimaging 27(2):232–236
33. Zanati Bazan SG, Braga GP, Luvizutto GJ, Trindade AP, Pontes-Neto OM, Bazan R (2016) Bihemispheric paradoxical cerebral embolism in a patient with pulmonary thromboembolism and presumptive fistula right-to-left shunt. J Stroke Cerebrovasc Dis 25:e95–e97
34. Del Sette M, Angeli S, Stara I, Finocchi C, Gandolfo C (1997) Microembolic signals with serial Transcranial Doppler monitoring in acute focal ischemic deficit. Stroke 28:1311–1313
35. Barbash GI, White HD, Modan M, Diaz R, Hampton JR, Heikkila J et al (1993) Significance of smoking in patients receiving thrombolytic therapy for acute myocardial infarction. Experience gleaned from the international tissue plasminogen activator/streptokinase mortality Trial. Circulation 87:53–58

25

Carotid intima–media thickness and cardiovascular risk factors in healthy volunteers

Birgit-Christiane Zyriax[1,3*], Kira Dransfeld[1] and Eberhard Windler[2]

Abstract

Background: Assessment of cardiovascular risk by scores lacks sensitivity and leaves the majority of future cardiovascular patients unidentified particularly individuals at low cardiovascular risk. The present analysis investigates into the correlation of carotid intima–media thickness (CIMT) and cardiovascular risk factors and derived scores as to the potential of improved cardiovascular risk prediction by combining the two.

Methods: The Stress, Atherosclerosis and ECG Study (STRATEGY) is a cross-sectional study of selectively healthy 107 women and 106 men without diagnosed and treated cardiovascular risk factors evenly distributed between 30 and 70 years. CIMT was determined by evaluating B-mode ultrasonograms offline according to a standardized protocol. The unpaired *t*-test was used to compare normal-distributed continuous variables, the Chi-squared test for normal-distributed categorical variables and the Mann–Whitney *U* test for non-normal distributed continuous variables. The association between risk prediction scores and CIMT was calculated by the Spearman rank correlation coefficient. Pearson correlation coefficient was used for the correlation between cardiovascular risk factors and CIMT. A multiple linear regression analysis was executed for the association of cardiovascular risk factors and CIMT.

Results: Age, systolic blood pressure, fasting glucose, total, LDL- and non-HDL-cholesterol and waist circumference were significantly associated with CIMT (each $P \leq 0.03$). The Framingham Risk Score, the Prospective Cardiovascular Münster Study Score and the European Society of Cardiology Score correlated significantly but only moderately with CIMT. The Framingham Risk Score considering BMI correlated most strongly and predicted 27% of the CIMT variance in men and 20% in women.

Conclusion: In individuals without overt cardiovascular risk factors and thus at low cardiovascular risk, CIMT and cardiovascular risk factors correlated only partially suggesting that combining CIMT and conventional risk factors or common derived scores may improve risk prediction in individuals at low cardiovascular risk. The clinical benefit as to cardiovascular events of such combined risk prediction needs to be explored in large prospective cohorts of still healthy low-risk volunteers. DRKS ID DRKS00015209 07/02/2019 retrospectively registered https://www.drks.de/drks_web/navigate.do?navigationId=resultsExt

Keywords: Carotid intima–media thickness (CIMT), Cardiovascular, Risk score, Atherosclerosis, Cardiovascular risk

Introduction

The early identification of individuals at risk for future cardiovascular events is of vital importance since early correction of emerging risk factors is more efficient than therapy of advanced atherosclerotic vascular disease. Risk assessment by scores lacks sensitivity and leaves the majority of future cardiovascular patients unidentified

*Correspondence: b.zyriax@uke.de
[1] Midwifery Science—Health Care Research and Prevention, Preventive Medicine and Nutrition, German Center for Health Services Research in Dermatology (CVderm), University Medical Center Hamburg-Eppendorf (UKE), Hamburg, Germany
Full list of author information is available at the end of the article

particularly in individuals at low risk without overt risk factors [1–3].

Noninvasive measurement of structural changes in straight arterial segments as carotid intima–media thickness (CIMT) is a well-established surrogate marker of early stages of subclinical atherosclerosis. It helps to identify individuals at risk of future clinical endpoints including coronary and cerebrovascular events earlier than established risk factors [4–7]. However, current evidence does not satisfactorily support the routine measurement of subclinical atherosclerosis in primary prevention [8].

The 10-year cardiovascular risk perception of widely used risk scores is mainly based on the presence of classical risk factors as lipid values, hypertension, diabetes, smoking, age and gender [1–3]. In observational longitudinal studies, a clear relationship was observed between scores and the incidence of cardiovascular events [3].

However, the predictive value is limited, as the majority of coronary events occur in individuals of low- and intermediate-risk based on risk scores [2, 4]. Since the absolute risk is low in these risk categories, it would be beneficial to improve the specificity of prediction to allocate preventive measures more efficiently.

Thus, the aim of the present explorative analysis of data from the Stress, Atherosclerosis and ECG Study (STRATEGY) representing a population at low cardiovascular risk that has not yet developed overt cardiovascular risk factors was to analyze the concordance of CIMT and common risk prediction scores regarding risk perception as to the possible benefit of combining the two.

Patients and methods

Design and recruitment

Methods applied in STRATEGY have been described in detail [9]. STRATEGY is a cross-sectional study of individuals without overt cardiovascular risk factors, 107 (50.2%) women and 106 (49.8%) men aged 30–70 years recruited in Hamburg through a health insurance by a flyer randomly included in regular mailings between September 2006 and March 2007. The data previously analyzed and published for other issues were re-used because of the low use of statins in primary prevention at that time and the opportunity to make use of the validated procedure of determining CIMT of the Study of Health in Pomerania. Participants without acute or chronic diseases, or any medication except for hormone replacement therapy or oral contraceptives and thyroxin for stably substituted hypothyroidism were invited for a visit. Up to at least 25 participants per age decade and gender were consecutively included. The data of 2 out of 215 individuals were excluded from the analysis because of missing data.

Data collection

Assessment of anthropometric and clinical data

All interviews and physical examinations were performed by the same trained investigator. Body height and weight were measured to the nearest 0.5 cm or 0.1 kg, respectively, body mass index (BMI) was calculated as weight [kg]/(height [m])^2. 'Smokers' refers to current smokers and 'non-smokers' summarizes ex- and never-smokers. A fasting morning blood sample was taken, immediately centrifuged at 4 °C and stored at 4 °C in tubes containing 1 mg fluoride per ml blood. Fasting plasma glucose, high-density lipoprotein (HDL-) cholesterol, and triglycerides were determined by standard techniques. Low-density lipoprotein (LDL-) cholesterol was calculated using the Friedewald formula. Blood pressure was taken in a sitting position in the morning three times in 1-min intervals after at least 5 min of rest. The results of the second and third measurement were averaged and used for the present analysis. Hypertension was defined as blood pressure $\geq 140/\geq 90$ mmHg [9].

Assessment of intima–media thickness (CIMT)

CIMT was assessed by the standardized method of the Study of Health in Pomerania (SHIP) as previously applied and reported [9–11]. IMT of the common carotid artery was recorded on both sides between the carotid bulb origin and a point 10 mm proximal using high resolution B-mode ultrasound (General Electric Vivid 3 Expert with a 7.5-MHz linear array transducer). The CIMT was assessed offline as the average of at least five consecutive measurements in 1-mm steps on both sides of the distance from the media–adventitia interface to the intima–lumen interface on the far wall in a region free of plaques—only one plaque in one participant was detected. The offline measurements were performed at the center of the Study of Health in Pomerania (SHIP), Greifswald, by a single reader, who was trained according to the standardized protocol of the study as reported in detail [9, 10].

Risk assessment by cardiovascular risk prediction scores

For each participant two variants of three established scores assessing 10-year cardiovascular risk were calculated [12–14] (Table 1).

Statistical analyses

The explorative analysis was performed on the entire study population and for each gender. Comparisons of means between groups were performed using unpaired *t*-test for normal-distributed continuous variables, Chi-squared test for normal-distributed categorical variables and Mann–Whitney *U* test for non-normal

Table 1 Predictors of cardiovascular risk calculated according to the Framingham Risk Score including lipids or body mass index, the Prospective Cardiovascular Münster Study Score including lipids or body mass index, the German version of the European Society of Cardiology Score including total cholesterol or total cholesterol/high-density lipoprotein

Predictors	FRS		PROCAM		ESC	
	Lipid	BMI	Lipid	BMI	TC	TC/HDL
Age, gender, smoking, systolic blood pressure	X	X	X	X	X	X
Diabetes	X	X	X	X		
Antihypertensives	X	X		X		
Family history			X	X		
Cholesterol, triglycerides	Total, HDL		LDL, HDL, Triglycerides		Total	Total, HDL
Anthropometry		X		Height, weight		
Calculated 10-year risk	Cardiovascular diseases		Myocardial infarction		Cardiovascular death including fatal stroke	

FRS Framingham Risk Score, *PROCAM* Prospective Cardiovascular Münster Study Score, *ESC* European Society of Cardiology Score, *BMI* body mass index, *TC* total cholesterol, *HDL* high-density lipoprotein

distributed continuous variables. The association between common risk prediction scores and CIMT was calculated by the Spearman rank correlation coefficient. Pearson correlation coefficient was used for the correlation between cardiovascular risk factors and CIMT. A multiple linear regression analysis was executed for the association between cardiovascular risk factors and CIMT. *P*-values of 0.05 were used as the cut-off for statistical significance. All analyses were conducted using SPSS 24.

Results

Baseline characteristics

Table 2 gives the characteristics of the population of the STRATEGY study. Compared to men, women were characterized by lower LDL-cholesterol, triglycerides, fasting glucose and blood pressure and higher HDL-cholesterol. However, on average most laboratory values were within the range of normal.

CIMT and cardiovascular risk factors

Similarly in both gender, the average CIMT was slightly elevated compared to 0.3–0.5 mm of infants [15–17] (Table 2). Age, systolic blood pressure, fasting glucose,

Table 2 Characteristics of the study population

	Men $n = 106$	Women $n = 107$	Significance *P*-value
Age [years]	49.6 ± 11.3	49.4 ± 10.6	0.893
Smokers [%]	8.5	11.2	0.505
Systolic blood pressure [mmHg]	129.2 ± 13.9	123.2 ± 17.9	0.007
Total cholesterol [mg/dl]	210.5 ± 35.7	207.1 ± 35.3	0.485
LDL-cholesterol [mg/dl]	124.1 ± 31.0	110.4 ± 32.2	0.002
HDL-cholesterol [mg/dl]	63.2 ± 15.8	80.4 ± 17.6	< 0.001
Total cholesterol/HDL ratio	3.5 ± 1.03	2.7 ± 0.72	< 0.001
Triglycerides [mg/dl]	116.6 ± 66.6	85.0 ± 36.6	< 0.001
Fasting glucose [mg/dl]	92.3 ± 9.5	87.5 ± 7.8	< 0.001
BMI [kg/m^2]	26.2 ± 3.2	23.9 ± 3.3	< 0.001
Height [cm]	180.6 ± 7.2	166.6 ± 6.8	< 0.001
Weight [kg]	85.6 ± 12.1	66.5 ± 10.0	< 0.001
Waist circumference [cm]	96.0 ± 10.6	81.6 ± 9.4	< 0.001
Carotid intima–media thickness [mm]	0.70 ± 0.1	0.68 ± 0.09	0.103

LDL low-density lipoprotein, *HDL* high-density lipoprotein, *BMI* body mass index

Table 3 Pearson correlation between single common cardiovascular risk factors and carotid intima–media thickness in men and women

Risk factor	Total ($n=213$)	Men ($n=106$)	Women ($n=107$)
Age	0.510 ($P<0.001$)	0.531 ($P<0.001$)	0.489 ($P<0.001$)
Smoking status	0.017 ($P=0.806$)	− 0.050 ($P=0.610$)	0.073 ($P=0.455$)
Systolic blood pressure	0.318 ($P<0.001$)	0.298 ($P=0.002$)	0.319 ($P=0.001$)
Total cholesterol	0.205 ($P=0.003$)	0.279 ($P=0.004$)	0.114 ($P=0.242$)
LDL-cholesterol	0.154 ($P=0.024$)	0.186 ($P=0.056$)	0.080 ($P=0.412$)
HDL-cholesterol	0.026 ($P=0.709$)	0.126 ($P=0.197$)	0.050 ($P=0.614$)
TC/HDL-cholesterol	0.116 ($P=0.092$)	0.098 ($P=0.315$)	0.040 ($P=0.682$)
Non-HDL-cholesterol	0.182 ($P=0.008$)	0.217 ($P=0.026$)	0.091 ($P=0.354$)
Triglycerides	0.127 ($P=0.065$)	0.167 ($P=0.089$)	-0.030 ($P=0.757$)
Height	− 0.014 ($P=0.841$)	− 0.140 ($P=0.152$)	− 0.124 ($P=0.202$)
Weight	0.048 ($P=0.489$)	− 0.053 ($P=0.592$)	− 0.926 ($P=0.926$)
BMI	0.075 ($P=0.274$)	0.024 ($P=0.808$)	0.060 ($P=0.539$)
Waist circumference	0.148 ($P=0.031$)	0.162 ($P=0.096$)	0.028 ($P=0.774$)
Fasting glucose	0.249 ($P<0.001$)	0.287 ($P=0.003$)	0.150 ($P=0.124$)

LDL low-density lipoprotein, *HDL* high-density lipoprotein, *TC* total cholesterol, *BMI* body mass index

total, LDL- and non-HDL-cholesterol and waist circumference correlated significantly though weakly to moderately with CIMT in the study population (Table 3). When analyses were considered separately for men and women, some correlations lost their significance probably due to small sample size.

Based on univariate linear regression, age explained 28.2% of the variance of CIMT in men and 23.9% in women. Systolic blood pressure predicted 8.9% of the variance of CIMT in men and 10.2% in women. In the total population 7.8% of the variance in CIMT was explained by total cholesterol. Based on univariate linear regression, age, systolic blood pressure and total cholesterol were the strongest predictors of the variance of CIMT, in men 28.2, 8.9, and 7.8%, respectively, and in women 23.9, 10.2, and 1.3%, respectively. Each year of life translated into an additional 0.004 mm CIMT, each 1 mmHg systolic blood pressure into an additional 0.002 mm CIMT, and each additional 10 mg total cholesterol correlated with a 0.007 mm higher CIMT in men and 0.003 mm in women. In a multivariate regression model the increase of CIMT was moderately predicted by age and systolic blood pressure, whereas all other common cardiovascular risk factors missed significance (Table 4). Since age may mask the effect of risk factors that increase with age, the multivariate regression was conducted omitting age, which revealed a stronger association of some risk factors with CIMT, particularly systolic blood pressure.

Table 4 Multivariate regression model of cardiovascular risk factors and carotid intima–media thickness considering and omitting age

Model parameters	Multivariate model including age		Multivariate model excluding age	
	Standardized regression coefficient	*P*-value	Standardized regression coefficient	*P*-value
Age	0.467	<0.001	–	–
Male gender	− 0.089	0.199	− 0.074	0.327
Smoking status	− 0.007	0.900	− 0.012	0.855
Systolic blood pressure	0.134	0.048	0.263	<0.001
LDL-cholesterol	− 0.078	0.262	0.069	0.342
HDL-cholesterol	0.033	0.663	0.142	0.086
Triglycerides	0.102	0.162	0.078	0.332
BMI	− 0.041	0.550	− 0.072	0.337
Fasting glucose	0.040	0.566	0.157	0.033

LDL low-density lipoprotein, *HDL* high-density lipoprotein, *BMI* body mass index

CIMT and cardiovascular risk prediction scores

Taking in account all major risk factors may have a stronger impact on the CIMT than considering each separately. Therefore, risk scores were calculated using the FRS, PROCAM or ESC and their respective variants (Table 1). The resultant scores were significantly higher for men than women ($P < 0.001$). Scores of FRS and PROCAM using weight and height (BMI) instead of lipids were significantly higher in both genders ($P < 0.05$). Still, both score variants and the ESC correlated strongly with each other ($P < 0.001$). Accordingly, all cardiovascular risk scores correlated significantly and positively with CIMT (Table 5). Compared to PROCAM the associations between ESC and the FRS and CIMT were slightly but not significantly stronger.

In univariate linear regression analyses positive association between calculated scores and CIMT were observed for all risk scores. Again, the associations were stronger for men than for women and FRS-BMI, which showed numerically the strongest of the quite similar association with CIMT, predicted 26.7% of the CIMT variance in men and 20.2% in women (Fig. 1). Assuming a close linear relationship each FRS-BMI score point translated into 0.006 mm CIMT in men and 0.008 mm CIMT in women.

Table 5 Spearman rank correlation between cardiovascular risk scores and carotid intima–media thickness ($P < 0.001$ for each correlation)

Risk scores	Total $n = 213$	Men $n = 106$	Women $n = 107$
FRS-Lipids	0.513	0.564	0.444
FRS-BMI	0.530	0.589	0.466
PROCAM-Lipids	0.464	0.509	0.437
PROCAM-BMI	0.479	0.543	0.447
ESC-TC/HDL	0.527	0.547	0.462
ESC-TC	0.507	0.561	0.410

FRS Framingham Risk Score, *PROCAM* Prospective Cardiovascular Münster Study Score, *ESC* European Society of Cardiology Score, *BMI* body mass index, *TC* total cholesterol

Discussion

The present analysis of the STRATEGY study demonstrates a correlation of CIMT with values of common risk factors within the range of normal and with deduced risk prediction scores even in individuals at low cardiovascular risk lacking overt risk factors. Yet, the correlations were modest. Thus, both, clinical risk factors and CIMT may separately reflect a contribution to atherogenesis. Since prediction of cardio- and cerebrovascular events has been shown likewise for risk factors or risk scores and for the CIMT, based on the results of this study of only partial correlation of risk scores and CIMT it appears reasonable to assume an additive predictive power for the combination of the two approaches in individuals at low cardiovascular risk according to their risk

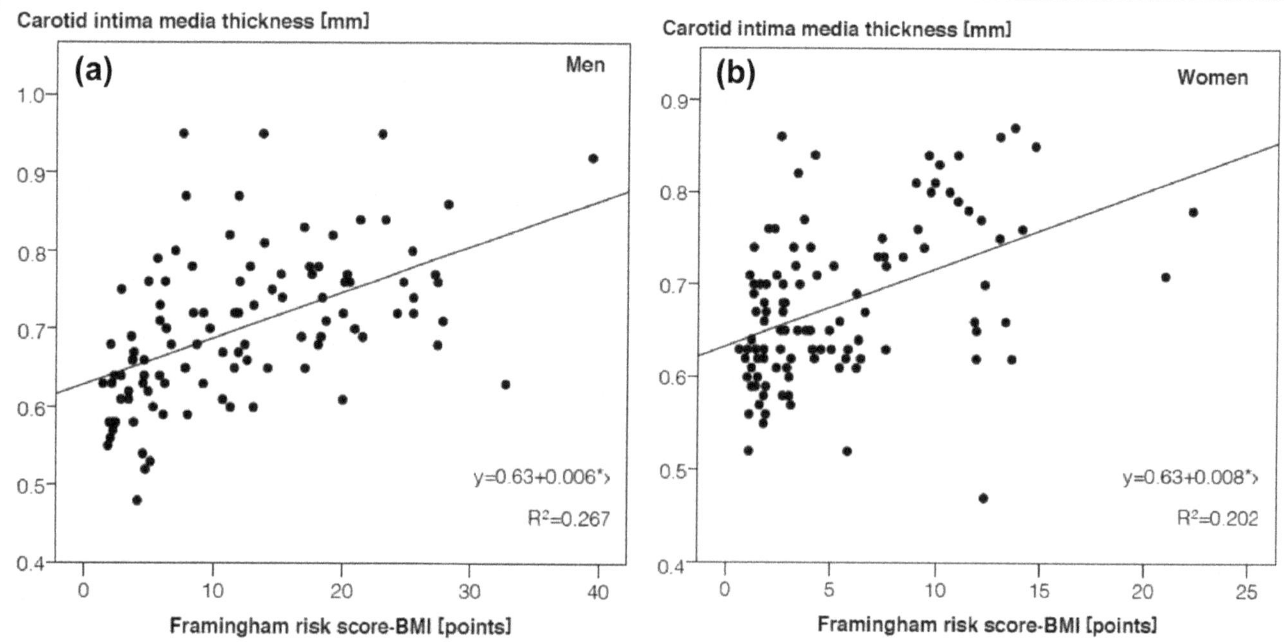

Fig. 1 Univariate linear regression analysis of Framingham Risk Score-BMI and carotid intima–media thickness in men (**a**) and women (**b**)

factor profile. The perception of CIMT as an at least in part independent cardiovascular risk factor rather than merely a reflection of the common risk factors is in line with findings in the general population including subjects at clearly increased cardiovascular risk. However, at that stage of overt risk CIMT appears to add little to the risk predicted solely by risk factors [18].

The data of Table 2 illustrate that the cardiovascular risk factors of the studied individuals were on average in the range of normal despite clear gender differences. However, considering the variance, in individual participants some risk factors reached elevated levels though not in the range supposed to require therapy, e.g., the systolic blood pressure reached on average already the range of prehypertension. Thus, almost 50% of men were prehypertensive which bears a substantial cardiovascular risk. Also, a considerable number of men and women had a fasting glucose above the limit of prediabetes, which corresponds to a markedly elevated cardiovascular risk as well. In addition, the standard deviation of the LDL-cholesterol indicates a prevalence of individually clearly elevated cholesterol levels. This may in part explain the somewhat elevated average CIMT in the studied population, considering that in male and female infants the CIMT measures 0.3–0.5 mm [15–17].

In line with the presumption that CIMT may increase due to the conventional cardiovascular risk factors, we found highly significant correlations of the basic risk factors systolic blood pressure, fasting glucose and cholesterol with CIMT. Though age reached the highest correlation, it may just or in part be a surrogate of increasing number and severity of risk factors with age. Similarly, weight may merely express the prevalence of components of the metabolic syndrome. In accord, waist circumference as a measure of central obesity reached a higher and significant correlation than weight and BMI. Multivariate analysis yielded a strong significant correlation for age, while among the modifiable risk factors only systolic blood pressure reached significance in line with previous investigations [19, 20]. Similar results were reported for the correlation of age, gender and systolic blood pressure with CIMT [21].

However, since age may confound the effects of the individual risk factors due to their increase with age, a multivariate analysis was performed omitting age. The correlation of blood pressure, LDL- and HDL-cholesterol and fasting glucose with CIMT increased, which was substantial regarding blood pressure and fasting glucose, the latter of which reached significance in addition to blood pressure. In total, this analysis indicates that the sum of the modifiable clinical risk factors has to be taken into account when comparing their effect on cardiovascular risk with that of CIMT.

The individual point estimates of the calculated scores showed a linear relationship with CIMT. However, the coefficients of determination were rather low indicting a vast variation. In other words, more aspects than the considered parameters of conventional risk factors are responsible for the increase of CIMT. Thus, in individuals without overt cardiovascular risk factors CIMT may well add to the information of the risk scores with regard to the prediction of cardiovascular risk, which needs to be shown in large longitudinal studies, though.

The present findings of the STRATEGY study have several limitations that need to be addressed. First, the analysis is confined to primarily quite healthy volunteers characterized by a healthy lifestyle and a low cardiovascular risk profile, while individuals with overt and treated cardiovascular risk factors were excluded. However, this low-risk study cohort has been deliberately chosen as it represents the target population for which risk prediction is important to individualize and initiate necessary measures to prevent cardio- and cerebrovascular events at an early stage.

Second, the sample size of the study is limited, thus, analysis of a larger population may have allowed to detect significant associations between risk factors and CIMT and their differences with regard to gender. Also, determination of CIMT has followed the protocol of the SHIP-study for matters of conformity and to allow comparison. Automated edge detection may provide more precise results.

Third, some risk factors are underrepresented, e.g., smoking, and thus may be underscored. However, smoking is an obvious risk factor and needs to be stopped in any event. This also applies to markedly elevated lipids and plasma glucose in the range of diabetes. Thus, the findings and derived conclusions may not apply to populations at clearly increased vascular risk.

Fourth, in this context it may be borne in mind that there are more parameters that may be worth considering as to cardio- and cerebrovascular risk as further laboratory values like lipoprotein(a), lifestyle factors, sociodemographic determinants and psychological characteristics, which may add significant predictive power. Although plaque thickness may be considered, plaques are rare in individuals at low cardiovascular risk as in this study [22, 23].

In summary, despite these limitations, our data provide relevant information about two screening methods that share some predictive power, but also suggests that a combination of both may add predictive value in individuals at currently low vascular risk according to conventional risk scores. Such approach certainly requires further confirmation in a prospective cohort not only to prove an additional prognostic value, but also benefit as to the prevention of vascular events.

Abbreviations

CIMT: Carotid intima–media thickness; LDL-cholesterol: Low-density lipoprotein-cholesterol; HDL-cholesterol: High-density lipoprotein.

Acknowledgements

N/A.

Authors' contributions

BCZ designed and initiated the study. KD analyzed the data and wrote the draft version of this publication. EW helped with designing and conducting the study and assisted the statistics and scientific writing. All authors read and approved the final manuscript.

Author details

[1] Midwifery Science—Health Care Research and Prevention, Preventive Medicine and Nutrition, German Center for Health Services Research in Dermatology (CVderm), University Medical Center Hamburg-Eppendorf (UKE), Hamburg, Germany. [2] Institute for Health Services Research in Dermatology and Nursing (IVDP), University Medical Center Hamburg-Eppendorf (UKE), Hamburg, Germany. [3] Midwifery Science—Health Care Research and Prevention, Preventive Medicine and Nutrition, Institute for Health Care Research in Dermatology and Nursing (IVDP), University Medical Center Hamburg-Eppendorf (UKE), Martinistr. 52—Bldg. N26, D-20246 Hamburg, Germany.

References

1. D'Agostino RB, Vasan RS, Pencina MJ, Wolf PA, Cobain M, Massaro JM et al (2008) General cardiovascular risk profile for use in primary care. The Framingham Heart Study. Circulation 117:743–753
2. Assmann G, Cullen P, Schulte H (2002) Simple scoring scheme for calculating the risk of acute coronary events based on the 10-year follow-up of the prospective cardiovascular Münster [PROCAM] study. Circulation 105:310–315
3. Conroy RM, Pyörälä K, Fitzgerald AP, Sans S, Menotti A, De Backer G et al (2003) Estimation of ten-year risk of fatal cardiovascular disease in Europe. The SCORE project. Eur Heart J 24:987–1003
4. Nambi V, Chambless L, Folsom AR, He M, Hu Y, Mosley T et al (2010) Carotid intima-media thickness and presence or absence of plaque improves prediction of coronary heart disease risk: the ARIC [Atherosclerosis Risk in Communities] study. J Am Coll Cardiol 55:1600–1607
5. Chambless LE, Heiss G, Folsom AR, Rosamond W, Szklo M, Sharrett AR et al (1997) Association of coronary heart disease incidence with carotid arterial wall thickness and major risk factors. The Atherosclerosis Risk in Communities [ARIC] Study, 1987–1993. Am J Epidemiol 146:483–494
6. O'Leary DH, Polak JF, Kronmal RA, Manolio TA, Burke GL, Wolfson SK Jr (1999) Carotid-artery intima and media thickness as a risk factor for myocardial infarction and stroke in older adults. Cardiovascular Health Study Collaborative Research Group. N Engl J Med 40:14–22
7. Den Ruijter HM, Peters SA, Anderson TJ, Britton AR, Dekker JM, Eijkemans MJ et al (2012) Common carotid intima media thickness measurements in cardiovascular risk prediction. A meta-analysis. JAMA 308:796–803
8. Goff DC Jr, Lloyd-Jones DM, Bennett G, Coady S, D'Agostino RB, Gibbons R et al (2014) 2013 ACC/AHA guideline on the assessment of cardiovascular risk. A report of the American College of Cardiology/American Heart Association Task Force on Practice Guidelines. J Am Coll Cardiol 129(25 Suppl 2):S74-75
9. Zyriax BC, Lau K, Klähn T, Boeing H, Völzke H, Windler E et al (2010) Association between alcohol consumption and carotid intima-media thickness in a healthy population. Data of the STRATEGY study (Stress, Atherosclerosis and ECG Study). Eur J Clin Nutr 64:1199–1206
10. Luedemann J, Piek M, Wood WG, Meyer S, Greiner B, John U et al (2000) Methods for quality assurance of medical examination in epidemiological field studies: the "Study of Health in Pomerania" (SHIP). Gesundheitswesen 62:234–243
11. Völzke H, Alte D, Schmidt CO, Radke D, Lorbeer R, Friedrich N et al (2011) Cohort profile: the study of health in Pomerania. Int J Epidemiol 40:294–307
12. Framingham Heart Study. Cardiovascular Disease (10-year risk) https://www.framinghamheartstudy.org/fhs-risk-functions/cardiovascular-disease-10-year-risk/. Accessed 04 Mar 2019
13. Assmann-Stiftung für Prävention. PROCAM-Schnelltest. https://www.assmann-stiftung.de/procam-tests/. Accessed 04 Mar 2019
14. Deutsche Gesellschaft für Kardiologie – Herz-und Kreislaufforschung e.V. ESC Pocket Guidelines (2017) Prävention von Herz-Kreislauf-Erkrankungen, Version 2016. Grünwald, Börm Bruckmeier Verlag GmbH
15. de Groot E, Hovingh GK, Wiegman A, Duriez P, Smit AJ, Fruchart JC et al (2004) Measurement of arterial wall thickness as a surrogate marker for atherosclerosis. Circulation 109(23 Suppl 1):III33-38
16. Doyon A, Kracht D, Bayazit AK, Deveci M, Duzova A, Krmar RT et al (2013) Carotid artery intima-media thickness and distensibility in children and adolescents: reference values and role of body dimensions. Hypertension 62:550–556
17. Kusters DM, Wiegman A, Kastelein JJ, Hutten BA (2014) Carotid intima-media thickness in children with familial hypercholesterolemia. Circ Res 114:307–310
18. Lorenz MW, Schaefer C, Steinmetz H, Sitzer M (2010) Is carotid intima media thickness useful for individual prediction of cardiovascular risk? Ten-year results from the Carotid Atherosclerosis Progression Study (CAPS). Eur Heart J 31:2041–2048
19. Azarpazhooh MR, Kazemi-Bajestani SM, Esmaeili H, Vedadian P, Ebrahimi M, Parizadeh SM et al (2014) Cardiovascular risk factors and nutritional intake are not associated with ultrasound-defined increased carotid intima media thickness in individuals without a history of cardiovascular events. Int J Prev Med 5:1412–1421
20. Maloberti A, Farina F, Carbonaro M, Piccinelli E, Bassi I, Pansera F et al (2018) In healthy normotensive subjects age and blood pressure better predict subclinical vascular and cardiac organ damage than atherosclerosis biomarkers. Blood Press 27:262–270
21. Hou Q, Li S, Gao Y, Tian H (2018) Relations of lipid parameters, other variables with carotid intima-media thickness and plaque in the general Chinese adults: an observational study. Lipids Health Dis 17:107
22. Amato M, Veglia F, de Faire U, Giral P, Rauramaa R, Smit AJ et al (2017) Carotid plaque-thickness and common carotid IMT show additive value in cardiovascular risk prediction and reclassification. Atherosclerosis 263:412–419
23. Naqvi TZ, Lee MS (2014) Carotid intima-media thickness and plaque in cardiovascular risk assessment. JACC Cardiovasc Imaging 7:1025–1038

Permissions

All chapters in this book were first published by Springer; hereby published with permission under the Creative Commons Attribution License or equivalent. Every chapter published in this book has been scrutinized by our experts. Their significance has been extensively debated. The topics covered herein carry significant findings which will fuel the growth of the discipline. They may even be implemented as practical applications or may be referred to as a beginning point for another development.

The contributors of this book come from diverse backgrounds, making this book a truly international effort. This book will bring forth new frontiers with its revolutionizing research information and detailed analysis of the nascent developments around the world.

We would like to thank all the contributing authors for lending their expertise to make the book truly unique. They have played a crucial role in the development of this book. Without their invaluable contributions this book wouldn't have been possible. They have made vital efforts to compile up to date information on the varied aspects of this subject to make this book a valuable addition to the collection of many professionals and students.

This book was conceptualized with the vision of imparting up-to-date information and advanced data in this field. To ensure the same, a matchless editorial board was set up. Every individual on the board went through rigorous rounds of assessment to prove their worth. After which they invested a large part of their time researching and compiling the most relevant data for our readers.

The editorial board has been involved in producing this book since its inception. They have spent rigorous hours researching and exploring the diverse topics which have resulted in the successful publishing of this book. They have passed on their knowledge of decades through this book. To expedite this challenging task, the publisher supported the team at every step. A small team of assistant editors was also appointed to further simplify the editing procedure and attain best results for the readers.

Apart from the editorial board, the designing team has also invested a significant amount of their time in understanding the subject and creating the most relevant covers. They scrutinized every image to scout for the most suitable representation of the subject and create an appropriate cover for the book.

The publishing team has been an ardent support to the editorial, designing and production team. Their endless efforts to recruit the best for this project, has resulted in the accomplishment of this book. They are a veteran in the field of academics and their pool of knowledge is as vast as their experience in printing. Their expertise and guidance has proved useful at every step. Their uncompromising quality standards have made this book an exceptional effort. Their encouragement from time to time has been an inspiration for everyone.

The publisher and the editorial board hope that this book will prove to be a valuable piece of knowledge for researchers, students, practitioners and scholars across the globe.

List of Contributors

Rosemary Thomas-Mohtat, Kristen Breslin and Joanna S. Cohen
Department of Emergency Medicine and Trauma Services, Children's National Medical Center, Washington, DC, USA
Faculty, George Washington University School of Medicine, Washington, DC, USA

Craig Sable
Department of Cardiology, Children's National Medical Center, Washington, DC, USA
Faculty, George Washington University School of Medicine, Washington, DC, USA

Jacqueline G. Weinberg
Department of Cardiology, Children's Hospital of Pittsburgh, Pittsburgh, PA, USA

Aparna Prasad
Department of Cardiology, Goryeb Children's Hospital, Morristown, NJ, USA

Lauren Zinns
Department of Emergency Medicine, Icahn School of Medicine at Mt. Sinai, New York, NY, USA

Pia Iben Pietersen
Department of Respiratory Medicine, Odense University Hospital, Sdr. Boulevard 29, 5000 Odense C, Denmark
Institute for Clinical Research, University of Southern Denmark, Odense, Denmark
Regional Center for Technical Simulation, Region of Southern Denmark, Odense, Denmark

Kristian Rørbæk Madsen and Bjørn Ulrik Nielsen
Department of Anaesthesiology and Intensive Care Medicine, Odense University Hospital, Odense, Denmark

Ole Graumann
Institute for Clinical Research, University of Southern Denmark, Odense, Denmark
Department of Radiology, Odense University Hospital, Odense, Denmark

Lars Konge
Copenhagen Academy for Medical Education and Simulation (CAMES), University of Copenhagen and the Capital Region of Denmark, Copenhagen, Denmark

Christian Borbjerg Laursen
Department of Respiratory Medicine, Odense University Hospital, Sdr. Boulevard 29, 5000 Odense C, Denmark
Institute for Clinical Research, University of Southern Denmark, Odense, Denmark

Silvia Mongodi and Anita Orlando
Anaesthesia and Intensive Care, San Matteo Hospital, Viale Golgi 19, Pavia, Italy

Giorgio Antonio Iotti and Francesco Mojoli
Anaesthesia and Intensive Care, San Matteo Hospital, Viale Golgi 19, Pavia, Italy
Department of Clinical-Surgical, Diagnostic and Paediatric Sciences, Unit of Anaesthesia and Intensive Care, University of Pavia, Pavia, Italy

Andrea Colombo
Department of Clinical-Surgical, Diagnostic and Paediatric Sciences, Unit of Anaesthesia and Intensive Care, University of Pavia, Pavia, Italy

Lorenzo Cavagna
Division of Rheumatology, University of Pavia, San Matteo Hospital, Pavia, Italy

Bélaid Bouhemad
Dijon and Université Bourgogne Franche-Comté LNC UMR866, F-21000 Dijon, BP 77908, Dijon Cedex 21709, France
Department of Anesthesiology and Intensive Care, C.H.U. Dijon, Dijon Cedex, France

Marco Baciarello, Elena Bignami, Andrea Bonetti and Francesco Saturno
Anesthesia, Critical Care and Pain Medicine Unit, Department of Medicine and Surgery, University of Parma, Viale Gramsci, 14, 431236 Parma, Italy

Rossano Girometti and Lorenzo Cereser
Institute of Radiology, Department of Medicine, University of Udine, University Hospital S. Maria della Misericordia, Udine, Italy

Ravita Chaichanalap and Tharangrut Hanprasertpong
Department of Obstetrics and Gynecology, Faculty of Medicine, Srinakharinwirot University, Ongkharak 26120, Nakornnayok, Thailand

Michael H. Walsh and Christopher J. Oleynick
Division of General Internal Medicine, University of Calgary, Calgary, AB, Canada

Kang X. Zhang, Justin M. Chen and Nicholas G. Cowley
Providence Health Care, Providence Internal Medicine Residency Spokane, Spokane, WA, USA

Emily J. Cox
Providence Health Care, Providence Medical Research Center, Spokane, WA, USA

Leo M. Smyth
Division of General Internal Medicine, University of Alberta, Edmonton, AB, Canada

Irene W. Y. Ma
Division of General Internal Medicine, University of Calgary, Calgary, AB, Canada
Department of Medicine, W21C, University of Calgary, 3330 Hospital Dr NW, Calgary, AB T2N 4N1, Canada
Department of Community Health Sciences, W21C, University of Calgary, Calgary, AB, Canada

Kathryn Malherbe
Diagnostic Imaging Solutions, Pretoria 0001, South Africa

Jack Levy, Devon L. Barrett and Nile Harris
Department of Dermatology, Emory University School of Medicine, Atlanta, GA, USA

Jiwoong Jason Jeong
Department of Radiation Oncology, Emory University School of Medicine, Atlanta, GA, USA
Department of Biomedical Informatics, Emory University, Atlanta, GA, USA

Xiaofeng Yang
Department of Radiation Oncology, Emory University School of Medicine, Atlanta, GA, USA
Winship Cancer Institute, Emory University, Atlanta, GA, USA

Suephy C. Chen
Department of Dermatology, Duke University School of Medicine, Duke Clinic, 40 Duke Medicine Cir, Clinic 3K, Durham, NC 27710-4000, USA

Renato Farina, Pietro Valerio Foti, Andrea Conti, Francesco Aldo Iannace, Isabella Pennisi, Luigi Fanzone, Corrado Inì, Federica Libra, Francesco Vacirca, Giovanni Failla, Davide Baldanza, Stefano Palmucci, Serafino Santonocito and Antonio Basile
Radiodiagnostic and Radiotherapy Unit, Department of Medical and Surgical Sciences and Advanced Technologies "GF Ingrassia", Via Santa Sofia 78, 95123 Catani, Italy

A. E. Schuitemaker, P. Schober and C. Boer
Department of Anaesthesiology, Amsterdam UMC, Vrije Universiteit Amsterdam, Amsterdam Cardiovascular Sciences, De Boelelaan 1117, 1081 HV Amsterdam, The Netherlands

P. R. Tuinman
Department of Intensive Care Medicine, Amsterdam UMC, Vrije Universiteit Amsterdam, Amsterdam Cardiovascular Sciences, De Boelelaan 1117, 1081 HV Amsterdam, The Netherlands

F. Daams and D. L. van der Peet
Department of Surgery, Amsterdam UMC, Vrije Universiteit Amsterdam, Amsterdam Cardiovascular Sciences, De Boelelaan 1117, 1081 HV Amsterdam, The Netherlands

H. R. Touw
Department of Anaesthesiology, Amsterdam UMC, Vrije Universiteit Amsterdam, Amsterdam Cardiovascular Sciences, De Boelelaan 1117, 1081 HV Amsterdam, The Netherlands
Department of Intensive Care Medicine, Radboud University Medical Center, Geert Grooteplein Zuid 10, 6525 GA Nijmegen, The Netherlands

E. M. Bronkhorst
Department of Health Evidence, Radboud University Medical Center, Geert Grooteplein Zuid 10, 6525 GA Nijmegen, The Netherlands

Viknesh Sounderajah, Sepideh Poushpas, Muzaffar Anwar and Usman Jaffer
Imperial Vascular Unit, Imperial College Healthcare NHS Trust, London, UK

Bilal Khan
Department of General Surgery, Kingston Hospital, London, UK

Pasha Normahani
Imperial Vascular Unit, Imperial College Healthcare NHS Trust, London, UK
St Marys Hospital, Level 2, Patterson Building, Paddington W21NY, UK

Giovanni Volpicelli and Thomas Fraccalini
Department of Emergency Medicine, San Luigi Gonzaga University Hospital, Torino, Italy

Luciano Cardinale, Marco Calandri, Clara Piatti, Carlotta Geninatti and Giuseppe Stranieri
Department of Oncology, Radiology Unit, San Luigi Gonzaga University Hospital, Torino, Italy

Frances M. Russell, Elisa Sarmiento and Benjamin K. Nti
Department of Emergency Medicine, Indiana University School of Medicine, 720 Eskenazi Ave, FOB 3rd Floor, Indianapolis, IN 46202, USA

Robert R. Ehrman and Jakob E. Ottenhoff
Department of Emergency Medicine, Wayne State University School of Medicine, 4021 St Antoine Ave, Suite 6G, Detroit, MI 48201, USA

Allen Barton
Boone County Emergency Physicians, Zionsville, IN 46077, USA

Cristina Ramos-Hernández, Maribel Botana-Rial, Manuel Núñez-Delgado and Alberto Fernández-Villar
Department of Pneumology, Hospital Alvaro Cunqueiro, Neumo Vigo I + I. Institute of Health Research Galicia South (IISGS), Xerencia de Xestión integrada de Vigo, C/Clara Campoamor 341, 36312 Vigo, Pontevedra, Spain

Rosa Cordovilla-Pérez
Department of Pneumology, University Hospital of Salamcanca, P.o de San Vicente, 182, 37007 Salamanca, Spain

Rajkumar Rajendram, Naveed Mahmood and Mubashar Kharal
Department of Medicine, King Abdulaziz Medical City, King Abdulaziz International Medical Research Center, Ministry of National Guard - Health Affairs, Riyadh, Saudi Arabia
College of Medicine, King Saud Bin Abdulaziz University for Health Sciences, Riyadh, Saudi Arabia

Arif Hussain
Department of Cardiac Sciences, King Abdulaziz Medical City, King Abdulaziz International Medical Research Center, Ministry of National Guard - Health Affairs, Riyadh, Saudi Arabia

Nobuyuki Takemoto
Department of Breast & Endocrine Surgery, Japan Medical Alliance East Saitama General Hospital, 5-517, Yoshino, Saitama-Pref, Satte 340-0153, Japan

Ai Koyanagi
Research and Development Unit, Parc Sanitari Sant Joan de Déu, Fundació Sant Joan de Déu, CIBERSAM, Sant Boi de Llobregat, Barcelona, Spain
ICREA, Pg. Lluis Companys 23, Barcelona, Spain

Masanori Yasuda
Department of Pathology, Saitama Medical University International Medical Center, 1397-1, Yamane, Hidaka, Saitama-Pref, Japan

Yuya Yamamoto
Department of Endocrine Internal Medicine, Japan Medical Alliance East Saitama General Hospital, 5-517, Yoshino, Satte, Saitama-Pref, Japan

Hiroshi Yamamoto
Geriatric Health Service Facility (COSMOS), Japan Medical Alliance Yokohama Stroke and Brain Center, 1-2-1 Takigashira, Isogoku, Yokohama, Kanagawa-Pref, Japan

Raham Bacha
University Institute of Radiological Sciences and Medical Imaging Technologies (UIRSMIT), Faculty of Allied Health Sciences (FAHS), The University of Lahore, Lahore, Pakistan

Iqra Manzoor
University Institute of Radiological Sciences and Medical Imaging Technologies (UIRSMIT), The University of Lahore, G 10\2 Canal Berg, Lahore 54000, Pakistan

Syed Amir Gilani
Dean Faculty of Allied Health Sciences (FAHS), The University of Lahore, Lahore, Pakistan

Jean-Eudes Bourcier
Emergency, Anesthesiology and Critical Care Department, Lourdes Hospital, Lourdes, France
Pôle Anesthésie-Réanimation-Urgences, Hôpital de Lourdes, 2 Avenue Alexandre Marqui, 65100 Lourdes, France

Emeric Gallard, Jean-Philippe Redonnet, Morgan Abillard, Quentin Billaut, Laura Fauque, Anna Jouanolou and Didier Garnier
Emergency, Anesthesiology and Critical Care Department, Lourdes Hospital, Lourdes, France

Luigi Vetrugno, Giovanni Maria Guadagnin, Alessandro Brussa, Daniele Orso, Francesco De Lorenzo and Tiziana Bove
Anesthesiology and Intensive Care Clinic, Department of Medicine, University of Udine, Via Colugna 50, 33100 Udine, Italy

Eugenio Garofalo, Andrea Bruni and Federico Longhini
Intensive Care Unit, Department of Medical and Surgical Sciences, University Hospital Mater Domini, Magna Graecia University, Catanzaro, Italy

Gianmaria Cammarota
Department of Anesthesiology and Intensive Care, Maggiore della Carità University Hospital, Corso Mazzini 18, 28100 Novara, Italy

Erminio Santangelo
Department of Translational Medicine, University of Eastern Piemonte, via Solaroli, 17, 28100 Novara, Italy

Andrew W. Kirkpatrick
Department of Critical Care Medicine, Foothills Medical Centre, Calgary, Alberta, Canada
Department of Surgery, Foothills Medical Centre, Calgary, Alberta, Canada
Synder Institute for Chronic Diseases, Foothills Medical Centre, Calgary, Alberta, Canada
Trauma Program, University of Calgary and Alberta Health Services, Foothills Medical Centre, Calgary, Alberta, Canada
Tele-Mentored Ultrasound Supported Medical Interventions (TMUSMI) Research Group, Foothills Medical Centre, Calgary, Alberta, Canada

Jessica L. McKee
Trauma Program, University of Calgary and Alberta Health Services, Foothills Medical Centre, Calgary, Alberta, Canada
Tele-Mentored Ultrasound Supported Medical Interventions (TMUSMI) Research Group, Foothills Medical Centre, Calgary, Alberta, Canada

John M. Conly
Department of Medicine, Foothills Medical Centre, Calgary, Alberta, Canada
Synder Institute for Chronic Diseases, Foothills Medical Centre, Calgary, Alberta, Canada

Lisandro Montorfano, Qian Yu, Stephen J. Bordes and Raul J. Rosenthal
Department of General Surgery, Cleveland Clinic Florida, 2950 Cleveland Clinic Blvd, Weston, FL, USA

Shankarapryan Sivanushanthan
School of Medicine, Georgetown University, Washington D.C, USA

Miguel Montorfano
Department of Ultrasound and Vascular Doppler, Hospital de Emergencias "Dr. Clemente Alvarez", Av. Pellegrini 3205, Rosario, Santa Fe, Argentina

Luigi Vetrugno, Federico Barbariol, Umberto Baccarani and Giorgio Della Rocca
Department of Medicine, University of Udine, P.le S. M. della Misericordia 15, 33100 Udine, Italy

Francesco Forfori
Anesthesia and Intensive Care Medicine IV, Pisa University Hospital, Pisa, Italy

Rodrigo Bazan, Gabriel Pereira Braga, Carlos Clayton Macedo de Freitas, Pedro Tadao Hamamoto Filho, Gabriel Pinheiro Módolo and Hélio Rubens de Carvalho Nunes
Department of Neurology, Psychology and Psychiatry, Botucatu Medical School, UNESP–Univ Estadual Paulista, Campus de Botucatu, Distrito de Rubião Jr, s/n, Botucatu, Brazil

Gustavo José Luvizutto
Department of Applied Physical Therapy, Institute of Health Sciences, UFTM–Univ Federal do Triângulo Mineiro, Uberaba, Brazil

Silméia Garcia Zanati Bazan and João Carlos Hueb
Department of Internal Medicine, Botucatu Medical School, UNESP- Univ Estadual Paulista, Botucatu, Brazil

André Petean Trindade
Department of Tropical Diseases and Imaging Diagnosis, Botucatu Medical School, UNESP–Univ Estadual Paulista, Botucatu, Brazil

Marcone Lima Sobreira
Department of Surgery and Orthopedics, Botucatu Medical School, UNESP–Univ Estadual Paulista, Botucatu, Brazil

João Pereira Leite and Octávio Marques Pontes-Neto
Department of Neuroscience and Behavior, Ribeirão Preto School of Medicine, USP–Univ São Paulo, Ribeirão Preto, Brazil

Kira Dransfeld
Midwifery Science—Health Care Research and Prevention, Preventive Medicine and Nutrition, German Center for Health Services Research in Dermatology (CVderm), University Medical Center Hamburg-Eppendorf (UKE), Hamburg, Germany

Eberhard Windler
Institute for Health Services Research in Dermatology and Nursing (IVDP), University Medical Center Hamburg-Eppendorf (UKE), Hamburg, Germany

Birgit-Christiane Zyriax
Midwifery Science—Health Care Research and Prevention, Preventive Medicine and Nutrition, German Center for Health Services Research in Dermatology (CVderm), University Medical Center Hamburg-Eppendorf (UKE), Hamburg, Germany
Midwifery Science—Health Care Research and Prevention, Preventive Medicine and Nutrition, Institute for Health Care Research in Dermatology and Nursing (IVDP), University Medical Center Hamburg-Eppendorf (UKE), Martinistr. 52—Bldg. N26, D-20246 Hamburg, Germany

Index

www.ingramcontent.com/pod-product-compliance
Lightning Source LLC
LaVergne TN
LVHW082148200926
848484LV00008B/2125